CW00517658

Looking Back
Moving Forward

Great teachers and practitioners of homeopathy, based in the UK, share their stories, wisdom, experience and insights

By

Rowena J Ronson

FOOD FOR THOUGHT PUBLICATIONS

Food for Thought Publications
Room 6, Concorde House
Grenville Place
London, NW7 3SA

Published by Food for Thought Publications
2007

Rowena J Ronson 2007

Rowena J Ronson asserts the moral right to be identified as the author of this work

ISBN: 978- 0-9547033-3-2

Printed and bound in Great Britain by RFD Print Services Ltd 2007
Book Cover Design by: RFD@ntlworld.com

Credits: Rebecca Knorr (for extensive editing and proofreading), Adam Samuels (for extensive editing, proofreading, attention to fine detail, the index and much, much more) and Francis Treuherz (for proofreading and allowing me to pick his brains for the bibliography!)

This book is dedicated to
the two constant lights in my life,
my sons, Josh and Theo

Contents

Preface			1-2
Chapter 1	Linda Gwillim and Bill Rumble	Monday 30 November 2004	3-23
Chapter 2	Brian Kaplan	Tuesday 11 January 2005	24-33
Chapter 3	Myriam Shivadikar	Tuesday 25 January 2005	34-45
Chapter 4	Ellen Kramer	Wednesday 9 February 2005	46-62
Chapter 5	Peter Chappell	Thursday 10 February 2005	63-77
Chapter 6	Robert Davidson	Saturday 12 February 2005	78-92
Chapter 7	Misha Norland	Saturday 26 February 2005	93-107
Chapter 8	Annette Gamblin	Monday 28 February 2005	108-118
Chapter 9	Francis Treuherz	Thursday 3 March 2005	119-135
Chapter 10	Charles Wansbrough	Saturday 19 March 2005	136-144
Chapter 11	Jerome Whitney	Monday 11 April 2005	145-161
Chapter 12	Mike Bridger and Dion Tabrett	Friday 15 April 2005	162-178
Chapter 13	Ernest Roberts	Tuesday 19 April 2005	179-188
Chapter 14	Gordon Sambidge	Wednesday 20 April 2005	189-199
Chapter 15	Sheilagh Creasy	Tuesday 26 April 2005	200-222
Chapter 16	Kate Chatfield	Thursday 28 April 2005	223-236
Chapter 17	Roger Savage	Wednesday 4 May 2005	237-249
Chapter 18	Subrata Kumar Banerjea	Thursday 12 May 2005	250-267
Chapter 19	Yubraj Sharma	Saturday 14 May 2005	268-278
Chapter 20	Kaaren Whitney	Thursday 19 May 2005	279-289
Chapter 21	Anne Waters	Saturday 21 May 2005	290-303
Chapter 22	Rebecca Preston	Wednesday 8 June 2005	304-310
Chapter 23	Martin Miles	Monday 27 June 2005	311-329
Chapter 24	Carol Wise	Saturday 27 August 2005	330-338
Chapter 25	Linda Razzell	Tuesday 13 September 2005	339-351
Chapter 26	Nicky Pool	Thursday 29 September 2005	352-359
Chapter 27	Lesley Gregerson	Thursday 13 October 2005	360-366
Chapter 28	Sue Sternberg	Thursday 20 October 2005	367-378
Chapter 29	Lionel Milgrom	Friday 28 October 2005	379-393
Chapter 30	Barbara Harwood	Thursday 3 November 2005	394-408
Chapter 31	Simon Taffler	Monday 28 November 2005	409-428
Chapter 32	Jeremy Sherr	Monday 5 December 2005	429-449
The Process			450-450
What I learnt – thoughts, reflections and questions for the future			451-452
Appreciations			453-454
Some words from Rebecca Knorr			455-456
Contacts			457-461
Index			462-490
Bibliography			491-497

Preface

The inspiration for this book came from an interview with George Vithoulkas during the summer of 2004 in Alonissos (the interview can be found at *www.vithoulkas.com/EN/interview_vithoulkas_philosophy.html.*[1]). My colleague, Nigel Summerley, and I asked him whom he thought were the current great teachers of homeopathy in the world and he did not come up with one UK based name. He felt that those he has taught over here have lost their way and are therefore not influencing homeopaths capable of sustaining our discipline into the future.

So what are we doing wrong in George Vithoulkas' eyes? Simply, he feels that we have strayed too far from the Hahnemannian path for us to be taken seriously. His aim is to see a meeting of the two disciplines - allopathy and homeopathy - to create a system where they are both utilised to optimum effect. But he questions how we can do that if we are unclear and unfocussed about how we are practising homeopathy and what we are teaching our students.

While reflecting on George Vithoulkas' point of view I thought it might be a good idea to interview our teachers of homeopathy here in the UK - to listen to their individual opinions on a variety of subjects including the future of homeopathy. I had spent the academic year leading up to the George Vithoulkas interview working as an education adviser for the Society of Homeopaths. As a team, the education department provides a liaison service for course providers whose full and part-time courses are recognised and recommended by the Society. My responsibility that year was for six of them.

As a classically trained homeopath I found myself in the exciting position of having three institutions with a nonclassical ethos under my wing. Once every couple of months I would visit one of the six during their college weekends, meet with the principal and core team, gain feedback from the students and observe classes. Nearly all the students I met were delighted with their choice of course provider.

So, it was not unfamiliar territory for me to then spend a year interviewing our forefathers and mothers. I felt that by hearing from our UK teachers we, as a profession, would be able to discover who and what is influencing the homeopaths of tomorrow. I had an endless list of names that I wanted to include but in the end I just ran out of time and pages! My original ambitious intention would have produced a book as big as the *Synthesis*[2] and included all the principals of our UK course providers and more. There were at least another twenty homeopaths that agreed to be part of this project but could not spare the time in 2005. Perhaps we will hear their stories another year and during a second pilgrimage.

However, this pilgrimage began at the end of November 2004 in Malvern. I attended a teachers' seminar held by the Homeopathic Symposium[3] and I spent those few days waiving about a synopisis for my book in the hope that those on my list would agree to an interview at a later date. You will see from the introductions to each chapter that many did and the first interview in fact took place in the bar on the last night!

This book is a record of my conversations with thirty four of the UK's great teachers and practitioners of homeopathy; a journey that opened my eyes in so many ways and a journey that I am excited to share with you. Within these pages hopefully you will find some nuggets to inspire you as well as provide you with an opportunity to observe the roots of the renaissance of homeopathy from the sixties through to the present day. My wish is for discussions to arise from these conversations and for us all to pull together as a profession to secure a continued and expanding future for homeopathy in the UK.

I have tried to make the book as consistent as I can in all respects. With this in mind I have spelt 'homeopathy' the modern way unless requested to do so otherwise, as you will see in Jeremy Sherr's interview. I would also like to point out that the chapters hold the opinions, perceptions and memories of the individual interviewees. I am aware some readers, especially the old timers or those interested in our history, might question these and perhaps even disagree. My aim is to establish a discussion group on the Internet but at the time of going to print this is a plan very much in outline. For further information please refer to www.lookingbackmovingforward.com.

I very much hope you enjoy reading this book. Long live homeopathy!

Rowena J Ronson
March 2007

CHAPTER 1: LINDA GWILLIM & BILL RUMBLE

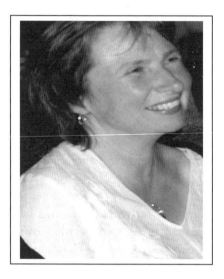 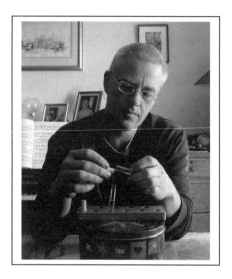

I met Linda Gwillim while working for the Society of Homeopaths and then I had the great pleasure of spending time with her and another of the core teachers/directors of the Welsh School of Homoeopathy, Bill Rumble, in Malvern at the teachers' seminar that I mentioned in the preface. In the afternoon of Tuesday 30 November 2004 we took to the bar with microphone and tape recorder in hand for a few drinks, lots of laughter and a great conversation. They are a truly inspiring partnership and I wished, at the end of this my first interview, that I could go back to college again now and do their entire course.

"Using a musical analogy, we teach them how to hold the instrument, to love the instrument and learn the chord structures, to enable them to improvise but also to enable them to find the 'blue note'. That for me is the analogy that I like to use. It is a note that doesn't exist other than in our soul, and that is what for me I aspire to send the students out with. Knowing the chords, loving the instrument, knowing how to fix it, how to tune it, but actually knowing how to find the blue note - the harmonic that resonates with their lives."
Linda Gwillim, November 2004

"If homeopathy is your 'calling' people get better, and if people get better they tell their friends and so on. If it is not a calling, it won't work out that way. But maybe the work we do will enable people to find out what their real calling is, because they will have been working with an amazing group of people for four years, in a way that everyone is on the same level."
Bill Rumble, November 2004

CHAPTER 1:   LINDA GWILLIM & BILL RUMBLE

ROWENA: I wanted to ask you both, what encouraged you to study homeopathy in the first place?

LINDA: Well my answer is very straightforward. I had a sick daughter of three and a half who received an immediate cure with homeopathy and I wanted to know more.

ROWENA: What were you doing at the time?

LINDA: I was a full-time mum. Before that I was a classroom music teacher; teaching piano and flute.

ROWENA: Where did you study homeopathy?

LINDA: I went to the College of Homeopathy (COH), which was run by Robert Davidson and Barbara Harwood at the time.

ROWENA: Same question to you, Bill.

BILL:. When I was twenty, I had a girlfriend who invited me in to her parents' home for a cup of tea. It was a grand house on the Regent's Canal, and in the living room was a huge, glass fronted cabinet full of weird bottles with cork stoppers. Upon closer inspection I read the names in copperplate script on the labels – *Argentum nitricum, Aconitum napellus* etc etc. I was transported into a feeling of awe and magic – like being in an alchemist's laboratory – time literally stood still for a few moments. "What are they?" I asked. "Homeopathic medicines," she replied, "My dad is an amateur homeopath."

I guess that is when the call came. Later, while at university when I was about twenty six years old, I went to see Peter Chappell and knew instantly that I wanted to practise. After I graduated I went to the School of Homeopathy in Devon in 1984 and I started practising and have been ever since.

ROWENA: Who inspired you the most while you were studying?

BILL: I was in an amazing position because the teachers at the School of Homeopathy were Jeremy Sherr, David Mundy, Murray Feldman, Janet Snowdon, Sheilagh Creasy and Misha Norland himself. They were a brilliant team and then I went off and studied with George Vithoulkas and Vassilis Ghegas in the late 1980s. I used to go to Holland three times per year and then organised for Vassilis Ghegas to come over here and run the courses in the UK. He was a fantastic teacher.

4

ROWENA: Do you feel you learned the most from him?

BILL: Initially yes, because he never thought psychologically. He would say that the patient didn't need to convey the meaning of how they felt. Do you know what I mean? The thing that has always fascinated me about homeopathy is that when you get to a point in the case when you don't know what is happening, you are really in the territory of the remedy. If you always have to explain the case to understand the dynamic, then you have not got down to the level of the inexplicable. Nobody knows how remedies work or indeed, how the vital force works either. When you enter that territory it is a mystery. Magic and synchronicities happen in that place and that is what Vassilis Ghegas taught me.

ROWENA: Do you angle your case taking, with that in mind?

BILL: Not really. I focus on the complete totality; a very Hahnemannian way of prescribing. I have always sought to emulate totality prescribing and not any other version of homeopathy. I prescribe on the symptoms that speak from the disease state.

ROWENA: The state that they are in at that present time?

BILL: Yes. I found Vassilis Ghegas' Kentian ideal of giving the remedy and waiting, hugely influential at the time. Not identifying with the victim, but identifying with the symptom maker. So you see what the symptom maker is saying and co-operate with it, and that involves less and less interaction. Every symptom has two parts – one is the part of the person who is suffering from the symptom and the other is the symptom maker, the vital force. If we identify only with the sufferer, we can miss out on the potential of the great mystery trying to unfold. If we enter into a dialogue with the symptom maker, the mystery starts to unfold. If you look at *Aphorism 7* of the *Organon*[4], Hahnemann says the disease will demand the remedy it requires because it is pointing out what it needs to transform itself into health. That is the basis of disease; it is trying to transform.

ROWENA: How do you do that in your case taking?

BILL: Complete relaxation until the point where the symptom maker reveals itself and then complete attention. There is a switch from total defused and relaxed attention to a sudden focus on the symptom maker and then it will reveal itself. The vital force has a hugely sophisticated energy; more sophisticated than any we have ever encountered.

ROWENA: How long did it take for you to get to the point that you are at now?

BILL: Since 1984.

ROWENA: So it has been your journey. Do you feel things have changed for you more recently?

BILL: Yes, because I am focusing on process rather than data. Hahnemann says in *Aphorism 104*[4] that once the image of the disease has been exactly recorded, the most difficult work is done. I teach my students to record the image of the disease. All the data is there, you don't need to memorise it in your head, but you do have to spend a lot of time going through the spadework and doing the digging. Recording the image of the disease is what we need to focus on in education - perceiving the image and developing skills to record it.

ROWENA: So you have a strong emphasis on practitioner development?

BILL: Yes.

ROWENA: Did you have that within your training?

LINDA: Within my training?

ROWENA: Yes.

LINDA: No.

ROWENA: So who inspired you when you were studying?

LINDA: I was taught by the same people as Bill; David Mundy, Tony Hurley, Misha Norland, Robert Davidson, Barbara Harwood, Ian Watson, Mike Bridger, all of them. I think for me the process work that Bill talked about has come more to me now through teaching rather than from my learning initially with those teachers, which is really interesting. So it is something that has evolved, rather than something that I was ever taught as such.

ROWENA: And has that been evolving more recently?

LINDA: Certainly for me the turning point was the proving of *Placenta humana*. That really changed my whole life, not in terms of the remedy but in terms of really understanding the homeopathic process. It also took me to a different place in terms of my process. Working with the students, it has just evolved. It is not something I learned, or that happened.

BILL: I agree. It is about arsing around with a group of people for a couple of days and seeing whatever comes up, allowing the process to express itself. A lot of energies come through people in that environment that they don't meet in the normal course of the day.

6

LINDA: Creating the space for magic to happen. And in doing that, that is where I have learned a lot and seen the students evolving. It is fantastic.

ROWENA: Do you do process work with the whole of the Welsh School intake or just one year?

LINDA: It happens throughout the whole course; it is an integral part of the whole four years.

ROWENA: Provings or the process?

LINDA: The process.

BILL: The more you focus on the process the more it happens. Patterns never emerge or reveal themselves when you try and get them to emerge. It is about engaging in the process in whatever is happening and reflecting on it.

ROWENA: And the provings, when do they happen?

LINDA: Students can do provings as part of their fourth year project. Bill has done one and I have done one so there is energy there, and they are keen to do it.

ROWENA: Do you use certain psychotherapeutic models for process?

BILL: I am very interested in Arnold Mindell's work - Process Orientated Psychotherapy - focusing on the body rather than the mind. I will give you an example. We had a situation in a class a couple of weeks ago that happened with a student. We were talking about the vital force and fields of energy and she said, "Oh my God, there is an incredible black cloud that has come over me and I feel really, really frightened." But she didn't leave the room, she sat with it and said she was really scared and I said to her, "Where do you feel it in your body?" She said, "I feel it in my legs." I asked her what it was like and she said it was intense pressure so I said, "OK, amplify it. What makes you feel it more?" and she said, "Pressing." I said, "OK, press", and she pressed as hard as she could and amplified it and then she said, "Oh my God, it has gone up to my head." She was in the moment and it just passed and then she said, "I want to sing and I want to dance."

It was such a great example of homeopathy. What the remedies do is amplify it. It was such a lovely, living example of amplifying a sensation and actually seeing what was really trying to come through, and it started as a black cloud. That is what I mean by process; taking whatever is there instead of trying to protect it or suppress it. Instead of saying, "You don't fit in this institution, people do not speak like that here", or whatever, instead of trying to sweep it under the carpet and keep everything normal, actually what we do is we seize creative potential. We encourage trouble.

ROWENA: Does that transfer to how you practise as homeopaths?

LINDA: Yes.

ROWENA: So how would you take those symptoms, and would you still take them if they resolved the issue within the consultation? If they were going through the process you described and had an experience and those feeling went away and, let's say they had insights and changed state, a) would you take those symptoms if they have shifted, and b) how would you take them?

BILL: Oh, that is a really good question. It is often not necessary. You can go through a process within the group and that is the amazing thing about working with groups of people. You don't actually need to give a remedy; just the work in the group resolves the problem.

LINDA: It is a huge part of the course.

ROWENA: But when that happens in a consultation and the issue resolves itself?

BILL: It depends on the situation.

LINDA: If that happens in a consultation with me, I will probably not prescribe straight away as they have had the remedy in a different form and they are already doing the process. I would like them to get on with it.

ROWENA: So you are practising this process way of teaching, but that is then transferred into the consultation? That is quite unique.

LINDA: It is about teaching what you do.

BILL: And as Hahnemann says, the patient should describe exactly the sensations where they occur. The patient needs to describe exactly what they are experiencing.

ROWENA: And this has evolved with you, it is not something you were taught?

LINDA: I wasn't taught it.

BILL: Nor me. It is taking the *Organon*[4] as a source, as it is all in there.

ROWENA: I am sure you are aware of the debate about homeopaths struggling to make a living. What skills do you think the students that leave your school need in order to be successful homeopaths? What do you think makes somebody persevere to practise at the end of their training?

LINDA: I don't know about what makes them persevere, but I would like to think that what students come away with from the course is a love of the subject and a respect for themselves as well as their patients. And an ability to look at themselves in response to what goes on in the case taking so that they can reflect on that and be in touch with that magic.

ROWENA: So the love of it?

BILL: Yes, and also the calling. Misha Norland said very accurately this morning that some people become homeopaths because they already are, and other people are there for their own internal process. But I believe in the calling, and I think what we both feel very passionately about this. When someone has the calling, we will try and create the environment where the calling can be explored creatively and in detail.

LINDA: It says in the prospectus that basically what we want to do is to lead the healer from within, out - and that, for me, sums up an overview of how I see the course.

BILL: The Latin word educare means leading out, and that is where the word education comes from.

LINDA: And I think that is the basis of how we set the course up.

BILL: And at the end of every academic year we run a summer school from a Thursday to a Sunday, in a three hundred acre organic farm and we all have incredible experiences there. We do classes in the morning and ritual work in the afternoon.

LINDA: We all camp out in the field and we have lessons in a beautiful geodesic dome, which is especially set up for the occasion.

ROWENA: Is the ritual side of things based on shamanism?

BILL: It can become that but we do not emphasise that aspect. As far as people are concerned, they are engaged in work that culminates on the Saturday with a ritual journey through a pathway in the woodlands and we light candles and people process through it on their own to an area where there is fire and drumming.

LINDA: And there is a gateway, a threshold, and they put some aspect that is no longer useful to them into the fire.

BILL: It is a powerful meeting with nature and everybody participates in the work and an awful lot goes on.

ROWENA: Do you do any work with issues of abundance, poverty consciousness and how we view money?

LINDA: That is not what it is about.

ROWENA: Do you feel your graduates are managing to practise and make a living out of being homeopaths?

LINDA: Ninety five percent of our graduates are practising to some degree, but obviously there is an element of struggle in setting up as there is with any profession; getting your name known and all the rest of it. They are doing it at the level that they can afford to.

BILL: That goes down to calling as well. It is how much you are prepared to sacrifice for your calling. If you look at people like Picasso, he sacrificed everything for his calling and other people do too.

ROWENA: Do you think we will ever get to a point where there are too many homeopaths?

LINDA and BILL: No.

ROWENA: There has been a lot of talk about that recently.

LINDA: The more there are, the more the profile of homeopathy is raised. Patients choose who they want to see, as an energetic response. I don't believe we will ever have too many.

ROWENA: There is confusion among patients that homeopaths prescribe in many different ways. How do you feel we can address that?

LINDA: We all prescribe in different ways because we are all individuals. I don't see it is a problem, personally.

BILL: I think with the emphasis on exploring the individual's process within homeopathy, they come to practise homeopathy in a way that really works for them. We encourage our students to explore practising in their own way.

LINDA: What is really interesting is that as clinical supervisor, I am able to see all the students' cases and it is brilliant, because you can see the individual coming out in the casework. They are going out to practise independently in their own way with a full toolbox knowing when to use the appropriate tool with each individual patient.

ROWENA: In terms of that toolbox, what is in it?

LINDA: There is obviously all the philosophy and materia medica, the knowledge and experience of provings, the peer group experience – that is very important as well. And there is the process stuff and the ability to reflect, and there are different methodologies and an eye for knowing when to use what.

BILL: It is not like a course where we say that we are going to explore all these different methodologies for you, but if something comes up we won't necessarily dismiss it as a system. Do you know what I mean? We don't have a rigid system.

ROWENA: Is it case-led, then?

BILL: Yes.

LINDA: The way we do it is that we have a lot of visiting lecturers and they are bringing their qualities in too. So in the fourth year Bill and I only see them once, whereas in the first, second and third year we teach them three times each. So in the fourth year, they are getting a much more varied input of teachers. You can see that reflected in their casework. They have someone teaching them organ remedies and all of a sudden you see different influences coming into their work.

From my perspective we give the foundation. Using a musical analogy, we teach them how to hold the instrument, to love the instrument and learn the chord structures, to enable them to improvise but also to enable them to find the 'blue note'. That for me is the analogy that I like to use. It is a note that doesn't exist other than in our soul, and that is what for me I aspire to send the students out with. Knowing the chords, loving the instrument, knowing how to fix it, how to tune it, but actually knowing how to find the blue note, the harmonic that resonates with their lives.

BILL: A lot of that comes through the teaching clinics, as well. We do video clinics where the students take the cases on camera and sometimes you can just see that someone has hit the blue note. They may not hit it again for ten years, but once they have hit it, everybody hears it. That is a lovely analogy.

ROWENA: Give me an example of that from your teaching clinics.

BILL: Okay, a couple of weeks ago we had a video clinic, and there was a boy of fourteen who was suffering from asthma. He had had a very traumatic background; his father was dabbling in shamanism and died in a sweat lodge and there was a lot of insecurity because of his unsteady history. It hadn't been a secure upbringing at all and he was very attached to his mother. The student who was taking the case said, "Do you have any fears? Any animals, perhaps?" and then she suddenly asked, "Insects?" Somehow she knew about the wasps; I don't know where it came from, and he went "Wasps!" He started to animate and actually he had been chased by a swarm of wasps when he was eighteen months old. Now that was the formative moment that impacted on his vital force; that was the moment when energetic impact occurred and she hit the blue note. From somewhere came the question, "Insects?" and he became completely alive in that moment back to eighteen months old; he re-experienced them. She tried to move on then, and asked about food desires and I intervened and said, "Stay with the wasps." That was one of those moments.

ROWENA: Do you think it comes from the source? Inspired?

BILL: Quantum physics calls it the field, homeopathy calls it the vital force, the aborigines call it the dreaming, and that is where it comes from, and it is a mystery; it is like the dark side of the moon, you don't see it. It is the field of the remedy. My own personal feeling is it is the entity. Hahnemann describes it as the disease attempting to communicate. In his time they regarded diseases as energetic entities, and I think he was right.

ROWENA: But another homeopath could take many, many cases and never get to that place where they get blue notes. So why is the disease state not speaking to those homeopaths?

BILL: I don't know; I cannot speak for them. But for me it is all about an awareness that extraordinary synchronicities are waiting to happen. Mysteries are waiting to unfold, if we let them. We just need to learn how to notice them, rather than go looking for them. We have an illusion in this profession, that we find the remedies. If we think that by thinking we can create the remedy, we are inflating our own importance because that energy has been there since the dawn of time and we must not fool ourselves that we create it through our thinking, our computer programme or through our knowledge. Too much knowledge is the biggest handicap. Sure, you have to get people to study and do the disciplined work because things don't come up if you don't apply yourself, but it is not the end in itself. The end is the blue note.

LINDA: It is about not trying too hard. I can think about another incident with a case taking where the student tried too hard instead of sitting back and letting it evolve, and it just wouldn't happen.

ROWENA: What about students knowing and owning their own issues? Do they notice their own blue notes? Does your course include space for students to understand what they might project onto their patients?

BILL: Well again, that is another huge advantage of group work because when somebody says something, before they have even finished they realise that they are describing themselves and not the being that is visiting them. Do you know what I mean?

ROWENA: Do you think that the Welsh School attracts people who may be a bit more spiritual?

LINDA: I think it attracts people who are geographically close to it!

BILL: Yes, but also we do have a huge range of different people, from all walks of life.

LINDA: And people who are aware of their blue note before they come and others who don't even know what a blue note is. But they are all drawn to finding it.

ROWENA: And that is good.

LINDA: Yes.

BILL: Very ordinary people.

LINDA: Extremely ordinary people some of them, and it is amazing watching them unfold.

ROWENA: Do you think that it is because you approach personal development in a way that it is not a hidden agenda?

LINDA: It is written into the prospectus. They know the very minute they come for the interview; it is very transparent.

BILL: Yes, but we never name it. That is the key to it, because if you name it, if you call it transpersonal or this that or the other, you are stuffed. You never name it.

LINDA: Everybody who experiences it will see it as something different so it is really important not to name it because otherwise it loses its individuality.

BILL: Some of the best things happen spontaneously and when they are least expected.

ROWENA: So even though people may choose the Welsh School because of the location, they are clear about what they are letting themselves in for. So they will either think, "This is for me", or they won't.

LINDA: It is clear from before they come how the Welsh School works, but it is not labelled as any particular thing. From the prospectus students can see that we are encouraging the healer from within to come out and that we work in a group so that everybody can learn from each other and share their life experience. It is obvious it is not chalk and talk and that we are not going to teach how to become a homeopath in that way, because that is not what we do.

BILL: It is non-modular.

ROWENA: So describe a weekend to me, then.

LINDA: Students have the same facilitator for the whole weekend, so that they can really get into process work; really get into the core of what they are looking at. You can go in there with an idea of what you are going to be doing and end up not doing it all because if something striking comes into the room, then what can you do but go with it?

ROWENA: Do you have assessments?

LINDA: We don't have a timetable so there is nothing like that at all. They do two pieces of homework a month. We might start the weekend with a case to teach a particular remedy but then we might deviate a little as this has resonated with an aspect of one of the student's own cases. It flows and there is never a stuck point or a boundary. It is very fluid and moves in the direction the students want it to go. Obviously we make sure that everything is eventually covered on the course but it happens in its own rhythm. It will happen differently with each year group as every group is different. This helps to keep the teaching alive.

ROWENA: And the anatomy and physiology?

LINDA: They do that as a correspondence course, but obviously if we have a case with severe pathology, it is all integrated.

ROWENA: What happens when one student demands a whole lot of attention?

LINDA: The group process comes in. We encourage the group to work through it – as Bill says, often the situation needs amplifying in order to move through to resolution. I see my role more as a facilitator in this process.

BILL: I must admit I have intervened recently in that situation and said, "Look, you know, hold your horses", but actually that ended up with...

LINDA: More process...

BILL: Yes. There are only two rules, one is to offer no solutions and the other is no physical violence.... That's a joke by the way!

LINDA: And own everything you say...

ROWENA: I have got a much better feel now of how it works at the Welsh School. How do you see the future of homeopathy in this country?

BILL: Well, we are in the Golden Age at the moment because we are working without having to be regulated from outside. A lot of people say they really want recognition for homeopathy; they really want us to be incorporated into the mainstream health care system, but I personally feel I like working underground.

LINDA: Same here; grass roots, quietly doing what we do and getting on with it.

BILL: We like working at grass roots and getting on with the job. We have been practising under common law since the nineteenth century and I am glad homeopathy is not acceptable to certain elements of the medical profession because to make it so would be very destructive; it wouldn't enable people to pursue their calling. For me, that is the bottom line. If someone has a calling, I will make it as easy as possible for them to be able to fulfil that calling because I am lucky enough to have had my calling made possible.

ROWENA: How easy do you think it is for homeopaths to make a living from practising?

BILL: We are all working within a system that actually works against us. I might sound naïve, but I still believe where there is a will; there is a way. I would be happy to go out and chop trees down at the weekend if I wasn't teaching, or do something else, if I had to, so that I could continue working with my calling.

LINDA: I was practising for some years before I started teaching and was busy. It was only because it combined my love of homeopathy and my love of teaching that I taught.

ROWENA: But then you are one of those homeopaths who started a long time ago and there were fewer homeopaths around.

LINDA: Personally, I don't think it is to do with that at all.

ROWENA: Do you mean because the increase in homeopaths should be counterbalanced in terms of demand because of the rise in consciousness and awareness?

BILL: If it is your calling people get better, and if people get better they tell their friends and so on. If it is not a calling, it won't work out that way. But maybe, just maybe, the work we do will enable people to find out what their real calling is, because they will have been working with an amazing group of people for four years, in a way that everyone is on the same level.

LINDA: Absolutely,

BILL: And maybe that actually will enable them to find their way through to somewhere else. Because invariably people have looked back, even if they decided not to practise, and said, "God, that was just an incredible experience."

LINDA: We have got people who have graduated who have found through doing the course that their calling is slightly different and have gone off and started that part of their journey.

BILL: That has actually clicked into place for me now and makes a lot of sense. Studying with us is just part of the journey; the destination isn't necessarily being a homeopath.

LINDA: No... we don't know what the destination is... we never know what it is...

BILL: That gives a whole different slant on this argument, doesn't it? We don't know what the destination is and what life has in store for us. We don't know because it is a mystery.

LINDA: And thank God for that.

ROWENA: So if it all changes and we end up working for the NHS, things would be quite different in this country.

LINDA: I wouldn't want to, personally. I want that freedom to practise in the way that I practise. It would be incredibly different working for the NHS.

BILL: And it might work for some people.

LINDA: Yes, for some people that might be their journey and that is not to say it is right or wrong, but it is not for me.

ROWENA: What skills do you think are crucial for a homeopath to learn?

BILL: Love yourself. You have to love everything about yourself and I don't mean to never deny yourself. Regard yourself with affection and humour.

LINDA: I know what you are saying. My slant is to be open hearted to everything, including yourself.

BILL: Yes. That is the same thing, isn't it? One of the incredibly interesting dynamics that I have been working on with groups recently is this idea that there is a part of yourself that views your life with curiosity and there is another part that gets involved emotionally and gets right in there and feels it and gets torn apart and tortured. The course is about training people to identify those processes and give them space to work with them. You can be completely involved with your patient on an emotional, open hearted and loving level and there is another part of you that is watching in the undergrowth for something to move. You know what I mean? It is like the hawk eye that sees it all. If you can get people to tune in that way as part of their training, they start tuning in that way as part of their lives, as well. I always use the analogy of Laurel and Hardy, "That is another fine mess you have got yourself into"? You know we have that voice which speaks...

LINDA: And we have been called Laurel and Hardy, as well...

BILL: And which one are you?

LINDA: We won't go there...

BILL: That is another fine mess you have got us into Stanley. I think this whole foolish thing about wholeness ... we should learn to be separate. To be a healer there is a part of you that engages on a soul level with people and there is another part of you that really sits apart and can actually spot things. And that is a lesson in whatever walk of life you are in and also in your own personal life too, to be really whole hearted in your acceptance of yourself and have that eye and listen to that voice. The eye is the one who walks beside you, the one you don't see but who occasionally you visit, and occasionally visits you. That is what it is all about, for me.

ROWENA: I wonder what interesting path I would have taken if I had come and studied at the Welsh School. Which books do you consider must reads for students and practitioners?

LINDA: The *Organon*[4].

BILL: I work entirely from the *Organon*[4] when I teach philosophy.

LINDA: If I were on a desert island I would take the *Organon*[4] and my repertory.

BILL: And Stuart Close's *The Genius of Homoeopathy*[5]. He is so humble and awestruck by homeopathy all the way through it; I think it is a lovely book. Also *Grimm's Fairy Stories*[6], it is all in there.

ROWENA: I am sure it is.

LINDA: It is, actually; the fairy tales contain all the archetypes.

BILL: And all the potentials because that is how we learn about the structure of the mind. I am very interested in mythology and in process work. *Working With The Dreaming Body*[7] and *Dreaming While Awake: Techniques For 24-Hour Lucid Dreaming*[8] both by Arnold Mindell are both fantastic books and are very interesting as well.

LINDA: I would also like to mention another important role that the Welsh School fulfils. We provide a community for the graduates to remain part of, so they get invited to both the winter and summer schools, any of the teaching clinics and we also run a Post Grad and Continuous Professional Development courses for them to come back to. Our graduates also go on to become supervisors for the Welsh School and run the Saturday 'acutes clinic'. There is something about community that is really important.

One of the students said to me, "It has been the best four years of my life and I don't want to leave and the nicest thing is that I know I don't have to" and for me I think that is really important; that there is that support network. Graduates are forever phoning me up wanting to touch base and we have a system where students buddy with someone a year or two below them, so that keeps them in contact with what is going on and I think it is a really important part of the process. I think a lot of homeopaths go under or stop practising because they haven't got that support or communication network.

BILL: That was the vision that I had at the beginning, this idea of a homeopathic community that was wild and loving and supported rather than uptight, tightassed, conformist and competitive.

ROWENA: Did you set up the Welsh School together?

LINDA: Adam Martanda set it up.

BILL: Adam Martanda had an idea to set up a school in Wales, a few people got interested and then he backed out.

LINDA: In the meantime, he had interviewed us as teachers, hadn't he?

BILL: Yes. What happened was, I rang him up and said, "What about my job? I have just committed five or six weekends". And he said, "Well, why don't you do it?" So I said, "OK."

LINDA: And then he phoned me and said, "If you still want to do it, phone Bill Rumble."

BILL: And you wrote to me.

LINDA: And then I got a phone call from you saying, "What are you doing tomorrow? We are going to Czechoslovakia!" That was my first conversation with you!

ROWENA: So why Czechoslovakia?

BILL: Oh, I was running courses for the London College of Classical Homeopathy (LCCH) over there at the time, so I was looking around for someone to go with me because somebody else had pulled out. We set the Welsh School up ten years ago.

ROWENA: So how many students do you have?

LINDA: We have a maximum of twenty in each year group but an average of fourteen. We bought our own premises recently in the middle of Carmarthen and can run the clinic from there, which is fantastic. My vision was to set up a low cost training clinic so that students have access to a wider variety of patient. It has been a fantastic asset and learning experience for the students.

ROWENA: And is it easy to attract patients into the clinic?

LINDA: The clinics are full. We run them every fortnight and there are almost too many patients.

ROWENA: Do you run them separately to your weekends, then?

LINDA: Yes, we run them on a Friday so that all the year groups can come and work together, which is another brilliant part of it as it encourages the community. I did one last Friday and some of the first years were there working with the second, third and fourths, and some post grads and it was just beautiful to see the interaction between them.

ROWENA: Do you have to market yourself as a school to get students?

LINDA: We do some advertising, but not very much, and *The Big Issue*[9] is the main place but our recruits are mainly through word of mouth via our students.

ROWENA: So how do you think we can stop homeopathy slipping into a dormant state again?

LINDA: By doing what we do, quietly, getting on with it.

ROWENA: And being in the present...

LINDA: And being in the present. Doing it and not trying to prove it.

BILL: I suppose really the basic underlying philosophy is to observe what is trying to happen and see if you can help it.

LINDA: Let it go where it is going.

BILL: Yes, and not be frightened of trouble... It is better to fail gloriously than succeed miserably.

LINDA: It is about being true to what you do, isn't it? Walking your talk and just doing it and not trying to equate it to anything or become evangelical about it or whatever.

BILL: And it is down to calling again because what we do is no more important than what anyone else does who follows their calling. You know what I mean, it doesn't matter if it is homeopathy or surgery or tree surgery or whatever. Do you know what I mean?

ROWENA: Who do you think are the great homeopathy teachers of our time?

LINDA: I think and hope that there aren't any.

ROWENA: I thought you might come up with something like that, which is why I asked the question!

LINDA: I have a real aversion to guru status. The students are great homeopathy teachers, the patients are great homeopathy teachers...

BILL: Life is a great homeopathy teacher.

ROWENA: Who would inspire you? Who would you go and see?

LINDA: I find that a really hard question to answer because I admire bits of everybody, but there's nobody I would elevate to the status of sitting at their feet.

ROWENA: I knew you were going to say that too.

LINDA: I admire many homeopaths and many teachers and so many of my students and patients have taught me so much. There are bits I take from everybody. I realise as I say all this that one of the people who really influenced me was Robert Davidson. If I am really honest, when I started my training I was one of the students who wanted to be spoon-fed; I wanted to be taught how to be a homeopath and how to do it. As a result Robert said some outrageous things that really made me think that I had to do this for me and it changed my life, because previously my educational process had been being spoon-fed and he challenged me to challenge him and therefore to challenge myself. I have to really honour that because that was a turning point for me. He gave me the confidence to actually know that I had the answers that I needed for myself, in me. He empowered me and taught me that and it was the biggest gift that I could have had at that time in my life.

BILL: Misha Norland had a huge impact on me as he always created the sense of wonder and he has never lost that. The man is a magician.

LINDA: Yes, that is the word for me, magic. We are all magicians and I think that is what I love about teaching; we are actually seeing the magician in all the students and what we are giving them is a few tips on all their spells, if you like.

BILL: The other focus is on having a healing art; you know Hahnemann often talked about the medical art. Anyone who has the capacity to bless, needs to be aware of their capacity to curse and if they don't know they have that capacity, they are in big trouble. So you have to be aware of that.

ROWENA: So knowing your dark side?

BILL: Yes, absolutely, and actually realising that most of our creativity comes from our dark side. The dark side of the moon, that's where all the creativity comes from and it only gets nasty if you don't listen to it. If you suppress it or it comes out sideways... you know...

LINDA: I would say that the work we do with the students is very much about getting the dark side out; shedding some light on it, looking at it and illuminating it. I think it is a very important part of who we are.

ROWENA: So do you use a lot of self-disclosure of your own experiences when you are working?

LINDA: We don't often have to because of the way the course is run.

BILL: I use self-disclosure in as much as I will often disclose my own blundering nature at the time. I am not frightened to blunder and blow it and I think that is really important.

Self-disclosure doesn't necessarily mean recounting endless regurgitated stories of childhood wounds, but actually not being frightened to be a fool.

LINDA: And not being frightened to say, "I don't know"...

BILL: If you look at mythology, the fool is actually always a great healer. So for me the self-disclosure is often just about not being frightened of that foolishness.

LINDA: The fool is the carrier of the knowledge.

BILL: It is the youngest brother or sister in all the fairy stories that makes it through to the other world because they don't know anything, they are innocent, and nobody expects anything of them.

ROWENA: That is really interesting.

BILL: And they always listen to the talking animal or the dwarf or the misshapen witch with the eyes moving in opposite directions. It is the fool in us that is the potential healer.

LINDA: Because they don't have that investment...

BILL: ...investment in what I have to be or whom I have to satisfy. You know, they don't have status.

LINDA: They do not have an inflated ego.

BILL: Yes, that is the aspect that is really important.

ROWENA: What do you think you offer to your students when you teach them?

LINDA: Space to explore, play, be themselves, be honest and provide the safety for them to go into that dark side.

BILL: And an extremely rigorous clinical training.

LINDA: Yes. Extremely rigorous.

ROWENA: Yes, because that is where your focus is, really.

LINDA: It is there where we really place emphasis because it is there where everything comes together.

BILL: And also a really sound and debated grasp of philosophy.

LINDA: And materia medica. I think it is all brilliant. I would love to be a student on the course!

BILL: You are a nutter anyway; a total nutter who doesn't need much sleep!

LINDA: No, I don't, but that is because I love what I am doing; that is what it is about. But coming back to Bill's point, if I want to stress anything, it is our really rigorous clinical training. I am proud of the clinical training that we offer.

ROWENA: And that is not just the clinics on the Fridays; it is the whole process that you are all going through throughout the weekends.

LINDA: Yes, it is part of everything.

BILL: In a New York theatre in the 1920s there was a talent competition and the host stood up on stage and said, "Now, Ladies and Gentlemen, I would like to introduce to you Miss Ella Fitzgerald who is going to dance. What? Hang on a second, ladies and gentlemen. What was that, Ella? Ah, she has changed her mind. She is going to sing." That is the calling... that is the moment... do you know what I mean? And she decided to sing...

ROWENA: So she really was going to dance?

BILL: She was going to dance and at the last minute she said, "I am going to sing, I am going to sing!" And she was the greatest jazz singer that ever lived. That is the calling. It just happens like that, and for me that is what it is all about.

ROWENA: Linda, Bill – what a great evening and a fabulous conversation. I feel I have learned so much from you both and I am so glad we found the time to chat together. It has been a real pleasure. Thank you.

CHAPTER 2:   BRIAN KAPLAN

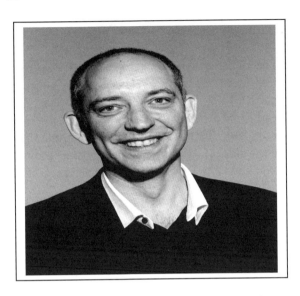

Tuesday 11 January 2005 took me to Harley Street to the clinic rooms of Brian Kaplan. I was a little nervous, it has to be said, not that Brian is intimidating in the least but this was my first interview since the teachers' seminar in Malvern six weeks earlier where my journey began. He was one of the speakers and gave us a really good insight into Provocative Therapy, a tool he uses quite separately from his homeopathy, to shift his patients back into balance. I had met him there and he had agreed for me to call him to arrange a conversation. He comes across as a little shy and extremely likeable – I would imagine I could happily tell him my case and feel safe, held and in good, knowing hands. His Harley Street rooms were impressive and expressed the professional air of a specialist in his field. As I waited a few moments in reception I had a chance to stare into his art therapist wife's abstract paintings adorning the walls and temporarily, I lost myself.

"Homeopathy is a very powerful tool but it is not an overriding system of medicine. If a person has got appendicitis, still the best treatment for them is an appendectomy. If they have raging meningitis, I still believe their best chance is with a lumber puncture (spinal tap) to find out if they have got bacteria which is causing the meningitis, enabling us to give them the right intravenous antibiotics. But in its place homeopathy is very powerful."
Brian Kaplan, January 2005

"From my perspective if I had to say what is crucial to learn, I would say an understanding of transference and countertransference. This is basic stuff in psychology and if we don't know about it, we can damage the patient by saying and doing the wrong things."
Brian Kaplan, January 2005

CHAPTER 2: BRIAN KAPLAN

ROWENA: How did you get into homeopathy?

BRIAN: I went to medical school to become a doctor because I had a very good experience with my GP - he had a fantastic bedside manner. He was a very humane, warm, loving person who told jokes. In retrospect I think that is what attracted me to medicine – the human side of it. But when I arrived at medical school for very classical training, each subject was regarded as a journey on its own. I found myself in a system that brutalised me with science. There was no human side of it and it was very depressing. But I stuck it out, thinking that hopefully at the end of it I would find something.

A natural path for me to follow would have been to go into psychiatry, but there it was even worse. I saw that this technical side and mechanistic approach to medicine was even more brutalising when applied to psychological disorders. In other words, if someone has got something mentally wrong then we must do something to their brain - we must drug or shock or cut the brain. So it wasn't a natural home for me either.

I was also interested in yoga, and I went into a yoga bookshop in the middle of Johannesburg and picked up a book written by Gordon-Ross called *Homeopathy an Introductory Guide*[10]. Looking through it, what attracted me was the human side; if the communication is there then the process works well and one can choose a medicine. What I learned from the book was that the quality of your bedside manner and your way with the patient would actually facilitate the prescription of the correct medicine. It was directly related.

ROWENA: So it has a very therapeutic effect?

BRIAN: Yes, I think the homeopathic way of taking the case history is one of the most healing approaches because it is so receptive. When you listen as an orthodox doctor most of what is said is pushed to one side. In homeopathy you cannot push anything aside. You must listen because even if one fact, one thing the person says doesn't give you a clue, it is repeated and that is the gestalt of it. You cannot ignore that. And that is what attracted me to the process. Homeopathy values a person's subjective experience of their disease, of their life and of their relationships with other people. I don't know anything else that places value in that way.

ROWENA: So you came into homeopathy via a very different journey to most professional homeopaths. Often it is because we have had our own healing response to homeopathy.

BRIAN: Yes, and it took a long time for me even to get an effect from a homeopathic remedy. When you have studied homeopathy you loose your innocence as the homeopathic patient. If you say something, for example, fear of darkness, then your homeopath is going to process that. So it is a big problem. I was found a constitutional remedy by a fantastic homeopath that was living with me for a while and so of course he observed me a great deal.

ROWENA: I liked what you wrote about taking cases of other homeopaths, and I know from asking homeopaths myself that there is a huge lack of trust within the community. Homeopaths just think that another homeopath will not get their case and prescribe the right remedy.

BRIAN: Homeopathy is not designed for people who know homeopathy inside out and there was a time when I thought "Hell why did I choose this? I should have chosen the Alexander Technique and then every day I would be getting an Alexander lesson!"

ROWENA: I think we have chosen a hard road; it seems that other therapists have it easier. Doctors are not so intimidated by acupuncture, for example.

BRIAN: Homeopathy is hard and it gets the most abuse as well. I don't encourage people to do it unless they have really fallen in love with it and nothing else will do, especially if they don't start young enough. You can do homeopathy at any age, but you need to be totally committed.

ROWENA: That was something I wanted to explore with you, the fact that there are so many homeopaths around and many are struggling to build a practice and make a living from it.

BRIAN: Yes, well there probably are too many. There are other things one can do that are much simpler, like colonics or reflexology. Well, you might not want to do them, but it is much easier to get a result. Every time you put your hands on, for example, you will get something. But with homeopathy, if it is the wrong remedy, it is quite hard.

ROWENA: So which homeopathy teachers inspired you the most?

BRIAN: George Vithoulkas. I think that the work that we did at the Homeopathic Physicians' Teaching Group (HPTG)[11],) in terms of supervising the case taking process, the relationship with the patient and getting behind the words etc - I think it was a contribution to homeopathy in this country.

ROWENA: Who did you do that with?

BRIAN: I was part of a homeopathic physicians group of doctors that met in 1991. All but one of our eight had studied with George Vithoulkas and Vassilis Ghegas. There was a famous course that was meant to start in London in February 1986. It was meant to be for three weeks, three times a year for three years. I signed up for the whole course but unfortunately it only lasted for the first three weeks. It just fell apart, but we still had those three weeks of training from George and it was excellent.

The founders of HPTG) were all members of the Faculty. In fact the history of the Faculty is interesting because it goes through high potency constitutional phases, and it goes through low phases. When Margaret Tyler was there it was very Kentian, but we felt it was becoming a bit wishy-washy and we wanted a more classical approach. We wanted to teach doctors a more classical type of homeopathy and that we did. So we set up this course in Oxford called the HPTG), and we eventually taught vets.

Only two doctors and two vets are left now and I am no longer involved, but we did good work, there is no doubt about it, and all the people who were a part of that would acknowledge this. The late Andrew Lockie was part of it too. We looked at the side of homeopathy that involves communication with the patient. I would like us to be remembered for our contribution at developing the homeopathic patient relationship, the transference, the psychological process that goes on as we went into that a lot. We would meet with a psychotherapy supervisor, a fantastic guy called Robin Shohet, who wrote a book called *Supervision in the Helping Professions*[12].

ROWENA: George Vithoulkas talked a lot about there being homeopaths that had learned with him, and then they had chosen not to follow his way of prescribing....

BRIAN: Well, I have actually stuck with him and I can understand that because I think I know what he means. I think he is very concerned about people who create a different way of looking at the materia medica altogether, say in the terms of the kingdoms. I have heard him say, "What does this patient look like to you - an animal, a snake, a mineral, a plant? You think it is an animal, well I will show you how I cured this person with a flower remedy!" I do sympathise with that, as I don't quite get that theory myself. In my opinion *Lachesis muta* can often be very close to *Phosphorus*, but they are on the complete opposite spectrums of the kingdoms.

I would say that if the patient is wearing a great big crystal, you don't give *Silica terra*. But if you take the case and you see the whole thing is *Silica terra* and then you see that she is wearing a crystal - it is like an elegant confirmatory feature. But to base the case around that - I am with George Vithoulkas. I like the way he still dissects the case like he is still in engineering training, and he listens and it is based on what the patient has said very strongly, and not his knowledge of the periodical table. To be honest I haven't gone so much down that route.

On the other hand I think we are wrong not to listen to what some of these people are saying, for example, a big influence of mine is Massimo Mangialavori. I never heard George

Vithoulkas teach that if the case looks like *Tarentula hispanica* one should look at all the other spiders. Yes, it may have many *Tarentula hispanica* features, but do you know which features are specific to *Tarentula hispanica*, or are they just spider features? So I think when Massimo says that just because you think it is *Lachesis muta* you should look at all the other snakes and observe the subtleties, we should listen.

This idea that it has to be the simillimum is ridiculous. If it is similar, it is going to heal and if it is more similar it is going to heal better. So if you give *Lachesis muta* and it was meant to be *Crotalus cascavella*, you may get some sort of result but you will get a better result with *Crotalus cascavella*.

I am worried that people are keen to learn more about *Chocolate* because it sounds more romantic than *Natrum phosphoricum*. Who can tell me the materia medica of *Zincum phosphoricum*? I think it is the last remedy in Kent but people don't know it, but they know *Eagle (Haliaeetus leucocephalus)* and *Scarlet Macaw*.

ROWENA: So how do you feel about polypharmacy and mixopathy?

BRIAN: You can get results doing that, but I feel you don't learn anything about the patient from it. I think if you give four remedies mixed together the remedy that is right will have the effect and the others may or may not interfere, but what you won't do is learn anything from it. You give two remedies, what you do learn? The patient is better but you cannot be sure which remedy helped them.

Using machines is also problematic. George Vithoulkas would definitely be against machines, even though he says it is possible that machines can do something. He made a simple craft and his rules of looking at everything are quite solid and based on what was traditionally done for a long time - the Kentian approach. But I sometimes wonder about him and Vassilis Ghegas, if they have another agenda - a spiritual agenda; a religious approach behind the scenes - but I don't feel it impinges on the type of homeopathy he teaches. He strikes me as somebody with a big mission and he sometimes looks egotistical, but I think ultimately he is concerned with homeopathy and the future of it rather than self-aggrandisement.

At a seminar once, I had a case I had presented to him, and he had been thinking about it, and when he spoke to me I felt a completely different presence. When he is in his own world, teaching homeopathy he is in a higher state, and I haven't met anyone else that I have learned from as much as I did from him when he was in that higher state.

For myself these days I have become much more focused on just a few symptoms. If I can just get a few very strong, individualising symptoms, that is my approach. I want a few very reliable things.

ROWENA: So is that keynote prescribing?

BRIAN: That is a good point. In some ways, I suppose I do use keynotes, as George Vithoulkas does a lot. Sometimes it is the gestalt, the addition of all the little things, but for me to look something up in the repertory, it would have to be very strong. I had someone today and she had tinnitus, definitely worse for motion. If she engineers the movement of her head, the tinnitus gets worse. That is a symptom. There were four remedies.

ROWENA: Do you let students sit in with you?

BRIAN: No, I don't. I used to at another clinic in Letchworth, but it is not that culture in Harley Street. The patients don't think of it as a teaching clinic. But I do work at the Royal London Homeopathic Hospital and teach doctors, but I don't have anyone sitting in my private practice anymore.

ROWENA: I think that that is another failing that we have within our profession - we don't really have an apprentice scheme, and so we come out of college and we know some but there is still so much to learn. So what is the training like for doctors now?

BRIAN: The most you can do is three months full-time with three months distant learning with video cases and stuff like that. That is what the hospital does, and then there are various other courses. You see, we created a classical course as an alternative to the Faculty and now there are several, and again now all the courses are struggling. There are too many of them but we started that. Now the doctors have become much more classical; we are responsible for that.

ROWENA: What were they like before?

BRIAN: There was only one, the Faculty. Now there are courses everywhere.

ROWENA: So did they advocate symptomatic prescribing?

BRIAN: The only thing it was; was cheap. It was two hundred pounds for six months because they were desperate for doctors to study homeopathy but I think it is three thousand pounds for three months now. At that time they got different teachers in and taught what they wanted to teach - there was no co-ordination. So I met some great teachers - my great mentor Eric Ledermann - and I met others like Ralph Twentyman, Marianne Harling, Donald Foubister and other famous homeopaths. I learned from some and I didn't from others. Some I found very inspiring and some I found very disheartening. I sat in with someone who just put on a fake smile when the patient came in. That is why I wrote about a fake smile in my book, *The Homeopathic Conversation*[13]. I just couldn't believe it really. I thought a certain personality went into homeopathy, but I realised there are all sorts. You see, there are some doctors who go into homeopathy because they couldn't fit in to the rest of medicine. The homeopathy profession needs to be careful as it doesn't want all the weirdoes and misfits.

ROWENA: So do you see homeopathy becoming dormant again?

BRIAN: I worry about the regulatory bodies, because what they want is evidence- based medicine for disease and a treatment. They don't buy into this idea that we are not treating the disease, that we are trying to stimulate the body's own natural healing ability to do something about the problem and in order to stimulate that we need to find a medicine that suits the whole human being. The more you regulate, the more you embrace a mechanistic approach to medicine. So I do worry that these regulations will favour only orthodox medicine. I always say that even if all of these regulations had been in place, Harold Shipman would have been excellent at ticking the boxes and pieces of paper and rubber-stamping.

ROWENA: So how would this affect you then?

BRIAN: I hope that homeopathy will be able to defend itself. There are a lot of pressure groups that support homeopathy, and were the government to crack down on doctors using homeopathy, I hope that there would be enough defence there to mount a serious protest.

ROWENA: Do you only practise homeopathy?

BRIAN: No, I do something called Provocative Therapy, which is I think homeopathic psychotherapy, because it encourages people to do more of what they are doing. I have noticed that when you provoke people in this way, you see them demonstrate stuff as opposed to telling you about it and there is a difference. And that is an interesting point about having a homeopath living with you as he is seeing you live, rather than you telling the story. A person comes in here and they are telling the story and in my mind I am seeing a movie, but that is not the same as seeing them do it. Sometimes I hear about people who were charming and then the receptionist tells me they were so rude!

ROWENA: I know what you mean. We need to take each detail into consideration from the first time they make contact. So on another subject, how do you think we can make money in homeopathy?

BRIAN: You see it is different if you are not a doctor because doctors offer a mixture of services. For example, I can take a blood test, I can do a physical examination, I can phone up a specialist. I would say homeopathy is not an easy way to make money because it involves a lot of time and the rewards are small financially.

30

Homeopathy is a very powerful tool but it is not an overriding system of medicine. If a person has got appendicitis, still the best treatment for them is an appendectomy. If they have raging meningitis, I still believe their best chance is with a lumber puncture (spinal tap) to find out if they have got bacteria which is causing the meningitis, enabling us to give them the right intravenous antibiotics. But in its place homeopathy is very powerful. Now if someone combines it with something else - does something else - I think that is what starts to make George Vithoulkas nervous. He wonders if they are really committed to homeopathy. I don't actually think it is a problem if someone does something else as well because in their mind, their system makes sense.

I have always said - and I know this could go down as quite a unique position - if you want to use machines, if you want to practise polypharmacy using a mixture of fifty different remedies - do it, that is fine, but as long as you have studied the classical approach as well, otherwise what the hell are you giving? You are giving a bunch of medicines, you don't know what they are doing and it is ridiculous. If someone has studied classical homeopathy and continues to educate themselves in classical homeopathy and yet does these other things, finds a role for these other things that is their business.

ROWENA: But the course the Faculty runs is only for three months. When I was studying homeopathy it was very much said, "Don't go to a doctor homeopath because they only study for a very short period of time and they cannot possibly know homeopathy as we do."

BRIAN: There are elements of truth in that.

ROWENA: I know that there are cases of arthritis at the Royal London Homeopathic Hospital being treated symptomatically with *Rhus toxicodendron*, for example.

BRIAN: Not officially, it depends on who you might meet. There would have been people who did that sort of thing, but it was not official policy.

What you hear from the doctors' side is that they will cite a case of malignant melanoma that was missed by a lay practitioner, or a person with renal failure where no one took a blood test, and the truth is that that is also true. But I also agree that there are doctors that are just resting on the laurels of being a doctor, who haven't done the years of study that every homeopath knows you have to do in order to get good at it.

ROWENA: Do you think that homeopathy is effective for treating people with cancer?

BRIAN: I have never seen a case, well maybe one, where you just treat the cancer with homeopathy. I think it definitely has to play a role in the treatment to get the immune system involved.

ROWENA: And you would do that constitutionally then?

BRIAN: Yes, treat the constitution of the patient is what I would do.

ROWENA: *Robin Murphy's tapes*[14] says the cancer layer is actually a layer in itself and so you are not achieving anything by doing that, and sometimes it is actually very difficult to see the constitutional picture when the cancer picture is so strong.

BRIAN: That is what I would do if I am honest, I would just treat constitutionally, look for a remedy that suits that whole human being, and see what remedies crop up that also suit the cancer, but I would be looking for a remedy that suits the case.

ROWENA: Would you do it gently along side their allopathic medication?

BRIAN: Yes. I might repeat the medicine in an LM potency on a daily bases for people having a lot of treatment with other things. I tend to repeat the remedy and keep just going with it. But I prefer to leave it to doctors who are specialists in treating cancers, as they are not my favourite cases to treat. I am not sure that homeopathy would be the most potent treatment you can use for cancer in the alternative world, to be honest. There are therapies like the Gerson diet, for example. Just pure homeopathy for cancer, I don't think so, but I think it can play a role, definitely.

ROWENA: What lessons do you think are crucial for homeopaths to learn Brian?

BRIAN: From my perspective if I had to say what is crucial to learn, I would say an understanding of transference and countertransference. This is basic stuff in psychology and if we don't know about it, we can damage the patient by saying and doing the wrong things. When taking a case you want their most intimate, most guarded information because that is going to be the centre of the case - the stuff that they feel most vulnerable about. If you are asking for information like that, you must know something about what happens to the person as a result of talking to you and what you can be left with. Homeopaths need to be supervised. They need to do psychological work on themselves so that they are able to cope with that stuff. It is a very lovely journey to make and you need to enter into this dynamic with the patient not being fearful of it. You might need to get supervision because you may be left with something from it that you churn over and over. It is important to have some model where you can deal with the stuff that is happening to you, because you are entering into psychological territory that is quite marshy and dangerous.

It is very difficult to be non-judgemental; you have to keep a hawk eye on yourself all the time. I remember one case that I had of a beautiful woman who trusted me and brought her child to see me. One day her husband came to see me also and during his case he told me that he sleeps with prostitutes. It was early in my career, but I felt the hackle. I thought, "What are you doing? You have this beautiful wife and child and why are you doing this?" And that was judgmental.

ROWENA: Absolutely. It is incredibly hard. I have written a teaching manual on practitioner development, and I ran a workshop for the principals and lecturers of our homeopathy colleges while working for the Society of Homeopaths. I gave them an exercise on prejudice and they all said, "Oh no, I didn't realise I still have prejudices too!"

BRIAN: That is what I say. I think Hahnemann is slightly joking when he says that all that is needed to make the correct prescription is to be free of prejudice. You would be an enlightened human being if you were free of prejudice; if you just see every other human being as a manifestation of spirituality and light camouflaged by a personality.

ROWENA: And if we are so obsessed with homeopathy then that is a prejudice in itself. If a patient says they took a paracetamol and our body language changes...

BRIAN: George Vithoulkas found a system and I am sure he has helped thousands and thousands of people but that doesn't mean that everyone has to emulate exactly that. If you force yourself to emulate that you might not be the best homeopath you can be. But I agree with him there are some people saying stuff that is a bit unsubstantiated. There is a time in homeopathy now where everyone wants to say something new, but how about we do a test and see how much everyone knows? Who can write the materia medica of *Natrum phosphoricum*? People want the new and the romantic, and there I agree with him that it is a problem. Why not learn all the basics well? I could still go to a lecture tomorrow on *Lycopodium* and someone could teach me something and then I would see *Lycopodium* in a different sort of person. I am more interested in that, to be honest, than new remedies.

ROWENA: Thank you very much Brian, for sharing your time, insights and experience with me.

CHAPTER 3:   MYRIAM SHIVADIKAR

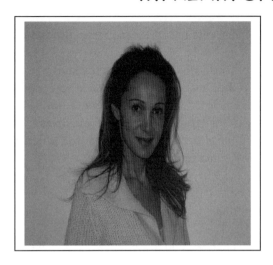

Tuesday 25 January 2005 took me to visit Myriam Shivadikar in Finchley, North London. Myriam was responsible many years ago for encouraging me to go and study homeopathy so I have a lot to thank her for! She is a very dynamic lady and is always developing how she practises and prescribes. She will be familiar to you if you have ever attended an Alliance of Registered Homeopaths' (ARH) conference, as she is the very knowledgeable and rather glamorous presenter. I found hearing her story really fascinating as I started to understand how and why she practises the way she does.

"I am still a classically trained homeopath; the shortest time I give for a first consultation is an hour and a half. But then, after taking the history, my only question is, "What needs to be cured?" and from there I work out the methodology. Homeopaths have many methodologies to choose from, for example, aetiology, Eizayaga's layers, constitutional, miasms, acutes or Kentian. There are so many different ways and none are right and none are wrong."   Myriam Shivadikar, January 2005

"When there is a lot of allopathic interference, you have to decide how to treat them and on what level and there is still no guarantee that the remedies will work. An allopathic drug may have blocked the remedies' action for whatever reason. Today, homeopathy is more challenging then in Hahnemann's times. There is a lot more pathology, especially in modern cities like London. In Iceland, India and Sri Lanka there are more clear-cut constitutions but that is not the case here and this creates a problem."
                    Myriam Shivadikar, January 2005

"I think that one of those absolute keys to being a successful homeopath is having a curiosity for knowledge. Once you think you know it, you haven't got it all."
                    Myriam Shivadikar, January 2005

CHAPTER 3:   MYRIAM SHIVADIKAR

ROWENA: So tell me Myriam, who has influenced your practise of homeopathy?

MYRIAM: Jan Scholten because what he says makes sense to me and like Rajan Sankaran, his talent is making remedies more practical, accessible and easy to understand via a system. Robin Murphy did a lot for me in another sense. He says that homeopathy is incomplete and is merely a therapeutic system of medicine. This made sense to me as I came from a Traditional Chinese Medicine background, which has eight branches to it - acupuncture, herbs, diet, massage, remedial exercises, moxibustion and surgery. Homeopathy is just one modality and we have borrowed anatomy and physiology from allopathic medicine. As a result it seems isolated, and to think we can just give a remedy and that is enough is a mistake.

People and the planet have changed and many homeopaths have realised that we cannot just give a remedy and wait for three months. Some colleges are therefore incorporating nutrition, diet, herbs and flower essences into their syllabi. Robin Murphy has said that homeopathy is part of a yogic branch of healing but now in the West all we have left of this yogic branch is the homeopathic element. So his input into our profession, apart from his book *Homeopathic Medical Repertory*[15], was to access all these old systems of medicines and bring them back. He works with astrology and homeopathy, for example, and his ideas are simple and can be found in his books.

ROWENA: I found Robin Murphy very inspiring on cancer. So tell me Myriam, how did your journey with homeopathy begin?

MYRIAM: My father is a medical doctor and during the 1970s my mother was ill. All the way through our childhood she was ill, as she was an epileptic. She was on all the drugs, bedridden and there was nothing that anyone could do for her with conventional medicine. It was horrible for my father, being a doctor and not being able to help his own wife. Then one of his friends said that he was going to go to Liverpool to learn acupuncture for two years and asked my father whether he fancied keeping him company and my father agreed.

After several months he started practising acupuncture on my mother and her epilepsy was cured – not palliated but cured! She came off all her drugs and my father was totally amazed. As a GP you cannot treat anyone in your NHS practice privately so he told patients who, for example, had neck and back problems that he had a new treatment for them. They would have to come off his NHS listing, enrol with someone else and then come and see him privately for acupuncture, but he would charge practically nothing, as it was practise for him more than anything else. So as kids we had all these weird people coming to the house. I always said I would never do this to my family, as we couldn't even come downstairs because there were all these strangers in the hall.

When it came to my A levels, I wanted to take loads of subjects as I was very academic and a bit of a nerd. My father wanted me to do medicine but I didn't. For him it was not up for discussion so I was forced to do the three sciences. After my A levels were finished I left home. I told my father that I loved him but that I really didn't want to do medicine; it just looked too boring.

In the early eighties, a Sri Lankan doctor called Professor Anton Jayasuriya started running some international congresses so that practitioners of every type of complementary medicines could unite. At that time homeopaths would scoff at acupuncturists and acupuncturists would say that homeopathy was psychojargon. Practitioners didn't understand each other's disciplines and Jayasuriya saw a gap in the market.

My father was the first British doctor to have a Bioresonance machine . It was invented in Germany and he was asked to teach how to use it in seminars and conferences because he spoke English. So in time he went to one of Professor Jayasuriya's conferences to teach about his machine and while chatting to him, my father mentioned me. Professor Jayasuriya suggested my father send me to Sri Lanka to learn acupuncture at university there. So a year after I had run away from medicine, I was on my way to study on a one month intensive course where all you do is live, breathe, drink, eat and sleep acupuncture! At the time, I had absolutely no interest in going, but I did it to make him happy and I thought it would make him leave me alone to get on with my own life. But the unexpected happened. I went there, fell in love with medicine and stayed six and a half years in Colombo!

Two weeks after I arrived, a war started. I was constitutionally *Carcinosin* at this stage and wrote letters to my mum saying that the war had nothing to do with me, that I hadn't started it and that I was not responsible – a real *Carcinosin* delusion! And then I got very ill, which is how I got into homeopathy. I was absolutely eaten alive by mosquitoes and the doctors there had never seen anything like it. My legs got infected and there was pus everywhere. It was terrible and I couldn't walk for two months. I was staying in the students' hostel and there was a German homeopath there that was learning acupuncture. People came from all over the world just to learn acupuncture for one month. It was a taster; it did not qualify you to practise it, but you would get an idea as to whether you wanted to study further or not.

ROWENA: Were they mostly medics?

MYRIAM: A lot were but there were lay people as well. So, this German homeopath was observing me in agony in the hostel but I wouldn't take the antibiotics because I never had had drugs in my life. I was flushing them down the toilet because of my principles. Everything hurt. Just negotiating to go to the toilet, which was a few yards, was agony. So I was not moving around much and he observed me and prescribed *Sulphur.* He had seen that I wasn't washing but hadn't asked me why. It was because I was in total agony not because I was worse for water! His observations led him to the wrong conclusion.

ROWENA: So he was assuming your skin was worse for washing?

MYRIAM: Absolutely, and assuming can stop you getting to the cause. Unfortunately the *Sulphur* gave me the mother of all aggravations but I was really impressed. The usual story is people say they went to see a homeopath and they had this amazing cure and then they were converted. I had an aggravation and I was converted! I was so surprised that this tiny little pill could cause all of this that I wanted to start studying homeopathy immediately, but because of the aggravation I could not walk for two months! Professor Jayasuriya sent a doctor round to dress my wounds because my legs were a real mess. There was a brilliant library in the hostel, and since I was housebound, I just worked my way through all their books.

In time, because I had studied more homeopathy than anyone else there, Professor Jayasuriya asked me if I would teach and that is how I really got into it. In Sri Lanka we were part of the state South Colombo General Hospital and we had our own acupuncture ward where we saw a thousand patients a day; not in a year but in one day. We had two clinics, one in the morning and one in the evening.

ROWENA: That is unbelievable.

MYRIAM: It was amazing and total chaos at the same time. Each patient got three minutes and they all sat in rows on chairs, mostly for acupuncture. We would get some symptoms and treat them. It was a free clinic and we got to see absolutely everything. We could send patients across the hall for blood test or an x-ray and get the results straightaway. It was very efficient even though it is third world country.

ROWENA: What modalities were used other than acupuncture?

MYRIAM: Many different methods of complementary medicines but the first one was acupuncture. Professor Jayasuriya invented a therapy called homeopuncture, and he used it originally on patients with vitiligo (white patches on their skin) who had not responded to other therapies.

ROWENA: Was the homeopathy case taking achieved in three minutes also?

MYRIAM: On a daily basis remedies were prescribed using Hering's three legged stool principle (at least three major keynotes of a remedy need to be present) but each patient was given, at some point in their treatment, a proper appointment in order to take a full case history. Sri Lankans are very laid back, they are Buddhist and generally they don't get cancer, multiple sclerosis or AIDS. Their beliefs make them very chilled and relaxed.

ROWENA: What diseases do they get?

MYRIAM: Climate related diseases such as asthma and rheumatism. Professor Jayasuriya was a rheumatologist and we learned a lot through him. They had been using homeopathy separately from acupuncture, but certain patients were still not improving and then he had the idea to take a remedy in liquid form, dip the acupuncture needle inside the remedy and then puncture the acupuncture points. When I went there in 1984 that was all they were doing. Later on we did laser therapy and after that an osteopath from England came over and taught manipulative medicine. They used all sorts of weird and wonderful therapies because Professor Jayasuriya was very inventive and creative.

I asked Professor Jayasuriya why they used homeopathy and not Chinese herbs, the obvious choice, as it is part of TCM. He replied that Chinese herbs are indigenous to China and he was really against destroying the planet. He was extremely environmentally conscious and said that if you eat a mango you have to go back and plant a mango seed. With homeopathy, you don't need to destroy a large amount of plants just for the medicine.

ROWENA: Good point. So the government funded this place?

MYRIAM: Yes, the hospital was government funded; however, the university I attended in Sri Lanka was a private establishment. In a third world country, you get so much experience and learn to make clinical decisions very quickly. At one point, I personally had a hundred patients a day with students following me around. At that time, I had no idea you could give homeopathy by mouth! I thought that the only way you administer it was by needle. When I came here I was horrified that patients took remedies orally. I was passionate about homeopathy and stayed there six and a half years. The university held four or five congresses on complementary medicine every year all over the world.

I came back to England in 1991 and even though I was a teacher in Sri Lanka, I was never trained officially as a homeopath. I realised that I needed to go to college here because I needed to learn homeopathy philosophy; there is no time for it in Sri Lanka. There had been a war going on while I was there and we just had to get on with it full-time, seven days a week, from seven in the morning until one or two in the afternoon. It is too hot to practise in the afternoon so we had a siesta and then we would work again from five until seven and attend lectures from seven until nine.

ROWENA: That is a really long day.

MYRIAM: It was great though and because of the siesta, it felt like two days in one.

So I came back in 1991 and realised I wanted to go a little bit deeper with this. I didn't know any homeopaths but was told through my connections with acupuncturists that one of the best colleges, politically, was the College of Homeopathy (COH).

ROWENA: Politically, why?

MYRIAM: Because my acupuncture colleagues were political people, they claimed that COH had a foot in the door of the government. Coupled with that, it was only down the road. At the same time as studying I was learning all about these machines from Germany. As I was treating patients already and I was given the option of what year to join as COH queried why I wanted to study anyway since I was already a practising homeopath. I decided to start in the second year, which is where the philosophy begins. It was a strange time in my life as I was also teaching in India and in various other places and I was already quite well known on the international lecturing circle.

As a student, I was fortunate because straightaway I could apply on a Monday morning to my patients what I learned over the weekend at college and see what worked. I attended seminars by Rajan Sankaran and George Vithoulkas and I met Eizayaga who was an amazing teacher. Alongside that I spent two years learning German because the Germans wouldn't teach about their machines in English at that point.

ROWENA: Could you explain to me a bit about the machines Myriam?

MYRIAM: When I actually came back to the UK for good I didn't have anything, so to make some pocket money I would help my dad in his clinic while I was learning German. I made his appointments for him and watched and observed him. In time I realised that the way he used his machine was not compatible with my style as we have different philosophies.

ROWENA: So are there doctors who use these machines?

MYRIAM: At that time they were only training doctors in how to use them. My dad was learning homeopathy German style. And not only German style but German medical style. Most of the remedies he used were in ampoules (an injectable form in a saline suspension that is isotonic to the body) so very little was in grains or tablets. He would transfer the information from the ampoules to the patient via injection. That is the German way of administering and it is very interesting.

ROWENA: Did he work constitutionally?

MYRIAM: He didn't understand that concept at that time.

ROWENA: Because he has only had a short training in homeopathy?

MYRIAM: Yes, because MDs only need a short training in order to qualify to practise, but fortunately my father has an enquiring mind and was mainly self-taught. While I was there I could help him but as an allopath, he didn't individualise. If I suggested *Causticum* for a stroke patient he wanted to give *Causticum* to all patients that had had a stroke. Consequently, I was tearing my hair out. Some doctors use the machine for desensitising patients with allergies against antibiotics so you can use the machine for pretty much anything. My father was doing cutting edge stuff just in a different direction to me. His background was in surgery.

ROWENA: Is he still practising?

MYRIAM: No, he is seventy five now and helps look after my daughter while I practise. There are many different types of machine and in some ways Anton Jayasuriya is absolutely right and so are the Chinese; barefoot medicine works. Why do you need anything more elaborate? But patients in Sri Lanka are not as complicated as over here; they are not interfered with so much. They haven't had antibiotics and chemo and radiotherapies and hormones and surgeries and vaccines. They also don't get stressed because even while I was there during a war they were just calm and accepting and just said that it was their karma. There is a war, curfews, the rainy season and no food, but it is still their karma. Amazing. Over here there are a lot more layers and this is why I use my machine - it helps me to sift through those layers.

I am still a classically trained homeopath; the shortest time I give for a first consultation is an hour and a half. But then, after taking the history, my only question is, "What needs to be cured?" and from there I work out the methodology. Homeopaths have many methodologies to choose from, for example, aetiology, Eizayaga's layers, constitutional, miasms, acutes or Kentian. There are so many different ways and none are right and none are wrong.

We tell our patients to take whatever it is that we give them and we might give them another remedy as a back up if the first doesn't work. We ask them to let us know in six weeks how they have done and then we reassess. If both don't work then perhaps there is something that is blocking the case like use of steroids currently or in the past.

ROWENA: So if someone is on steroids, would you give them *Cortisone* to clear the layer?

MYRIAM: Yes, or perhaps *Apis*. Checking out the regular remedies with my machine, I would be able to see that they didn't work because the cortisone was creating a block. *Cannabis* also blocks remedies from working.

ROWENA: So do you give *Cannabis* in the same way, to clear that block?

MYRIAM: Sometimes I just give it and wait. I find the remedies don't work otherwise.

ROWENA: In what potency would you give *Cortisone* or *Cannabis* under those circumstances?

MYRIAM: Sixes or thirties, it depends on what effect it has had on them. Sometimes it will be as my first prescription but my style is always changing and developing. When there is a lot of allopathic interference, you have to decide how to treat them and on what level and there is still no guarantee that the remedies will work. An allopathic drug may have blocked the remedies' action for whatever reason. Today, homeopathy is more challenging then in Hahnemann's times. There is a lot more pathology, especially in modern cities like London. In Iceland, India and Sri Lanka there are more clear-cut constitutions but that is not the case here and this creates a problem.

ROWENA: So let us say somebody comes to you with cancer. How do you approach their case?

MYRIAM: I would take the history with a timeline because we need to understand where, how and why the 'dis-ease' originated. In cancer cases or cases with mixed pathology, I see the case in layers as this approach breaks the case down into bite sized chunks. I would use my machine as a tool because it is important for me to know which organs are affected and how much pathology there is.

ROWENA: How does the machine tell you that?

MYRIAM: The type of machine I use is meridian based technology. There are many channels of energy or meridians, which travel all over the body and these channels end in the fingertips and in the toes. A circuit is created when the patient holds a brass electrode connected to the machine, which has a dial from which you can get readings. What is being measured is the electrical resistance of the acupuncture points and when there is a disorder the resistance reduces. Each machine is calibrated so that the readings are from zero to one hundred. A reading of fifty is fine but with a child it may be sixty as their vitality is stronger. We can actually measure the vital force of a patient using the machine.

Measuring each of these points on the hands and the feet takes less than five minutes and then I will make a note on their card of the state of their organs. If the reading is only thirty five or forty for the large intestine, I will underline it. If it is really low I will underline it twice and circle it; just like when we use the repertory and we see remedies in plain, italic and bold. The readings provide useful information for me.

Using a patient with cancer as an example, although his case has serious pathology, this still could be a Kentian aetiology as there is a strong emotional component that could have triggered his illness. His wife had thrown him out, they got divorced, he has restricted access to his children and he has to now pay for two mortgages and sort his health out alone. He is angry about the injustice, is feeling like a victim and it is likely I would think about giving him *Staphysagria* or *Carcinosin* as a top layer. Then from the readings if his liver or kidneys are really low then I would give him remedies to support, detox and drain those organs. These remedies I supply in a separate bottle and they are usually a combination of herbal tinctures.

For homeopaths there are many different ways to treat a patient. Everything you do is based on your perception, knowledge and observation at that point in time. The machine gives you an objective tool to assess the state of the organs and this may influence your prescribing but it doesn't mean that you don't use your normal methods as well. With a tool like this we can see how much pathology there is and how much change has occurred when they come back for a follow up sessions. A patient could come for treatment for headaches but with the machine as a tool you can assess clearly where the condition is originating from and see if something more sinister is going on.

ROWENA: Which is an area we could be weak in if we didn't pick up the red flags. If your patient had had chemotherapy, for example, would there be a specific remedy that you would prescribe first?

MYRIAM: Cadmium sulphuratum deals with the side effects of chemotherapy beautifully so I would give an individualised drainage tonic with specific herbal tinctures and tissue salts so that the patient can take it frequently to give organ support and I would include the *Cadmium sulphuratum*.

ROWENA: In low potency?

MYRIAM: Yes, a 6C. The tonic drains the liver, kidneys and lymph and the *Cadmium sulphuratum* is for toxicity but it might not work for all patients. It is also good for assisting patients to stop smoking.

Once we have worked out what needs to be cured and what sort of remedy we are going to prescribe, then we can check the remedies on the machine. What I have explained to you so far is the diagnostics aspect. My particular machine also provides an electromagnetic treatment. Patients hold the brass electrodes and place their feet on brass footplates. This creates a closed cybernetic circuit within them, and uses their energy and modifies it. It works by taking harmonic, healthy waves, and amplifying them to make them stronger. At the same time the disharmonic, unhealthy waves are inverted in order to cancel out their pathology.

ROWENA: Like cures like?

MYRIAM: Yes. It is like making a nosode in a way. The machine separates out what is healthy and what is not healthy and there are two different waveforms. Diseases don't just happen; they start off with biophysical changes and then they turn into chemical changes and then into pathology. Often, when people come to us, we get the end stage of their rheumatoid arthritis or Crohn's but it has taken time to develop.

The machine has a honeycomb testing plate named as such because it has little holes where you can put remedies. Anything you put on this testing plate will go into the circuit and then you can see what influence a particular substance or remedy has on the patient. With the remedy on the testing plate you can then recheck their points. You might think that your patient needs *Calcarea carbonica* in low potency repeated often so you might place a 6C on the testing plate and check their weak points, which you already ascertained at the beginning of the consultation. You then look to see if the remedy has pushed the readings up and if it has then it is a good remedy for them. If it brings the readings up and then the needle goes down again it means it is good but it is not going to hold. I then will try a 12C and 6C together and I keep doing this until I have two or even three potencies of one remedy all together and the reading holds. I give all my patients remedies in water as I find that medium much softer.

ROWENA: So do they bang it on their hand like LMs?

MYRIAM: If the remedies are in very low potency, yes.

ROWENA: So they would be plussing it.

MYRIAM: Yes. Hahnemann said you should never repeat the same remedy twice. Diseases are dynamic, so their cure should be too. I feel that homeopathy can work very much preventatively and if you see a constitution we can predict what might happen next. We might recognise what acute remedy a patient might need by using the relationship of remedies. For example, a patient who resonates with one of the Mercury remedies constitutionally will need *Pulsatilla nigricans* in an acute. They might also go into a *Rhus toxicodendron* acute and get stressed out and have joint pains or they might also need *Syphilinum* because that is their genetic, miasmatic remedy. They will also need a tonic because that group of remedies reflects a very toxic state. As a result my patients go away with three or four spray top bottles of remedies.

ROWENA: The main criticism of polypharmacy, which I am sure you are aware, is….

MYRIAM: How do you know which remedy has done what?

ROWENA: So how do you know?

MYRIAM: I don't regard my prescribing style as polypharmacy.

ROWENA: So what is the technical term for when you prescribe lots of different remedies at the same time?

MYRIAM: It is the same remedy but in different potencies at the same time and that will be their main remedy. The tonics are on a herbal level to support the organs. Here is a typical example of how I prescribe. Let us say that the patient is tubercular and has come to see me with recurrent coughs and colds. Having taken their case I might find that genetically or constitutionally they are one of the tubercular remedies like Tuberculinum bovinum, *Calcarea phosphorica* or *Phosphorus* but because of the nature of tubercular types and their sensitivity, they cannot take their constitutional too often. On a tonic level they will need remedies to support their lungs. For some patients, when the lungs are affected, so is the skin and bowels. In Chinese Medicine these organs are related.

Nothing deep goes into the tonics; perhaps I will use *Lobelia inflata*. For a lot of people I use *Iodium* for coughs, which is effective and mild, and with the tubercular types it covers a lot of thyroid gland issues. I might use *Berberis* if they have eczema as a result of their lungs being messed up. And then of course I look at diet and life style.

ROWENA: And you put your remedies on your machine which checks out all its ingredients and how the patient will respond to it.

MYRIAM: Yes, I call it cooking or alchemy. Do they need more of this? Do they need more of that? It cooks until it is beautifully tailored to the patient.

ROWENA: It is really great talking to you Myriam. Your description of how you prescribe, I hope, will answer a lot of the questions from homeopaths and patients who didn't understand it before, as this is not the way some of us were trained.

MYRIAM: Homeopathy is a very old system of medicine. They say the Egyptians used it as well as Paracelsus and then Hahnemann came along and created a system; after all he is German and they are very good at that! He did all the groundwork for us and developed the principles and worked out the provings and potencies. And he changed his mind many times as he refined it and carried on evolving through his many editions of the *Organon*[4]. In the last edition, for example, he went on to create the LM potency because he found through trial and error that LMs were the most gentle of all potencies. He was always looking to make things as refined and precise as possible. If he were alive today he would have developed homeopathy even further.

ROWENA: So tell me where you teach Myriam?

MYRIAM: I teach homeopathy in various colleges, the College of Practical Homeopathy in the Midlands (CPH Midlands) and the Practical College in Iceland and the Lakeland College of Homeopathy. I also teach at the School of Shamanic Homoeopathy and the London College of Traditional Acupuncture. I think that one of those absolute keys to being a successful homeopath is having a curiosity for knowledge. Once you think you know it, you haven't got it all.

ROWENA: Myriam, thank you.

CHAPTER 4: ELLEN KRAMER

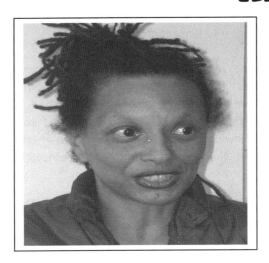

Wednesday 9 February 2005 took me back to the College of Practical Homeopathy (CPH). I had been there the year before in my role as education adviser for the Society of Homeopaths and met with Ellen Kramer for the first time then. CPH in London occupies a whole floor of a building above a shop on the High Street in Finchley. It was a student clinic day, but Ellen managed to maintain her focus with me and illustrated, yet again how enthusiasm, dedication and ambition play a large part in the successful career of a homeopath. Ellen fixed her deep and intense brown eyes on me and I knew that hour I would spend with her would shake my classical foundations and leave me breathless.

"Homeopathy works – it is easy and it is simple. You just have to know the art of application. And the methods are a guide. They guide you to that application. Practical homeopathy is the practical application of different methods according to each patient. So it is the patient who tells you what to do, not you trying to apply something to a patient."

Ellen Kramer, February 2005

"Homeopathy is a safe system of medicine; it is gentle, it is effective, and you get excellent results. If you are not getting the results, it is because you are not applying it properly."

Ellen Kramer, February 2005

"If you think you are going be a homeopath without evolving in some way you are mistaken, because your patients will take you down places you don't want to go. People change subtly; they don't realise they are doing it. But you have some people who find practitioner development a bit challenging for them so they try and sneak off, but I know who they are and unfortunately they are the very people who need to do it the most."

Ellen Kramer, February 2005

CHAPTER 4: ELLEN KRAMER

ROWENA: What brought you into homeopathy?

ELLEN: We had a tenant who was studying to be a homeopath at the College of Homeopathy (COH). The first time I came across homeopathy was through him when I was pregnant with my daughter in 1987. I had very, very bad morning sickness and he prescribed some remedies that worked. And then I went off to the Clissold Park Natural Therapy Centre in Stoke Newington and saw a homeopath there, and after that I didn't have morning sickness right the way through the pregnancy. I thought, "This is really interesting!"

I decided that I wasn't going to vaccinate my daughter. I had been vaccinated all my life and my immune system was shot, and I could see it was devastating. I already had two boys that had been vaccinated, and I could see the effect. And in fact it was my father, when I was taking my younger son to be vaccinated, who asked me "Why are you doing this?" And I said, "Oh because you've got to." He said "No you don't." He said to me, "Do you know as a child we never got vaccinated, we all got measles and mumps and all these things." He was brought up in South Africa and he said "We were fine. It's not a good idea to keep doing this." And I thought to myself "Oh you batty old man!" So I didn't take any notice of him until my daughter was born, and when she started suffering from earaches I took her to an acute clinic at Clissold Park.

This was like the turning point of my entire life. She was screaming and yelling and doing a complete *Chamomilla* child. And the homeopath there was looking in her book which I later realised was Kent's *Repertory*[16]. She flipped through it, and then she looked through another book, which I later realised was a materia medica. And she put her hand into the drawer, came out with this set of little pills, she popped one in Zoë's little mouth and it was like a miracle. Five seconds later Zoë was out like a light. She must have been about nine months at the time. Then she gave me a bag of little pills to take away and it was miraculous. I couldn't believe that something did that, and I knew that the kids had never responded to Calpol or anything in that particular way. So I went home and I got very excited about homeopathy and I actually found out from her that she was doing some tutorials in homeopathy, so I signed up for those.

I was going to Ghana and she did me a whole travel pack as I refused to take the conventional vaccines. It was the first time I had taken my daughter and my husband, and I went for it. I decided then that we would not be having our vaccines or the antimalarials, and everyone was going "You're going to die, what about polio, what about this, what about that?" I bought this whole set of remedies, she gave me this list of what to do with malaria if you got it, and I ordered them all from Ainsworths. I started taking *Malaria officinalis* once a week, and I gave that to my daughter and my husband, too. We were out on holiday with my sister, who was pregnant, and she was actually taking the antimalarial. And I said to her, "You know, you shouldn't be taking that while you're pregnant, it's very dangerous." And she said "Oh you don't know what you're talking about." I said "Fine." She got malaria and actually was hospitalised when she came back from Ghana.

That was it; I knew homeopathy worked. When my husband was ill, the GP said to him that he had contracted dermatitis and suggested to him that he go and see a homeopath. He saw Brian Kaplan and that was it; I was just hooked. I wanted to treat the kids homeopathically then. And I remember we got in contact with this great Indian homeopath in Baker Street, and we went to see him. He was a Sikh and he was fantastic. You would get there and there would be a queue of patients waiting to see him - they were all Indian. We had got really run down and had continuous colds and chest infections. He wasn't a classical homeopath but he gave us a couple of pills, which we took, and we felt great. Then I got a kidney infection and I went to see him again and he gave me some more pills and I got better. And there I was, absolutely hooked on homeopathy.

I started buying my own remedies, and at the time we were really broke and I couldn't afford to see a homeopath regularly, except for acute illnesses. And I thought to myself, if the homeopath at Clissold Park can do homeopathy from looking in a book, I can do it! It cannot be that hard. So I got myself David Gemmell's *Everyday Homeopathy*[17], and got started.

If the kids were unwell, I would prescribe for them. And I began thinking that I needed to do a course in this, because there was something else going on as we kept getting these acute illnesses. I applied for classical training in homeopathy at the London College of Classical Homeopathy (LCCH) in Morley College.

I was working as a hair and makeup artist, I had my kit, and I was prescribing remedies to everybody on the shoots. I had some fantastic experiences with different people on different shoots. And all I had was this book. And everything I gave worked. That is how I got to know my acute remedies - through friends, family and work colleagues. People would say, "Go and see Ellen, she has got a remedy for you." On several occasions when I was on a shoot I saved the day by having the remedies.

We were shooting a commercial for Saudi Arabia and the star model on the commercial suddenly got really ill with a very, very bad sore throat. We were having lunch and it looked like we were going to have to stop. She was going down rapidly and the producer there said to me, "Ellen, haven't you got one of those things you keep in your bag?" So I spoke to her and looked at her throat and I could see that her tonsils had swelled and had all these white globules on them. I used to carry this huge kit around with me and from it I prescribed an alternation of *Aconitum napellus* and Mercury (*Mercurius solubilis*). One of the things you will know about me is that I never forget what I give people; I never forget a case. And she got better and I just thought, "Good God, it really works."

ROWENA: What made you alternate? Where did you get that idea?

ELLEN: I got it from doing it with the kids at home.

ROWENA: But was that in one of the books?

ELLEN: No. The reason why is because, when I was taking down symptoms for acutes I wasn't quite sure exactly which remedy it was. All I could see was that it seemed to look like two particular remedies so why not give both remedies and alternate and see.

ROWENA: Rather than sit there for hours trying to work it out exactly?

ELLEN: Yes. And the other thing about David Gemmell's book, *Everyday Homeopathy*[17] was that he would say, in acutes give the remedy every hour for six hours and reduce as symptoms improve. So that is what I followed and that is how I still do my acutes. I give the remedy every hour for six hours, so when I alternated I would be alternating hourly.

So I had spent, before I actually decided to do the course, about five years prescribing at home for friends and family, until it was actually getting beyond a joke in terms of dealing with people's minor problems. But I could see that there was more to it than just the acute symptoms that people were presenting to me, because the remedies would clear it and then they would go off and they would have another acute and things like that. So that is what inspired me to do the course.

I had got a sense when I went for my interview at LCCH that it felt all wrong. They were talking about how you weren't allowed to prescribe remedies. And I had been for five years, and they were going on about how dangerous it was and all this stuff. I remember thinking that I mustn't tell them I was prescribing. I had also met a student from there, who was a model, and she had a baby who had severe eczema, and she had been using homeopathic remedies that had been prescribed. She was seeing a homeopath and the eczema was getting so bad, and I asked her why she didn't give remedies herself. She told me that she wasn't allowed to at college. And she was so fearful.

When a friend said that he didn't think LCCH was the college for me, I just thought to myself, well maybe he is right. He said he knew a friend, who was setting up a college in Hackney. His friend was Robert Davidson and I thought he was the scariest guy in the world; he even grunted. Their College of Practical Homeopathy in the Midlands (CPH Midlands) was already going, and they had now decided to open the London one.

I thought that it was all kind of dodgy, but I enrolled anyway as on another level it felt right. On the first day I arrived early as the college was local to me, and there was David Howell manoeuvring these tables and hoovering. And I said, "Well, I've come for the college." He said "Yes, well you can start hoovering now as you've got here so early." I thought to myself, "What kind of an outfit is this? The first thing he asks me to do is hoover!" So I found myself hoovering and then helping to lay all the tables out. And that was it, the college started, and I was just totally and utterly into it. It was so bizarre; it was almost like I knew this stuff before and I had come home.

It was the first course I had ever been on that I understood anything that they were telling me, because I am very severely dyslexic and found that it was such a handicap when I was at school. And most of my school life was spent looking out the window, because whatever people were talking about made no sense to me. And when I was at CPH it did make sense to me, because it was practical.

The minute I was encouraged to see patients that was it, I was on a roll. I was so enthusiastic I talked of nothing but homeopathy to anybody who wanted to listen to me. When I was on a shoot every model that came to see me for their makeup ended up having homeopathic remedies. And I had some interesting cases. I had one model that was sweating profusely from her hands and arms, they would just pour water. She had had this very serious car accident where she had been concussed, and she was going to have an operation to remove the sweat glands because it was so bad. And I suggested to her to try *Opium* because it is a big head trauma remedy and it has profuse sweating.

So she bought *Opium* 6C from Ainsworths and I recommended she take it twice daily and see how she got on before the operation, as it would be very bad to suppress it. It was about nine months to a year later when I saw her again. She said, "Thank God I saw you, I took that *Opium* 6C and it all went. The profuse sweating just went."

I ran my practice out of CPH student clinic. I was just so enthusiastic. I would go up to people on the bus. I remember this child that was covered in eczema. I just couldn't help myself, I just said, "You don't have to suffer, why don't you come to our college clinic as we treat eczema." I would tell everybody and I had some great cases. When I left college I continued to treat them and I built up my practice from there.

Before we left college Robert Davidson told us about a payment scheme for our patients. Because I had been self-employed for about nine years, I was really getting fed up of living from hand to mouth. So I listened to this, and one of the things I am quite good at is taking ideas and turning them into working models. I went home and I couldn't sleep, I was so excited, and I started calculating how many patients I needed to run the scheme, and what I would do to run this payment scheme. What I realised was that the biggest obstacle to developing one's practice is fear of not having enough money and not being able to pay your rent.

ROWENA: Because it gets in the way?

ELLEN: Yes, and also it puts patients off. Nobody wants to come and see someone who is fearful, nobody wants to come and see somebody who thinks that they haven't got enough money. So I thought to myself, if I could get enough patients on the payment scheme, I would be earning so much regular money a month. So I wrote all these ideas down and I went back to college and I said to Robert Davidson "Can you explain to me exactly how you did this?" He said "Oh, go away and work it out yourself." So I went away and I worked it out myself.

Just before I graduated, I wrote to all my patients and said that I was setting up a practice in Gaskin Street in Islington. There was a little clinic there called the Islington Green Centre of Complementary Medicine and it was going to cost me thirty pounds for half a day, so because I am in business I knew that I needed to make that pay for itself. I told them that I was setting up this new scheme, which they could go on to by standing order. I would be offering them a service, they could come and see me as many times as they liked for that payment.

For fifteen pounds per month they could come to see me as many times as needed, or my normal fee was twenty five pounds a session. I had ten patients who decided they would like to go onto the payment scheme and follow me from college. So that was the basis of my practice. I now knew that I had enough money each month to actually pay for my clinic. And the scheme really took off; I actually had loads of patients on the scheme. One of the things that I recognised was the eighty/twenty principle; eighty percent of people came once or twice and that was it; they didn't come back again. And then they couldn't be bothered to cancel the scheme.

The other twenty percent gave me the most aggravation, so they are the ones that I worked really hard with. They went on the scheme and they milked it. But I didn't mind because the other eighty percent didn't. It is the same scheme that health centres run - eighty percent of the people who join never, ever, go and twenty percent of the people go regularly and trash up the equipment, but it doesn't matter because the other eighty percent don't.

ROWENA: But you're not doing that payment scheme now?

ELLEN: No I am not.

ROWENA: If you were, how much would you charge a month?

ELLEN: If I were doing it now I would charge about thirty to thirty pounds a month for it. I worked out the details of what they got, and basically they got a bargain and a lot of people were really pleased about being on the scheme, because at that time there was no *Homeopathic Helpline*[18]. So people would call me up on the phone at all hours. I was running a busy acute helpline for my patients with *Everyday Homeopathy*[17] as my materia medica and repertory. It was fantastic, and from there my practice flourished. This was in about 1996 and I had qualified in 1995. 1996 also gave me the opportunity to go and work in Romford, which is the best place in the world to work. People come on so many different allopathic drugs. They are drugged up to the hilt.

ROWENA: Why particularly there?

ELLEN: God knows. It is the suburbs; they drug people up there. And they are the sort of people you never see in Islington, because in Islington people were attracted because they wanted an alternative. The people that I saw in Romford were the desperate. They were on many, many drugs, especially people in their sixties and seventies. I remember asking one man to bring in the drugs that he was on. He brought me in a full carrier bag. And I then had to work out how you wean people off their drugs. And that is how I learnt all about tautopathy, which is one of the methods of using the drugs back in potency that have caused the symptoms. Every time a patient came in with their drugs, I would take a sample of the drug and then I would send it off to be potentised. I have got a huge drug pharmacy. Tautopathy also helps those stuck on recreational drugs. The same system applies.

ROWENA: So if someone comes in on Cannabis you would give them *Cannabis* homeopathically? Nothing else?

ELLEN: Until they get to a point, and then slowly help them to reduce it. So I worked out all different ways of doing this with drugs, because in Romford you have got two chances of getting it right, and if you don't start getting a result they don't come back. And if you get a result they bring loads of other patients. So I had to learn quick, quick, quick, sharp, sharp, sharp. It wasn't easy, I had my disasters, you know. And that is where I learnt the folly of totality prescribing. Looking for totality prescriptions for patients when they are not ready, adds to their problems. It doesn't help.

When people are highly toxic from the drugs that they are taking; the main organs that are affected are the kidneys and the liver. I remember I had a lovely case of a lady who was suffering from hot flushes. She couldn't go on to Hormone Replacement Therapy because she had had a stroke but she was really suffering with the menopause. She was in a wheelchair so she couldn't come and see me. So I went to her and I looked at the case and it was a classic *Natrum muriaticum*. Her stroke had started within a year of her husband dying. Unfortunately it was a complete disaster, her symptoms became much worse; she was in a right state.

Then I went on a classic remedy hunt, I thought it has got to be *Lachesis muta*, because she is loquacious and all this sort of rot. I gave her *Lachesis muta* and it just got worse and worse, to the point where I just said to her, "Look, I don't think homeopathy's for you. I think you should see a nutritionist and a herbalist, thank you very much, goodbye." I felt I was just adding to her problems. Now in hindsight, I would never, ever, ever start a case from that perspective. I would actually look at what was presenting. She was on about seven or eight different drugs. She was on blood thinners and drugs for high blood pressure. Now I would have started her off with a detox therapeutic, organ drainage and nutritional support. And then I would be looking at which drugs are causing the main symptoms.

ROWENA: So when you get a patient who comes to you with side effects of Tamoxifen after breast cancer and has had radiation treatment – and has a history of the Pill and Hormone Replacement Therapy – would you give *Tamoxifen* in potency to start the case?

ELLEN: Yes, you can buy Tamoxifen and give it back to them in potency. It works. I have had patients that come and say that they just want you to help with the side effects of Tamoxifen. I think, "Well thanks for your money, here's *Tamoxifen* back in potency." I tell them to take less of it because they will become more sensitive to its action. Tautopathy gives the patient maximum therapeutic value from their allopathic drug. So they just need to take less of it, otherwise they can go into overdosing. You sensitise the vital force to the drug so they need less of it. You can use tautopathy to wean people off their drugs, so if they are taking *Thyroxine*, in time they are only taking one *Thyroxine* a week and the rest of it they are taking homeopathically, and that one *Thyroxine* a week is enough.

ROWENA: So when you get patients that have come to you for something else and then they tell you that they are on *Thyroxine*, would you go with the *Thyroxine* first?

ELLEN: No, not unless it is a problem. If people are on drugs I leave them alone until it becomes a problem. I know if they are on good homeopathy, within about a year the drugs will be a problem. Because the liver starts to clean up; it gets more sensitive to the drug and the vital force will not tolerate a poison any more.

ROWENA: Yes. And when you get alcohol out of your system, if you then go back and have one glass, you are drunk.

ELLEN: Yes, it is the same principle. The best notes are the ones you get at CPH. If you are not a practical homeopath, you don't actually understand that you can treat anybody you like; it is the method that you choose to treat. You know the method you use will give you access into the repertory and the materia medica. The method you choose will mean that you will either choose to do a drainage remedy or not.

I find it very difficult to understand how people are so hung up on a methodology that suits nintenth or early twentieth century patients. It is just not applicable to twenty first century patients. You get the odd twenty first century patient who you can apply that method to. So it doesn't surprise me that you get a whole load of homeopaths that say you cannot make money out of homeopathy; there are not enough patients. I just think to myself, good; if that is your belief system, stay there. I don't believe that, I know homeopathy works; it is just how you apply it. Homeopathy works – it is easy and it is simple. You just have to know the art of application. And the methods are a guide. They guide you to that application. Practical homeopathy is the practical application of different methods according to each patient. So it is the patient who tells you what to do, not you trying to apply something to a patient.

It is like having tools in a toolbox the classical method is one method. I really understand where Kent was coming from, because I would say in observing people, eighty percent of their sickness comes out in mental and emotional stuff. Now, the simple question is this, can I cure that now? If I can, there are no drugs, there is no suppression, there are no obstacles to cure - and then a Kentian totality prescription will work.

If you have a mental/emotional causation, you can see that their pathology is coming out of that, but they have spent twenty years on Amitriptyline and have got loads and loads of other stuff, or their diet is so appalling they are nutritionally depleted, can you give them that? No, you cannot. Unless you want to enjoy a good aggravation, and then tell your patient it is a healing crisis when it is not. It is inappropriate prescribing because you don't understand what you are doing. Okay, if you can see it is coming out of a mental/emotional causation, there are no obstacles to cure, and if you go back to the *Organon*[4], what did Hahnemann say? He says remove the obstacle to cure. What is it that needs curing? What needs curing is the cause of those symptoms. If you can cure that straight away, then what we call here at CPH 'the whole patient methods' will work.

If there are obstacles to cure, then you are basically looking at what we call 'part patient methodologies', that is, organ drainage, tautopathy, aetiology, sequential, nutrition, cell salts and polypharmacy. Those are your toolbox and you will get a result with your patient.

ROWENA: Everything you have said makes perfect sense. I think if somebody sat down with you who practised in a different way to you, if they heard that, they would understand it. But I am wondering if people attract what they can treat; do you know what I mean? Because I do think that there are a lot of classical homeopaths who have very successful practices and they don't practise the way you do, so I am wondering if they just attract those patients that they can help. I am not saying that there is some that they cannot but...

ELLEN: Listen, what you do in life is you get what you are open to learning, and I am very happy for people to do that. I think, if that works for you, it works for you because you are a great homeopath. It didn't work for me; it didn't work for loads of my patients.

ROWENA: It doesn't mean that you are not a great homeopath.

ELLEN: No, I had to find a different way of getting round the problem. So wherever people are and what they do in homeopathy, I applaud them. But I know that what I do works for me and I am very, very, very busy. When I was at my practice in Islington, which I have cut down to once a week now, the receptionist used to say to me, how can you see seventeen people in a day? How do you do it? I can do it because I know exactly what I am looking for. I know how to apply different methods to different people, so everybody who comes to the door, as far as I am concerned, is my teacher. They teach me homeopathy and I just have to be sharp, sharp, sharp, on how I apply homeopathy, and if they come to me and I think that all they need for the first month is nutritional changes; that is what they get. And I am happy for them to go away and make those dietary changes.

ROWENA: How do you know that they need dietary changes? Is there a questionnaire that you give?

ELLEN: No, I can tell by the symptoms they are presenting that they are depleted in all sorts of things.

ROWENA: And that you had as part of your training in homeopathy as well?

ELLEN: No, I picked that up, I had to. Most people are so fearful. If they get it wrong they think it is the end of the world. Do you know, when I was a student I used to go to tutorials and they used to say, "You did what?" I said, "Yes, I did that." "You aggravated what?" I said, "Yes, I did." I aggravated everybody; I spent a good year as a student aggravating everybody who came into contact with me.

I used to dread eczema patients as I had the worst aggravations with them. I had one mother who brought her husband with her, shouting at me because their daughter came with two bits of eczema on her elbows and was covered from head to foot in it now. She looked like somebody had taken a blowtorch to her, and that was on *Sulphur* 12C, once a day. What did that mean? That meant that I had inappropriately prescribed. I didn't understand what was going on; I didn't see that the cause was the vaccinations.

ROWENA: But *Sulphur* is worse for vaccination so it might have been the right remedy. So did you go with the vaccines in potency?

ELLEN: I did all of that, but what I didn't understand was the relationship between the skin and the bowels. Vaccines produce an incredible level of toxicity, they weaken the liver, the liver governs the digestive system, and the large intestines become extremely sluggish, and so on. You give something like *Sulphur*, which is a big liver remedy and it stimulates the liver. Then if the lines of elimination are blocked, where is it going to come out? It is coming out in the skin. So when you see eczema you know that the lines of elimination are blocked, that is the bowels, and that is why this stuff is coming out in the skin. You can see the cause, the toxicity from the vaccine, so what are you going to do? You need to start with the bowels first, you need to get those bowels moving; you need to get the bowels clean. So a healthy bowel movement is every time you eat your main meal, within half an hour to an hour or so, you should want to pass a stool. That is a healthy bowel movement. Most people are constipated.

ROWENA: So then what do you recommend?

ELLEN: You have to put them on to a complex carbohydrate, high roughage diet. Encourage them to eat more fruit, cut out refined carbohydrates and get them off dairy products and excessive wheat. And that is what I do; you know. Patients come in, they bring their kids with their skin and I say, "This is where we are starting. Before we go into energy medicine we have to start with what is not physically functioning properly, and we start there."

ROWENA: What happens if it is an emotional causation that is causing their bowels not to move?

ELLEN: If it is an emotional causation and there is no obstacle to cure, then you can go and do your classical case. If there are no steroids, for example, you can go straight in with your classical case, and guess what; you will get an excellent result. But I have seen very few children who have come to me that way. I have teenagers that come to me for acne, and I sit there and I say to them that we are going to start with opening their bowels.

ROWENA: And you do that via the diet?

ELLEN: Dietary recommendations and I use a lot of tinctures.

ROWENA: Specific to the organs?

ELLEN: Specific to the organs to get them to function properly. I look at what organs aren't functioning, what ones I need to nourish with different tinctures, and then I use diet and recommended supplements for them. So I start with where the patient is. I don't delude myself that I know the answers but I think, "This is going to be interesting." But I have got the tools, so nothing is a great challenge, and if I do get an aggravation I think, "What did I miss?" And most people are so busy telling me how unsafe homeopathy is, and I say to them it is because they don't know how to use homeopathy. They do not understand how to use homeopathy; that is why they think it is unsafe.

Homeopathy is a safe system of medicine; it is gentle, it is effective, and you get excellent results. If you are not getting the results, it is because you are not applying it properly and you do not understand how to apply it. And that is it. It is not the tool you are using that is at fault. It is not the patient. It is the person who wields the tool that lacks the knowledge. And so people learn homeopathy, and they take with them from their course all the fears and they never move beyond those fears.

And there is nothing to be afraid of when you are dealing with patients in homeopathy, because you should have an insight into vital energy that doctors don't even understand – they have no concept of vital energy. You are in a fantastic position. You cannot even begin to come close to the incompetence of your local GP when it comes to irritating and suppressing the vital force. Even if you were the most useless prescriber on this God's earth, all you would do is have constant aggravations, and if you are so stupid you cannot actually look at your aggravations and learn from them, then you deserve to stay stuck, poor and fearful.

At CPH we talk about the 'pigeon shit method'. It is when people say to me that they feel the patient needs *Lachesis muta* and I say "Why?" So they respond by saying that she was wearing an open top, she was very loquacious and she has got red hair and freckles etc. I just say to them, "That's interesting, I'm glad you know *Lachesis muta*. Now, where and why is this? Where have these symptoms come from? Why is the patient doing this? Justify it to me. Show me the evidence in your case that this is so. When you have found the evidence and you understand what needs to be cured..."

ROWENA: Then you will change your mind and not give *Lachesis muta* probably!

ELLEN: Yes. And I say that is just pigeon shit! So sometimes the students say to me "Actually, I think this is the pigeon shit method that I am using but I really don't know what to do." I respond by saying "Fine, at least you know it's that."

ROWENA: I want to know who has influenced you the most.

ELLEN: Robert Davidson because he threw me in at the deep end and forced me to figure it out for myself and Robin Murphy because I admired him so much as a homeopath and out of all the seminars I went to, he was the only homeopath that actually made any sense to me. Oh, and Ian Watson too. You know, I just looked at Robin and thought, that is the kind of homeopath I want to be, and he is talking in a way that I understand.

If I choose a seminar to go to, I am going there for a specific reason, there is something I don't understand that is going on with patients, and I need to go there and find out what others have to say. It is like when I went to A.U Ramakrishnan's seminar on cancer. There was something I couldn't quite understand, because I was taught for cancers, like other pathologies, you use low potencies, and yet he prescribes 200C plussed. And that is what I was experiencing in clinic. That actually my patients needed the 200C potency. The tumour is like an acute; it is sucking all the energy out of the patient. All the energy is actually in the tumour. So if you go low you are not matching the energy of the tumour. So that is how I look at seminars. I think actually there is something here, how can I apply this to one of my patients? And his method works.

ROWENA: It does, I know, as I have been working with cancer patients too, and I have been getting good results. Another question for you Ellen, how do we avoid homeopathy becoming dormant again?

ELLEN: You have to look at the patient. The thing that fascinates me about human beings is how they are stuck on what doesn't work, and they keep preaching it and trying to teach things that don't work to people. And I just think to myself how stupid it is for a whole group of people to follow what isn't working for the patient. You should be looking at your patients and then dump what doesn't work and looking at what does work. And students come back and they tell me these funny stories.

One student said she joined this tutor group and she was the only practical homeopath there, and there was a case that the homeopaths were looking at and she could see quite clearly that the patient was toxic. He has loads of bowel stuff going on and they had given him a remedy and he had aggravated horribly. So they asked her what she would do and she said that she thought he was toxic and she would use a part patient method of organ drainage and recommend linseed and high roughage to get the bowels moving. And they say to her, "Well, that is not homeopathy; it is naturopathy."

So she came back and told me this and I said, "Let's have a look at Hahnemann. Where do you think Hahnemann started? What do you think Hahnemann did with his patients? He always looked at their diet. Why do you think he gave *Sulphur* to everybody? He gave *Sulphur*, because they were relatively healthy people, he stimulated the liver, and *Sulphur* got the bowels going. He prepared his patients. So, you are doing homeopathy."

Practical homeopathy means you have to do a thorough investigation of your patient; you have to find the evidence to justify what you are doing. You need to know where you are working with your patient, and what you want to achieve with your patient. You have got to adapt to every patient that walks through the door. Every patient will tell you what you need to do.

ROWENA: I learnt a lot from working with cancer, actually. That was a big turning point for me because I could see that some cases were totality and Kentian, and others weren't.

ELLEN: Working with cancer you can see that nearly all my cancer patients have got a core mental or emotional issue. I can see a totality remedy and I have tried it. Don't think that I am telling you all this because I didn't try it. I tried it but it made no difference; they just died. I didn't do anything for them. They just died off and I just thought I was a crap homeopath or that homeopathy doesn't work.

ROWENA: So, why CPH? Why are you here?

ELLEN: I am here at CPH because it has allowed me to put into practise what I see has worked in practise for me. When you look at my career as a homeopath it has been very, very quick. Within three years I was setting up the Centre for Homeopathic Education (CHE).

I had a vision of education quite clearly in my head; of the process you need to go through in order to train people. And I knew that I could train really good homeopaths, and CPH has offered me that opportunity to put it into practise. And I have changed the curriculum; I have changed the way we do things here, and I have seen students change, and my thing was that the person who is our highest achiever, who is doing homeopathy naturally, you want to really inspire them to go even further, and the person who is the lowest, you want to inspire them to work towards the highest, not to lower everybody's standards to the lowest. You have to support students to achieve the highest that they are capable of doing in terms of seeing patients and evolving as practitioners.

So this was like the ideal opportunity. I know that I can take anybody off the street and turn them into a fantastic homeopath. I know I can do that. And that is why, running the two year full-time course, yes, we get drop outs, we get people moving into the part-time course because they cannot take the pace. Because I will not let the students get away with shoddy stuff. I will not let them guess. I want evidence for everything that they say.

In that respect people say to me "You're really scientific and you're quite academic." And I say to them, "Well, if science is about clarity of thought then I suppose I am. And if you call it academia - justification for what you are doing - then I suppose, if that is what you think then it is." I just think that it is clarity about what you think, what you say, what you do. And I will not accept shoddiness from anybody here, I will not.

So, I think I am here at CPH because it is the right time. It is the right time to take practical homeopathy to a different level. I think Robert Davidson started a process off and I am here to take action for him.

ROWENA: Is he not around so much these days?

ELLEN: He comes and he teaches quite regularly.

ROWENA: And he teaches up at CPH Midlands and Iceland as well?

ELLEN: Yes he does. The students absolutely adore him. He has a lot to teach and has an incredible amount of wisdom. I think now, by getting more clarity, they really appreciate what he is saying and what he is teaching to them. Because I think a lot of the time it used to go over their heads, but now they really, really do value what it is he has to say, and it's very valuable stuff, because I think that his way of trying to look at the practicalities of applying homeopathy. He was way ahead of his time. And he should really be honoured for that. For actually trying to break away from the one method mentality and I totally applaud him for walking before me and doing that.

When you are here at CPH you think that everybody is a practical homeopath, but we are a real minority of people. A lot of the methods are limited and it is how you justify your way out of those limitations that gives you clarity about what you are doing. Different people devised the methods in different times in our homeopathic history, to suit the patients they were treating. And so they are of value, but you need to know where they are limited. And if you don't apply methodologies properly or you don't understand them properly, you won't understand those limitations; you won't understand how to use them.

I am well aware that you teach people all this stuff, but the important issue is that it is a foundation. They learn to then adapt and they are not in that place of fear, and what happens when you're out of fear is you become creative. So I am expecting the future practical homeopaths to develop more and more methods, as people get sicker and sicker.

ROWENA: So if they are sitting at computers and using mobile telephones there is probably going to be something that is going to be created to antidote those effects before anything else will work; that kind of thing?

ELLEN: Yes, and you have got to understand what made the person sick. You are a detective first and a homeopath second. You have to do the detective work and put your symptoms into the right context. Putting them into context makes you understand. You should never pick up the materia medica first; it should be the last book you look at. You should have decided your method, which will guide you through the repertory, before you pick up the materia medica. And then you should be able to differentiate, according to what caused that person to be sick. And sometimes the best materia medica is the *BNF*[19] because it has got all the drugs there.

ROWENA: And I met you in the early days of that, when I came here, and I thought, "Wow, what a lady", and I didn't know this place before and I didn't know you before, but I knew you were going to do great things. It was just obvious; you have got that energy.

ELLEN: It is just clarity and vision.

ROWENA: And being in the right place as you say, because if you are in the right place everything can happen.

ELLEN: And the other thing is; it should be fun. I wouldn't do this if I couldn't have fun doing it. I don't need to be doing this; there are other things I could do with my time, which are less time consuming. But the important thing for me is that I am really having fun watching it unfold and looking at things and thinking, "Actually that doesn't work, lets dump it next year" or "That really works, we must do more of that next year." What I am enjoying the most is producing the material, because it is helping the students; they just download it off the website.

Because our job here at CPH is to teach you how to use this information, your time shouldn't be spent getting information; it should really be spent teaching you how to use it. And that is why I can teach homeopaths in two years how to do homeopathy, because they spend their time being taught how to use the information. We are the only college that does it.

Also I say to the students, "If you don't turn up for your practitioner development, you are throwing your money away. Because if you think you are going be a homeopath without evolving in some way you are mistaken, because your patients will take you down places you don't want to go." People change subtly; they don't realise they are doing it. But you have some people who find practitioner development a bit challenging for them so they try and sneak off, but I know who they are and unfortunately they are the very people who need to do it the most. At key points in the programme you know that they will have issues that come up, and they need to look at these issues.

I am challenging them all the time. They come up with their, "I cannot do this" and I just say, "How interesting for you, you are absolutely right, you cannot do it, and so you're going to stay there, aren't you". And I just challenge them on it, and they grow. One of the students said to me, "What is it about you? Whenever I come to see you I always end up crying and having a breakdown." And I said, "It is only because I am just challenging your beliefs about things."

I have to say that is one of the wonderful things about Robert Davidson. He challenged all your belief systems and you either loved him or hated him. I left college hating him! It was only about two years after leaving college that I thought actually he was right!

ROWENA: I would have liked that. I enjoy being challenged. I will let you know whether I like being challenged by him after Saturday, as that is when I am interviewing him and he will probably challenge the living daylights out of me!

ELLEN: So, that is it. I am at the right college, doing the right thing at the right time and having fun. I will leave you with this Rowena: homeopathy is easy, simple and great fun.

CHAPTER 5: PETER CHAPPELL

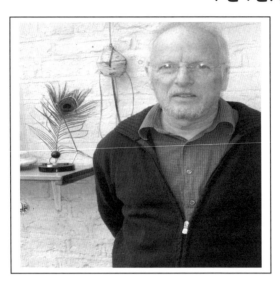

I found myself on Thursday 10 February 2005 taking the tube down to Shepherds Bush, West London, to the home of Peter Chappell. I had attended a lecture of his a few weeks earlier on his new remedies and I was keen to learn more about them and hear his story. He has been practising as a homeopath since the renaissance, he studied with Thomas Maughan, he was a founder member and is a Fellow of the Society of Homeopaths and he has a lot to say! It was a fascinating few hours.

"I have to say one of the weaknesses I perceive in homeopathy is that homeopaths are not sufficiently trained; they haven't done enough internal, therapeutic inner training. The world is emotionally illiterate and I think emotional intelligence in homeopathy is still limited."   *Peter Chappell, February 2005*

"I think that all colleges suffer from one big problem; they cannot educate properly because they haven't got the funds and if they charged the fees to do it properly, they would never get any students except the very rich ones. There are not enough funds to do the clinical training properly and there is not enough emphasis on self-development."
                                        Peter Chappell, February 2005

"It takes a long time to mature as a homeopath. It takes a long time to get good enough to earn a living and it is a lot about intention too. Many practitioners don't need to make a living, because they have got a supportive partner but if you want to make a serious living, it is hard I think, and this is not just a homeopathic phenomenon. Many people who train part time in therapies don't make it into practise, because they are not adequately trained."
                                        Peter Chappell, February 2005

CHAPTER 5:   PETER CHAPPELL

ROWENA: So let us start with how you discovered homeopathy - the beginning of your journey, Peter.

PETER: I split from my wife because I had a deep trauma, which affected my marriage. I didn't know it at the time, I didn't know it for thirty years, but it did. We had a daughter who was born but died at birth and we didn't have a funeral. That created in me a scenario that I never understood, but I kept seeing my wife as a burnt corpse, a burnt small corpse. I didn't associate the two. I split from my wife because I thought I couldn't keep having images of her like a burnt corpse; it just wasn't right. So I did some sculpting and I made images of her and this lead me into co-counselling, and co-counselling lead me to explore all the things I didn't know about myself.

ROWENA: How old were you?

PETER: I was twenty eight and suddenly I was living on my own in house with six empty bedrooms so I decided to put all the co-counsellors that I met, whom I felt were interesting, into the house. Even with hindsight now, I have to say, they were very weird people. But the truth is; I think I was too. I got to know them and I tried to find out about what these people knew that I didn't. I was an engineer and knew the conservative, conventional world of engineering, research and invention, but I didn't know anything about anything else. I was what I would call a nerd in the classic sense. I had a very technical skill base, but I was hopeless at interpersonal relationships.

I went on and discovered all sorts of things, including homeopathy and I went to one of Thomas Maughan's classes and thought that this was the first man that I had ever met who I regarded as a true man. Men are often boys really, despite what they might think. They have often not grown up yet and I think that is what women experience quite a lot too. One reason for this, in my opinion, is partly because men don't have any rituals. Whereas women menstruate, and have babies and go through the menopause so they have systems for maturing and recognising their milestones.

I feel there are a lot of issues around loss of culture; Christianity suppressed culture over thousands of years. The two world wars took the lives of millions of people. It took out the best men; the bravest and the strongest went to the war and many died. And those that were left, especially the men, suffered enormous wounds. The ones who survived came back and didn't talk about it so somehow we got crucified; the men and women got seriously damaged. So this process rolled up into me.

When I met Thomas Maughan he was teaching homeopathy one Saturday evening a fortnight. He had these classes in a middle sized Victorian terraced room. It was full to the brim of people sitting on benches, stools and the floor; anywhere they could, making notes. He just read out materia medica; he didn't do much else.

ROWENA: Really? What kind of books?

PETER: He read from his own materia medica, which we did try and publish at one point but we never got very far because it wasn't particularly brilliant. He wrote it based on his experience. He didn't teach about repertory, anybody else's materia medica or any systems. He just inferred that all you needed to learn was materia medica. Most importantly he was inspiring. While studying with him I didn't even know about the *Organon*[4]; no one ever mentioned it or taught it. Kent's *Repertory*[16] was around, but I didn't know about it. It was just too complicated even to understand, since no one taught it. What we did was to make a repertory ourselves, based on *Thomas Maughan's Materia Medica*[20]. I took every single line out of it and put it somewhere in my index so I could access the information.

ROWENA: Who was studying there at the time?

PETER: Robert Davidson, Martin Miles, Kaaren Whitney, Mary Titchmarsh, Jerome Whitney, and Michael Thompson. Misha Norland turned up a bit later on and various other people as well. There was another group in North London run by a man called John Damonte who trained Misha and a few others.

So that is how I got into homeopathy; I fell in love with Thomas Maughan; a most amazing man. Of course I had treatment with him. He gave me *Sulphur*, which gave me a very deep spiritual experience. The remedy made me see myself exactly as I was - a very ordinary, poorly developed individual with endless weird thoughts and failings. I recognised a big long list of them and felt stripped of all pretentiousness and defences. I saw that I was perfectly alright just as I was. That experience and process lasted about ten years.

First of all, Thomas gave me *Morgan* followed by *Sulphur*. He then gave me the tissue salts *Natrum phosphoricum* and *Kali phosphoricum* alternating to take three times a day. That was his first prescription and he had a routine. He said not to give the indicated remedy if you could spot it but to wait until you had worked on other levels first. Basically he knew about toxicity and detox, so he detoxed the body first, tuned it up, and got the person functioning better. Only then would he prescribe a constitutional remedy. He would know it by then anyway, or have a pretty good idea at least. This obviously had many advantages including stopping you needing to be spot on right at the start of treatment and to fully and deeply understand the person.

ROWENA: So was it because he wanted to get to know the person slowly?

PETER: No, he just wanted to make sure that they were ready for the remedy. His perspective was that if you give the indicated remedy when your patient is congested, for example, it isn't going to have much of an impact because it cannot drive through the shit. If they are really full of toxins the indicated remedy won't work properly so he prescribed routinely at the start of treatment using remedies to warm the person up.

He was inventing combination remedies at the time, which are still being used by homeopaths in the UK today. At the College of Practical Homeopathy (CPH) they talk about *Ambra grisea*, *Anacardium orientale* and *Argentum nitricum* in combination as *Triple A*. In those days he would think them up, order them from Galen's pharmacy, and just see what happened. They have become folklore since but he was really just playing about.

He gave me *Triple A* once and one of them opened up my heart and had a very profound effect on me. I could argue for *Anacardium orientale*, I could argue for *Argentum nitricum* and could even argue for *Ambra grisea*, but one of them really deeply affected me and I will never forget it. It made me feel incredibly loving, as if my heart had opened and something shifted inside me. I think he christened it 'the Love pill' based on my response and that of others.

By the time I was about thirty I was starting to practise and I think it must have been around 1970. I didn't know anything really but I thought you gave everybody remedies either in a 200C potency or 10M as their first prescription as that is what Thomas used to do. He would use a 200C for bowel nosodes and detox remedies followed by a 10M polycrest. I started practising using this system until I found my feet.

ROWENA: How long did you have to study with him?

PETER: Well, I didn't have the opportunity to study any length of time, because after about two years he was dying; he even treated us in his pyjamas and dressing gown. He had very severe lung cancer, but he just didn't want to give up smoking. I took him to see an acupuncturist in the final stages of his cancer and he was very impressed.

He used to love going out for the day; he didn't drive at that point. We often went for breakfast to Galen's, a homeopathic pharmacy in Dorset. He liked to leave at seven o'clock in the morning from South London before the rush hour and speed at ninety miles an hour along the not yet motorway roads to get to Galen's pharmacy for ten in the morning to collect his remedies instead of having them posted to him. He just loved the idea of going out for a trip and he also gave me driving lessons. Because he was the Chief Druid of England at the time, he was a very heavy-duty spiritual teacher. He had a long white beard and he looked like the Asterix Druid.

When we drove to Dorchester, the roads were bad and if we didn't overtake, the journey could take us all day. He would make me overtake on blind bends with only a fraction of a second's notice to pull out. He was teaching me about consciousness; he was saying, "You have got half a second and if you take that half-second we could be out and back in before they know it" and I could. Just occasionally we would go around a blind bend and there would be a tanker coming towards us, and I would slam on the brakes and would just make it back in again in time. But those who drove him never had any accidents with him.

ROWENA: Why do you think he wanted to teach you that?

PETER: It was to sharpen up our minds. He came from the Golden Dawn Tradition; the true mystical and magical tradition of England. He knew a lot and had done a lot of things. He said he had to climb down several levels of consciousness before he could make contact with the people of my generation as they were pretty much wiped out by drugs. Even then he was having a hard time finding anybody to teach anything to. Anyway he was my introduction to homeopathy, and I just loved him! He also ran rituals in Druidism and other classes so I just queued up and took the whole lot. And while he was alive it was totally fantastic. It was quite good afterwards but his presence was all I really cared about.

ROWENA: Peter, could you tell me some more about the Druid Order?

PETER: Essentially, it was a spiritual self-development organisation that used philosophical methods and rituals. For example, every fortnight at a certain time in the evening a group of people got together to do a healing ritual. There were never any exceptions and it still goes on now. The ritual is always the same and it includes sending healing to a list of people. For example, one time we were told of a child who was suffering at Great Ormond Street Hospital. They had an undiagnosed situation, the child was dying and they didn't know what to do about it. So we put the child on the healing list and the next morning the specialist knew what to do. He had woken up in the night and had realised what the problem was and did a simple test to confirm it the following day. So the Druids gave me a spiritual foundation, but we hadn't particularly trained as homeopaths. We had studied a bit, but we couldn't really learn a lot, as the foundations weren't in place.

ROWENA: How did you learn all the rest of it?

PETER: One time while I was meditating I got the 'instruction' to form the Society of Homeopaths. So I called a meeting and formed it and I was one of the driving forces in various guises for about five years. I looked around before we started the Society, but all the other homeopathic organisations weren't going anywhere significant. Later Robert Davidson and Martin Miles started the College of Homeopathy (COH) and gradually we built up more budding homeopaths and a larger body of knowledge.

Theoretically there were a few old homeopaths out there in the world and in the UK who could have been interested in forming an organisation, but when we actually tried to contact them they didn't like it at all. I think they considered us upstarts, and refused to join in. I was the one with business skills, so I said, "Let us start with a clean sheet", and gradually we got enough people so that we could afford to bring in teachers. We got George Vithoulkas and Vassilis Ghegas to come over first. Vassilis was George's number one pupil. Roger Morrison was also a student of George Vithoulkas at that point, and he came too. Vassilis had to learn English first, so for him teaching was tricky and quite a strain. Vassilis gave a most magnificent lecture the first time he came. He just radiated gold so we called him the golden man; he had a beautiful golden aura around him and he absolutely knew his stuff. His lecture was on *Aurum metallicum*.

Gradually we got the numbers and finance together so we could call in people from all over the world. We had Eizayaga from South America visit us and he brought with him another form of homeopathy, his layers approach, and I thought afterwards that I needed to balance out what I then called the Eizayaga effect. As a result I invited Candegabe from Argentina, I wrote him a letter saying that we would like him to come for a seminar and we would pay him five thousand pounds because we could afford it. We could guarantee to get a hundred people to a seminar, and if they all paid fifty pounds we could afford the five thousand pounds. It was as simple as that. The sums were very easy to do.

And then of course Rajan Sankaran arrived and he was ace for me. He was about thirty then and it was like sitting at the feet of a master. He knew so much more than I did and he was stunning out there; honestly, I just lapped him up. He sat in a room for four days and we gave him all the difficult cases of Europe to treat. The patients would come in and sit down and he would then write the remedy on a piece of paper, screw it up and give it to us, not to open. Then he would take the case for an hour and go through it with us, explain all the rubrics and then we would open the screwed piece of paper up and there was the name of the remedy. He had already worked it out in one minute. He did that routinely, virtually every time. And he got it right and the results panned out just by making observations when the patient walked through the door.

He was really funny in those days. He would not look at the patient at all, he would just listen, and he would write down the rubrics as they came out in the case in the side margins and doodle on the main pages. He had no eye contact and we had to warn the patients about this. We learnt a lot from him, and he solved our difficult cases and made them look easy. Obviously over twenty years he has evolved and every time he writes a book he says it is a work in progress, which it is. Nowadays his focus is on the patient's gestures so it is completely different. He has been going steadily step by step, and in Mumbai he has built up a base of people around him and they are all involved with each other.

I have never been to Mumbai, but I think that there is a great group of practitioners on the same wavelength who all work with his methods and they get good results. He says to understand the real person, watch their hand movements and their body language, and don't take much notice of what they say. As I understand it, if you want to know their unconscious processes, their deepest forming forces, or the shape of which they really are in a primitive way, you need to look at their gestures, because sign language came before verbal language. If you watch their hands you get the sign language; if you listen to their voice you just get the chitchat. Obviously, that is a simplistic version of what he does, but it conveys the depth to which he now goes.

He has taken individual homeopathy, what I call the first simillimum, to its peak. If I was practising now I would spend some time getting myself to grips with Rajan Sankaran's new system, so I was up to date. I would say that is where the energy is, if you want to be the best. Obviously, you can learn a lot from Rajan, from Jan Scholten, from Jeremy Sherr and all sorts of other people, who are great teachers.

Having said that, I think what I have discovered is what I call the second simillimum, which is possibly the biggest step forward in homeopathy since Hahnemann. It is like the next step after Hahnemann because up until now what everyone has been actually doing is refining Hahnemann. However, no one had any idea about how you treat diseases. It is my conclusion that individual homeopathy never treats diseases, it treats people, it removes obstacles to vital energy flowing, which allows the disease to be overcome, but it doesn't treat the disease. Now some very obvious remedies have affinities with diseases or certain types of pathology. *Aurum metallicum* and testicles, *Sepia succus* and fibroids, but that is because there is a relationship between the individual remedies inside a person and the disease simillimum.

For the first simillimum you must stick to the individual, and I would say you can forget anything in the repertory that has anything to do with pathology because it is at best only a confirmation and materia medica likewise. You can say it has got some indications in that way, but fundamentally you need to stick to the individual.

ROWENA: But that doesn't fit in with, say, the *Ramakrishna method*[21] of treating cancer?

PETER: I think that the big hole in homeopathy is that the individual approach is fine, but it ignores the disease as a valid entity. I think I have now solved the problem of what was missing in homeopathy; what to do about pathology. There have been endless teachers of homeopathy dying of cancer, for example. It is normal, because we know that a certain percentage of the population will always die of cancer. But homeopathy doesn't address cancer properly.

To say the medical profession has got it wrong, going down the diagnosis route, is to dishonour God, because God is everything. You cannot say that God is just on the side of homeopathy, or say that the medical people have got it completely wrong; you have to look at the progress allopaths have made since Hahnemann, in terms of diagnosis and surgery. All we are complaining about is that their therapeutic medicines are suppressive, palliative or ineffective. Even at best it is incredibly mechanical. If you provide insulin, a basic ingredient for life, to a diabetic, it keeps the person going but it ignores the bigger picture.

I think pathology is the great big hole in homeopathy; we ignore it because the medical profession has focussed on it. We have gone the opposite way and treat the person not their disease and I did that for thirty years too. When I went to work on AIDS in Africa I took seventy cases and I wouldn't treat anybody who didn't have AIDS. I don't think that most homeopaths have ever taken seventy cases of any disease consecutively. It is a very salutary experience, because I realised that these people were Sepias and Aurums and whatever else, and also they have got AIDS and it is nothing to do with them; it is nothing to do with the individual.

Now I know that that is the theory; it is in the *Organon*[4], *Aphorisms 100 to 104* - in an epidemic like measles or smallpox, don't treat the person, treat the disease and take the totality of that disease. With that in mind, you realise that the individual remedy is there in the individual and that the disease is nothing to do with that individual. There is no connection between the two in an epidemic so you can ignore all the individual's reactions to it.

People react in two ways - according to the disease and according to who they are, and the two are completely separate; they are nothing to do with each other. There might be a correspondence, but in an epidemic everybody has susceptibility. You have just got to have sex with the wrong person and you are in business. Even if you only sleep with your husband or wife, if they have slept with someone else, if they have got it, you have got it, end of story. And this confirms that it has nothing to do with the individual. So diseases reflect societal events. Diseases, like AIDS, represent a different level of consciousness; they have their own consciousness, they have purpose and they are part of the divine plan.

ROWENA: So what do you think is the purpose of AIDS?

PETER: That is a tough one, but it does teach about honesty, commitment and truthfulness. There are too many sexual diseases around and it is dangerous to the evolution of the human race to have unprotected sex without recognising the diseases you are likely to get. People with AIDS will often have gonorrhoea, syphilis, herpes, chlamydia and all sorts of other sexually transmitted diseases. I don't know if that is the whole story, but there is a big story about AIDS.

ROWENA: And the purpose of cancer? Perhaps you can put a moral twist on AIDS, but what about cancer?

PETER: Well which chakra would you say affects cancer the most?

ROWENA: I would say the heart.

PETER: I would think so too. The disease holds the energy of compassion. I think cancer is about compassion and pathological oversensitivity.

ROWENA: And suppression?

PETER: And suppression of that; suppression of love, I would say, is part of cancer. But if you have lots of cancer patients you can figure this out, it is not so complicated. I don't know all the answers. Pathology is the bit that is missing in homeopathy, and all those combinations of remedies and all those intercurrents; they are basically an attempt to fill a void or shadow that we don't know what to do with.

Now people have talked about miasms and *Carcinosin* as a remedy for the cancer miasm but cancer is not a miasm because it is not an epidemic disease. All the other miasms are based on epidemic diseases. I have renamed them actually, and call them CEEDS - chronic effective epidemic diseases. So miasms are based on epidemic diseases, which are based on micro-organisms. For the first two billion years of human evolution that was all that existed so we evolved from protozoa, bacteria, viruses, in other words, micro-organisms, and as a result they are very fundamental to our makeup. They are even more primitive to our makeup than minerals because they were the earliest forms of life and they are very powerful.

ROWENA: As in *Syphilinum* and *Medorrhinum*?

PETER: Yes. There are as many miasms as there are epidemic diseases, and there are technically thousands of epidemic diseases. So Psora is all the other miasms, which we haven't identified. I think there are probably at least fifty main ones, of which we have identified, at least five or six. Rajan Sankaran has recognised nine in his system, and you will notice he does not have Psora. Where the individual approach of homeopathy doesn't work, there are all sorts of 'unlike' treatments within homeopathy to try and compensate for that. As I am sure you are aware, Ian Watson wrote a book, *A Guide to the Methodologies of Homoeopathy*[63] about all these different methodologies.

In my opinion, all chronic diseases are unique combinations of epidemic diseases. Epidemic diseases exist inside the same person for a long period of time; for example tuberculosis (TB) and malaria coexist together in Africa inside many people, it is just normal. There is

71

no way that you can have only one disease at one time; everybody has got lots of miasms running all at the same time, it is just impossible for them not to. It is just a question whether the immune system keeps them under control or not. But if the person has AIDS or is subject to enormous trauma, the miasms start becoming active; the vital force cannot keep them under control and they just start to manifest.

Hahnemann says if you have got no symptoms, you have got no disease and there is no way that this can be true. That is only an ideal. There are lots of things that are wrong with what Hahnemann said, but you know he wrote the *Organon*[4] two hundred years ago, for heaven's sake, and things have moved on. I have written a book called *The Second Similimum*[22] and in it I have pulled homeopathy apart, reformed it and said what I think about it. I might be completely wrong in some of my formulations, but I had a go at it based on my experience of homeopathy.

What I observed was that things join together in the microcosmic world by symbiosis, and in the real world they do too. Turtles have fish that swim with them to keep them clean. Buffalo have birds that sit on them to keep them clean and eat the flies. Symbiosis is everywhere. Inside our guts we have enormous numbers of bacteria to help us eat and snails have certain animals inside them to help them eat too and without those they couldn't live. I think diseases are combinations of miasms and therefore you can treat diseases like chronic miasms; you just take the totality of a disease and you find the remedy and prescribe it.

Carcinosin is not a miasm; it is the first example of a disease remedy. I am not breaking new ground here. Donald Foubister said how brilliant *Carcinosin* was in treating incipient cancer, and it is pretty close. It is brilliant and totally curative at times. I have a case in my book, *Emotional Healing with Homeopathy*[23], with a seven year follow up; complete cure of diagnosed cancer based on one dose of *Carcinosin*.

ROWENA: Is that because it matched the situation?

PETER: Yes, but it should do. Unfortunately, the reason why *Carcinosin* generally doesn't work is because there should be a hundred different samples in there of different types of cancer. Or you could take a *Carcinosin* made typically from ten people with a typical cancer you are working with. You could have cancer of the testicles or cancer of the prostate. Ten different men with prostate cancers from around the world, all samples mixed together at the same time by some intelligent process and made into one remedy. Then you have got a remedy that has got a possibility. At the moment we have one remedy for cancer and it clearly doesn't work. If it did then the *Ramakrishnan method*[21] wouldn't have evolved. So I have worked out a different way of making remedies, which does work, and I now have remedies for miasms and remedies for diseases.

ROWENA: So have you been using your *Cancer* remedy to treat people with cancer?

PETER: Well I don't treat people except in Africa; I wait for other people to get me the evidence. Also it is more convincing if other people do so. Disbelief was a real issue for me in Africa with my remdy for AIDS, *PC1* remedy, so it was good that practitioners other than me treated patients and they got the same results. So my system seems to work and I have got enough results now to show that it seems to work across the board. There are results for cancer treatment documented on my web site with two year follow ups, but not enough results by a long way.

ROWENA: Are your results mainly for your AIDS remedy then?

PETER: My early results are all AIDS. Later I started work on chronic diseases. While not everybody gets a result the first time they used one of my remedies, sometimes they get a fantastic result beyond anything they have previously experienced. In some cases practitioners have given patients who have been treated for twenty years without a very satisfactory result, one of my remedies and they have responded very dramatically and successfully.

A homeopath reported back that the *Diabetes* remedy looks fantastic. She said she has patients with diabetes who are so much better as a result of taking it. Their energy levels are up and their insulin levels have dropped and all the things that you could expect to have happened have happened; it is a fantastic result. And now, she says, "I am looking for gold. I want to see if I can get the remedy to cure diabetes completely; to get people off their insulin completely." I think that is pushing our luck.

So I think I have discovered the most significant improvement in homeopathy since Hahnemann. But actually I think it is bigger than that, because once you look at the implications, diagnoses and difference in remedies, it doesn't take a lot of genius to work out that this could create a problem; a big problem. It means that doctors could use it and get good results, which is fantastic. Just imagine if doctors could prescribe the second simillimum. They couldn't do the first simillimum because they are not trained as homeopaths and they don't have the time, but they could do the second easily. There is a huge amount of skill involved in getting a diagnosis, but once the diagnosis is worked out everybody could do it.

ROWENA: How do you feel about that?

PETER: I feel a bit weird being in a position where I have got something, which could cause a massive upheaval in human consciousness and it works!

ROWENA: How did it come to you?

PETER: Well, after I had got all my seventy AIDS cases, I just realised homeopathy doesn't have the answer to this and nor does any system. I didn't know what to do. I didn't have a lot of money, I had to have a solution, and I had to have it quickly because otherwise I would run out of money and I wouldn't get to the point of trying anything else. I thought, "I have only got one shot at this, and I have got to get it right."

I took eight weeks pondering over it around Europe and came to England and talked to my friends and my mentors but I saw that no one had ever thought deeply about it; no one had ever faced the issue. And I knew the issue because it had gone inside me; the seventy cases were inside me. I knew every single one of those individuals. In Europe people don't know about AIDS so much; it is not seen as a problem. In Africa it is life and death.

The people I have come across who understand the AIDS issue are people from Africa. Jeremy Sherr is South African, for example, and he understands it. Everybody in Africa has lost a relative in the family; it is that simple. We don't have that problem. To give you an idea of the size of the problem, in every extended family one person would have died of AIDS. And no one talks about it in Africa, because of the stigma; of the twenty five million people or so who have died, only very few have officially died of AIDS. That is the reality of Africa.

I didn't really think I could do this job but I focused in and thought, "Well Peter, you are good at inventing things and this is the job for inventors; it is a new path." So I thought, "I know where I want to get to and I know what I want to solve, but I don't know the connection between the two."

Many years ago, I did a postgraduate course at Cambridge University and my professor was solving a particular equation with the assistance of two computers, one analogue and the other digital. The analogue was very expensive and would fill up the whole of this room and the garden and cost ten million pounds. My professor had already been working on it for six months and I put the equation up and solved it in one afternoon. I just literally put it on the computer and played around with it to see what it did. I looked at the equation on the computer, using it as a microscope like device, saw it moving and said it does this. He worked from first principles. We both agreed with the solution to the equation but I used a modelling tool - the Buckmaster Fuller method - and he used a theory. And that is my approach to life. So when it came to solving this problem I just thought, "What can I do about it? How can I get around this problem?"

The issue as I saw it was how do you formulate the disease into one coherent pattern; how do you take those pieces of diverse information and form them into a spiritual essence? In a way what we are talking about is spiritual mathematics. I did manage to do it, but I want to prove that I have done so and therefore I have to do a lot of research. I want a theoretical mechanism for describing what I have done and I need some research tools. I know what I need, but I am not going to get them in a short period of time. I know which universities could offer me the research facilities and I know how much money is involved but it is not my top priority at the moment. If I am successful, people will throw money at me and then I can do it. And if I am not successful, no one is going to give me the money and it won't be needed! So I had better build a success base and evidence first and then think about the research later.

On a different subject, I have to say one of the weaknesses I perceive in homeopathy is that homeopaths are not sufficiently trained; they haven't done enough internal, therapeutic inner training. The world is emotionally illiterate and I think emotional intelligence in homeopathy is still limited. The results of critical life events and emotional trauma are often in the way when we are seeking the individual simillimum and we shouldn't be giving an archetypal simillimum at that time, but a traumatic one and that is usually enough. Most people go back to functioning okay when they have dealt with their trauma.

There is a constitutional pattern below the trauma that is archetypal and comes from the animal, mineral or vegetable kingdom and it might be a very satisfactory life pattern and doesn't always need treating. You could treat it, and it will open up a whole lot more if the life pattern is too constrictive. You often see by giving the remedy for that life pattern, that the person will open up and their energy will flow more efficiently. But the traumatic pattern is often laid on top of that, and I think homeopaths are not trained enough in that area and they don't understand themselves sufficiently, and therefore they don't understand this. You cannot understand other people without understanding yourself; that is a given. What is often not recognised is that the trauma miasm - if we can call it this - is in the way of the deeper archetypal remedies and the trauma needs to be treated first. Traumas pass down from generation to generation, as I have shown in my book *Emotional Healing with Homeopathy*[23]. It is common and is a dominant part of human make-up.

Sexuality is such a good example of an area where there is insufficient training. If a group of homeopaths went on a weekend course in sexuality training, I bet you on Monday morning when their patients sit in front of them again they would be asking questions they have never asked before. And they would be getting information or responses they have never had before, because they would then be much easier with the subject. And that is the same with all these areas.

Another area where homeopathy is relatively undeveloped is belief systems. I figured out that there are a whole lot of remedies out there in the 'belief structures realm', which are different from anything that we have proved before, because we don't deal with belief structures. You can give people really good remedies but their beliefs won't change. All sorts of other things change, but their beliefs stay the same. I have developed remedies that work on that level too.

My thought process behind this is based on my perception that the spiritual realm is the only solid reality; the rest of it is rolled out by our mind and is not grounded in reality. Being in a physical body is an enjoyable learning experience but it is not solid reality. The spirit is what is solid and we choose to roll out a body every now and then by a process we have evolved. So I started rolling out remedies for belief structures, and a simple but profound example is fat and famine. My *Fat* remedy is brilliant because there is a belief structure that there isn't enough food to go around. That is an easy one to understand.

ROWENA: So you wouldn't give it necessarily to someone who was overweight, because there are lots of different reasons why people are overweight, only if they have that belief system in their consciousness?

PETER: I would prescribe it when there is an eating disorder related to there not being enough food. But the whole human race has been through that issue as poverty and malnutrition were epidemic for centuries; you don't have to go back too far before people were dying because they were starving in the winter. In a way, it is a trauma miasm. They wouldn't be aware of it; it is completely unconscious and there is no way that you can approach the consciousness of that one. You can acknowledge that you are fat but you won't know that it might be because of a very deep issue.

I think that all colleges suffer from one big problem; they cannot educate properly because they haven't got the funds and if they charged the fees to do it properly, they would never get any students except the very rich ones. There are not enough funds to do the clinical training properly and there is not enough emphasis on self-development. And it is very hard to push people through a fixed programme of self-development, because actually each person needs their own system. So a college would need to have, say, ten self-development modules out of which students have to do their choice of three. There ought to be development modules in spirituality, psychological, sexuality and psychotherapy and half a dozen others.

The students would choose which ones to do with the support and guidance from the college, perhaps in the form of a counsellor, who would help them identify their issues and the areas where they are weak, so they could do training in those. The courses would be run independently of the college, to help students become more rounded individuals. A lot of us need psychotherapy; we need to develop and find out who we are. I would say that homeopaths should have at least a year of weekly therapy, with a good therapist, just to deal with their own issues.

I would also like to see a module that focuses on the work of Bert Hellinger[24]. He helped give me understanding to the meaning of unresolved deaths in the family and lack of closure. That issue has dominated my whole life so it is important to know how to give people funerals with homeopathy. People have so many unconscious, unrecognised and unresolved issues in their lives. Homeopaths need to know the purpose of funerals and how to achieve them. My observation is that none of the colleges provide adequate training in these areas and this is partly because they focus on the homeopathy and they do not provide enough time and space for the self-development of the person.

Another problem with our homeopathy education system is that we can never offer enough clinical training. Often it is the blind leading the blind. If they have their recent graduate students supervising the clinics it is a complete disaster. Graduates need to form really good support groups so they can partake in peer supervision as well as bring in experienced teachers to support their development and progression. Doctors don't leave the nest until they are thirty minimum and even then they receive enormous support and career structures.

It takes a long time to mature as a homeopath. It takes a long time to get good enough to earn a living and it is a lot about intention too. Many practitioners don't need to make a living, because they have got a supportive partner but if you want to make a serious living, it is hard I think, and this is not just a homeopathic phenomenon. Many people who train part time in therapies don't make it into practice, because they are not adequately trained. It is very easy to learn homeopathy theories but it is a much bigger task to learn the practice and be wise enough to do the practice.

It is lovely going to college for three or four years. You hang out with a nice group of people; you study an interesting subject and learn lots of fascinating things. But to do homeopathy for a living, that is a different story all together. As I said before, the support structures are not there therefore it takes a lot of willpower. Even the idea of being self-employed is not natural to most people. My parents were self-employed so I was brought up with that mentality. Self-employed people, in general, come from self-employed families.

I have to say that when I was in Africa working for nothing, and even giving my patients money so that they could eat, I loved it. I loved the fact that I didn't have to charge them any money at all.

ROWENA: What an interesting conversation Peter. Thanks so much for your insights and good luck with your new remedies.

CHAPTER 6:   ROBERT DAVIDSON

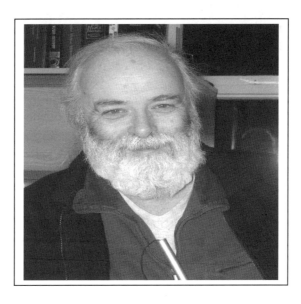

I had a hell of a journey to see Robert Davidson in Milton Keynes. It was a windy winter's day, Saturday 12 February 2005, and I felt like my car was going to be blown across the motorway. I heard he was a little scary too, so even though I was keeping calm on the journey there, the wind upped my stress level and I needed to take some *Rescue Remedy* in order not to project my nerves of driving on to the interview! I had nothing to worry about though - Robert turned out to be the pussy cat those close to him had said he was, and very funny and entertaining too. The most interesting looking homeopath I had met so far, complete with piercing eyes and long pony tail; he showed me into his clinic room where I was introduced to his various machines.

"Homeopathy is the reason you prescribe. It is not what you prescribe and it is not how you do it. Homeopathy is a principle. A principle is a vague idea, a kind of overarching vague idea. Anything specific in it is an interpretation of principle, which can only be judged by effectiveness in the world."   Robert Davidson, February 2005

"Homeopathy is a technology, it is not a science. It will probably be another couple of centuries before we have anything close to a science that explains it. Somebody fell over it, picked it up and wondered what the hell this is and found it worked."
                    Robert Davidson, February 2005

"My fundamental social role is that of disruptor and I have faithfully stuck to that over the years and, as such, those who have an agenda don't like me because I will disrupt it."
                    Robert Davidson, February 2005

CHAPTER 6: ROBERT DAVIDSON

ROWENA: I wanted to start with how you got into all this. I know you studied with Thomas Maughan, but what inspired you to even go to him in the first place? Tell me your story.

ROBERT: In 1971 I was living in a macrobiotic communal house in Ladbroke Grove, London. I was just sitting there in the lounge reading a paper one Sunday afternoon. One of the people who had left a few months earlier came back for a visit. She was talking to someone else about a particular gentleman and inadvertently I heard the conversation. He was in his seventies and his wife was pregnant and a few other things like that. I thought I should talk to him but I had no idea why. So I phoned him up and said, "I would like to talk to you". He asked me, "What about?" I said that I didn't have a clue and he replied, "Right then, tomorrow at three in the afternoon." And that was that. I had no clue about homeopathy; I didn't even know anything like that existed. This was in the early seventies and it actually hardly existed at all.

ROWENA: And what were you doing workwise at that point?

ROBERT: I was very bored repairing extremely primitive telephone answering machines.

ROWENA: And how old were you?

ROBERT: In 1971 I was twenty five. I am only twenty seven now; it is amazing how slowly it has gone. After a couple of months or so I turned up at his homeopathy classes and this whole universe opened up. I was this complete nutcase who wrote down absolutely everything he said. I was watching everyone else at the table. They knew that they would never forget what he said and they didn't write anything. Ha Ha.

ROWENA: Oh, I would have done what you did.

ROBERT: You can get wrist muscles the size of an elephant, you know.

ROWENA: Did you know what remedy he was? You observed him so much.

ROBERT: Thomas was undoubtedly *Arsenicum album*. He probably started off in his youth as *Nux vomica*, and there is a rare constitutional progression from the *Nux vomica* who lives life so intensely that they become different. Most people's lives are too dull, boring and protected for them to change constitutions. How long will it take a *Calcarea carbonica* to get enough life experience to need to evolve? So the *Nux vomica* just goes in there, head down; usually goes through *Ignatia amara* and gets into *Arsenicum album* in old age.

So many homeopaths actually turn into Arsenicum albums. It is more the nature of the work that they do. They often get ....

ROWENA: Obsessive?

ROBERT: Anally retentive. Thomas held the homeopathy classes on Saturday evenings. It was very simple. On the first evening the theory took an hour and a half, just the once. I liked that. After that we did materia medica before tea, and cases after tea. And that was it. It was about a three and a half year cycle. We just went through all the remedies and everything was fleshed out with our own real cases. And as you went along, you gradually got cases and you just ended up doing it. It was an evolution.

ROWENA: How many of you were there?

ROBERT: Not that many. There was a flow through; people would come and go. The classes were once a fortnight. It totally ruined my social life, but there was nowhere better to go so it was fine. When he died in 1976 I naïvely started teaching his Saturday night classes and at the end of 1977 I got the idea for the College of Homeopathy (COH), and set that up to start in September 1978. I had a lot of encouragement like, "Who is going to go? You will never get people. Oh, that is far too much money, nobody will pay that." It was an exciting time, but it was the same thing in 1985 when I started the first full-time course, "Oh, nobody can come full time; you are charging too much money." Yes, right. I like the beginnings of things, when they are usually impossible. When it gets administrative and 'corporate' I am out of there.

ROWENA: At the time that you studied was there the classical/practical issue being discussed?

ROBERT: Oh, no. I started that one and here is the story behind it. Thomas had a particular way of practising; he used the totality remedy. However as there was almost always a difference between the organ and the organism, because of modern drugs, lifestyle, foods, sugar, alcohol and all the rest of it, often the organs would be specifically damaged out of proportion to the organism. For instance, if you prescribe for the organism - the totality - and it starts to repair the totality at a rate of twenty miles an hour, say, and the organ can only do ten, then you will either have prolonged aggravations or problems with pain and all sorts of other stuff. His skill was to be able to help the limited organ do twenty miles an hour and keep up with the organism. So with his way of prescribing you didn't get the aggravations or the prolonged discharges. It was a very high level of skill and I don't know anybody who has replicated that yet. And, naïvely again, that is what we taught at COH from 1978 through to about 1981-82.

It was about 1982 and 'Greeks bearing gifts' started to arrive. When George Vithoulkas first came over what he found, in his own words, were the best homeopaths that he had so far come across. Then he decided that, of course, like everybody else except him, we were doing it the wrong way. By that time, the interpretation of what George Vithoulkas was saying was about essence; that there was the central core, this absolute essence. Find that; prescribe the 'right remedy' and everything cascades better. This is not actually true in these benighted times, except in rare circumstances.

ROWENA: So what is true?

ROBERT: In extremely rare cases, in a healthy culture, with sunshine, fresh air, bare feet on the ground, eating fish out of the ocean, ripe raw foods etc, then you will get that kind of possibility, of undisturbed integration. But what you had in this country were practitioners, some of them are quite famous now, doing that with a hundred percent of their patients. They did not individualise. Everyone got the same methodology, right or wrong. And the 'essence' concept survived on fanaticism for a while, because it was 'right.' The righteousness that came with it was intoxicating. To have the absolute truth of it was powerful. And it still exists, unfortunately worldwide now.

ROWENA: Do you think they were having successes?

ROBERT: Some, I guess. Those who had been 'Georged' then went through several other teachers, after that too, jumping from guru to guru. Their need for truth from external 'exotic' set up the whole guru system essentially – you know making money and getting laid; that sort of thing.

ROWENA: For men maybe, I don't think women quite see it that way. I don't think they study homeopathy in the hope that they are going to get laid more. Do carry on…

ROBERT: That was so close, I nearly opened my mouth and said something there, but luckily I made a complete recovery.

ROWENA: Go, on, I heard you were really challenging; I was quite looking forward to it.

ROBERT: Oh no, no, I will be nice. I will be boring; it's alright. So what happened was in 1982-3 George Vithoulkas arrived in the UK, to bring homeopathy to the UK and introduce it here. He presented in this huge hall down in Victoria to thousands of people. And everything became 'classical'.

What he did to capture his audience was fascinating and it was all in the language he used and still uses. It's very clever and I don't think he knows he does it. He says something using 'implicate' language. You accept this, then he says something else, and then something else and you get pulled through it all. But what you have done is you have gone along with his unspoken assumptions, the hidden assumptions, to get from one spoken part to another spoken part. You agree with his implied assumptions just to follow what he is saying. And you never get to challenge that; he doesn't like it when you do. It is one of the reasons he doesn't like me, because I wouldn't just sit and listen and agree. I used to tell people, don't go to his seminars - listen to his tape recordings. If you go there you will be 'got'. They all said "Oh no, I will not be affected. Not me." And they were all 'Georged'. It is quite astonishing and he creates that atmosphere from a place of certainty and by a subtle way of intimidating uncertain or innocent practitioners.

I remember one occasion, it was much later on, he met the heads of most of the colleges in the UK. He kept us waiting an hour and a quarter and then he kind of waltzed in with this phalange of German doctors. It was almost pantomime. He sat at the head of the table, with these doctors behind him and I thought, "What is going on here?" George Vithoulkas had a bit of a reputation at this point. He would get popular in the USA and then he would leave. Then he would get popular here, and leave. He would get popular somewhere else and leave. Eventually he gave up plans for world domination and then he went to Greece and let people come to him.

I remember one of the stories he told us that day. He was talking about this child who was sick, and no one could work out what was going on. She had been to all the diagnostic experts. No one could work out the disease. Finally George Vithoulkas recognised what the disease was, and from that basis they were able to work. So I asked him, "Does that mean we have to know more than all the specialists in all the specialities of medicine?" because that is what he had assumed. That was the intimidation. Everyone had swallowed it. Everyone else had just taken that on, that that is what they had to be able do. The intimidation of that is so huge it is almost violent. So I challenged him on that and the phalange of German doctors glared at me like I had just tried to urinate on their God or something.

But, it is fascinating - because of the way he structured it everybody just took it. All these Heads of colleges just took it; they were passive. I could not believe it. He never got challenged - he never does.

I remember in the late nineties he came over and tried to correct the obvious detrimental consequences of his visits in the early eighties. George Vithoulkas had become more unpopular here but his methodology hadn't. Classical was King. It had shifted though and other people took over the same mantle, the same singularity and hierarchical point of view about how things are. The higher up this hierarchy you go the more powerful it is, but in fact the evidence is to the contrary. At one point David Howell and I started the 'Not Just Classical Club'. Just to ruffle feathers and validate those who were actually practising the 'medicine of their own experience' rather than the 'medicine of what someone else says'.

I saw the devastation that was happening in UK homeopathy with George Vithoulkas, et al, in the eighties because people were abandoning what worked for them to do what didn't work for them. It just meant they had to do the next seminar. On seminars you get a kind of lift up to the perception place of the person who is guruing. You can see everything clearly for a short time and it's wonderful. Then on Monday morning there is just you alone with the patient - and you cannot do it. A guru teaches people what he does; a teacher teaches people what they can do. And, of course, people like the guru better!

ROWENA: Why do you think that is?

ROBERT: Glamour. They get visions of possibility. Pity its not their own.

ROWENA: Narcissism?

ROBERT: To an extent yes. Watching Rajan Sankaran's convulsions through the decades; he comes up with one thing after another after another just to stay ahead of the crowd. It is fantastic; like a Pied Piper. People like anything that has a methodology - a complete little paradigm, which is rigid and right - they love it. It means they don't have to think for themselves. And they don't critique it or themselves; they will just move to the next one.

ROWENA: When it doesn't work for them?

ROBERT: No, when the next one comes along. By this stage it is not about whether anything works or not; that is long gone. By the mid to late nineties you are hearing things like, "it is the patient's karma that they are not willing to get well". "I gave them the right remedy, they didn't respond". (Pardon? I mean just think about that for a minute) "You may be dying but you've had the right remedy so you will be born healthy in your next life."

ROWENA: Do you mean what is implied is the patient is their own obstacle to cure?

ROBERT: Yes, but we know that the right remedy is the one where there is a response. The whole idea that it was the fault of the patient had the usual 'spiritual' characteristics of being a convenient excuse; just an arrogant, vicious excuse because it condemned patients to the practitioners own limitations.

ROWENA: When was this?

ROBERT: It has been going on since probably the mid 1980s but it just gets worse and worse, as each generation of practitioner comes through.

ROWENA: So you set up COH. How long were you there for?

ROBERT: For a little while; ten years.

ROWENA: So what was it like?

ROBERT: It went though many periods of turmoil. Sometimes it was really bad. For instance, a teacher who had been to George Vithoulkas; seminars standing up and telling the graduating year, two months before their graduation, that everything they had been taught was wrong and that they didn't know the basics. It completely destroyed the students. What these teachers were doing, and there were quite a few of them, was so righteous, so hubris. They were so right that it was, and is, okay to attack, kill and destroy the 'wrongness' when you are in a position of knowing absolutely what is right. That, of course, is the single largest source of human conflict and mass murder. The levels of insanity that were going on were huge but not unusual for the species.

ROWENA: At that time who were you influenced by? Obviously Thomas Maughan, but later on?

ROBERT: Well, I listened to all of George Vithoulkas' tapes in the late 1970s[25].

ROWENA: So you were influenced by him?

ROBERT: Sure, long before all that stuff started. I listened to it mostly while driving and what he said worked reasonably well. I basically pinched a lot of it and included it in the course at COH. Of course the 'prophet in his own land' syndrome endlessly stalked me. So whenever someone foreign came over and introduced exactly the same thing as I had been teaching them, it was greeted as something new and fascinating. It actually used to piss me off insanely.

This classical fanaticism started to appear in the early eighties and it had the seeds of huge destruction. Having listened to *Robin Murphy's tapes*,[26] I got him to come over and had him do some seminars and that kind of broke it up and put the split in because it was important there was a split.

ROWENA: Why?

ROBERT: So the lunatics could die - either from poverty or from their self-righteousness. If you stand still long enough your own despair catches up with you. They have to keep moving and eventually they just move away. So, one of the reasons I got Robin Murphy over from the USA was because what we needed to introduce were methodologies. The concept didn't exist before then.

ROWENA: What was it like then if there weren't methodologies?

ROBERT: It was just 'what we did'. A lot of people still practise that way, saying there are no methodologies, there is just homeopathy. Which is true, as homeopathy is similarity. But homeopathy isn't what you do; homeopathy is the reason you do it.

ROWENA: Okay, explain that a little bit to me.

ROBERT: Well, homeopathy is the reason you prescribe. It is not what you prescribe and it is not how you do it. Homeopathy is a principle. A principle is a vague idea, a kind of overarching vague idea. Anything specific in it is an individual's interpretation of principle, which can only be judged by effectiveness in the world. (Read that one again..!) So the purpose of creating methodologies and distinct ways of doing things is that you create a set of rules within its own patient specific universe. Like Eizayaga's layers methodology, which has rules that are completely the opposite of Kent's? The methodologies contradict, but only if you use them to treat the same patient. That is one of the reasons I think there should be no philosophy in homeopathy; I am with Samuel on that.

ROWENA: He said that too?

ROBERT: Yes. He said 'have no theories'. Of course he then went on and had a theory but, hey, he's human too, maybe. Essentially homeopathy is a technology; it is an application of principle. The philosophy is not philosophy at all; it is actually just rule systems. And the rule systems apply individually within each distinct method. So the methods are defined by the rules you use, and what you need to do is retain integrity in your method and not jump from one method to another to another. That is why we ended up eventually creating distinct methodologies - aetiologies, Kentian, physical generals, layers and sequentials. Each methodology has its own rules and expectations. Each, if you like, has its own philosophy. What you do is individualise the methodology to the patient. That is the bit most homeopaths are missing. Almost no-one, worldwide, is teaching how to find the most appropriate method for each individual patient.

Survival (and health) is the ability to adapt to changes. Extinction and disease are the inability to adapt to changes. The righteous have no capacity to change. If homeopathy doesn't get that it has to be methodologically adaptable to the individual then it becomes extinct. It dies because its practitioners have never given up the allopathy in their soul.

Classical homeopathy is much closer to allopathy than it is to anything else. They don't individualise a patient; they just look for the symptoms which support the classical methodology. They don't even look and see if a patient is weak, strong, damaged or poisoned. It is like the person comes in and you do your thing with them. And your thing is to find the symptoms appropriate to finding a 'classical' remedy and the theory being that the 'right' remedy will then fix everything. This is pure fantasy ninety five percent of the time.

As I said, homeopathy is a technology; it is not a science. It will probably be another couple of centuries before we have anything close to a science that explains it. Somebody fell over it, picked it up and wondered what the hell this is and found it worked. It is a bit like somebody from medieval times stumbling over an electric torch; you pick it up; accidentally push the button and wow. Okay, it works but how does it work. Duh? It is a bit like Shakespeare watching television and wondering how the little people got in the box. The intervening evolutions and their changed perceptions aren't there. The glorious and amazing homeopathy simply becomes more sophisticated, over time, in what it does.

The uniqueness of homeopathy is that nothing ever developed becomes redundant. It never goes out of date. The monumental significance of this escapes most people. It is the one observation that makes science look like the kiddies playing in the puddles. With homeopathy you don't have to change fundamentals and you never have to throw away anything developed from experience. I can take a materia medica published in 1830, put it on my desk and use it. What has changed? Nothing. Homeopathy doesn't change because it is based on what is real. All the rest of it, science and all the other illusions of our time are based on what is not real. If science was true it would not be changing all time. It would be refining and exploring what is true, not scrabbling around looking for this week's truths and hoping to get next year's grants out of them.

ROWENA: Okay, I am following you.

ROBERT: The problem with science is that it can only deal with one thing at a time; therefore it has to pretend that only one thing exists at a time. So what you then have is the concept of repeatability, that if something is repeatable it must therefore be real. Science was invented to work out the difference between fantasy and reality. Previous to that we used things like *the Bible*[27], Aristotle or some reference source and it would tell you what was real. So you thought that if it doesn't say so in *the Bible*[27] it is not true. And if you say it is different we will just burn you, is that all right with you?

And it is a similar thing with science now. If it is not 'scientific' then it is not true. Science has the same limitation as everything else human. It has this deluded concept of repeatability. Think about this for a second. In the real universe nothing is repeatable. The entire universe changes all the time, every nanoinstant, so nothing can ever be repeatable. The only way you can find anything repeatable is if you create a small segregated artificial enclosure every time so that nothing appears to be changing. This system of science means that you cannot have a scientific evaluation of a complex system, such as a human being. I love this because it makes the whole of allopathy wrong. Science is so not up to the task of dealing with a complex individuality that if you 'get it' you should be rolling around on the floor laughing so hard it hurts. Or shocked to the core at how deep our delusions and enchantments can be.

I am not a fan of science however it is fun to play with. I like the toys, they help technology develop. But basically everything that is 'invented' is going to kill us, from control of fire onwards. Everything they ever invent creates a crisis, which needs a solution, which creates a crisis, which needs a solution, and all the time we are just heading deeper and deeper in our own excreta, until we drown in it. (As we are now. Remember, no fish in the ocean in fifty years. Oops.) Science is not a methodology that works for finding what is true - because it has scientists in it. You know, people with mortgages, ambitions and hubris, are open to corruption and the highest bidder.

Homeopathy is probably a future science because it is a science of complex systems. The only way you can deal with complex systems is individually and uniquely. There are some statistical methodologies you can use to help, such as the Inergetix Diagnostic and Treatment Technology. Mostly though, homeopathy is an idea whose time has not yet come because people are too enchanted; spellbound by the evolving stupidities of an ever narrowing current science to be aware that the "Emperor has no clothes".

ROWENA: Did you always think this way?

ROBERT: There were long periods of time when I was really happy and didn't think at all.

ROWENA: So what got you leaving COH and starting the College of Practical Homeopathy (CPH)?

ROBERT: It is a complicated story. Let's say there were reasons I left but one of the major ones was that the thing was so huge it was like a dinosaur and you couldn't change anything.

ROWENA: How many people were there?

ROBERT: Hundreds. In the early 1980s we had about one hundred and fifty people in the first year.

ROWENA: That is amazing.

ROBERT: And we kept most of them. Increasingly through the 1990s, (after I had left) they would have a large intake but lose far too many of them. This made it more manageable. But it was still too huge and quality control became a big and expensive issue. It was difficult to change or innovate anything because all the teachers would have had to change. No-one can pay hundreds or thousands of pounds a day to get teachers to come in for a seminar.

The College of Practical Homeopathy in the Midlands (CPH Midlands), started in 1988 and was something entirely new. I wanted to live in the USA for a little while and commute back here. So I needed a way to pay for my airfare. I had a look around and realised that there was this big black spot called the midlands. I had known David Howell for some years and thought 'he could do the work and I could just swan around and plan it, really'. So he and I started CPH Midlands. It worked really well. By about the third year it was getting too popular and expanding incredibly fast. Immigration had been sniffing around where I was in the USA so I came back to this depressed, grey, obnoxious, smelly, narrow, dirty little country.

ROWENA: Where were you born?

ROBERT: Ayrshire in Scotland. I spent most of my summers in the ocean. It was many, many years later that I realised that less than a mile and a half down from the beaches and tidal fence swimming pools that we used to play in all summer, there was the chemical industry's explosives factory. It was seven miles long and they used to just shove all this garbage into the ocean. I seem to have survived that reasonably well.

CPH Midlands just got busy and I came back and we just ran it. In 1993, because I was going to the midlands all the time and living in London, I thought I would start one in London. We took a lot of students from existing colleges, which terrified them and they never forgave us for that. It showed them that their foundations were less stable than they thought. In 1993, I also got a phone call from Iceland saying that they wanted someone to come and teach homeopathy there and what were we like – they had apparently phoned around. We got the 'deal' and started a college in Iceland as well, which is still going strong.

The country has less than three hundred thousand people in it and we are now, thirteen years later, starting to get a socially significant number of homeopaths. One of the graduates over there, who is extremely good at politics, has just helped draft a new law, which gives homeopathy and the alternative therapies most of what they want. We will have to see if their parliament messes it up, but it is extremely unlikely as the committee doing it said that, in their opinion, it was the finest piece of legislation that had ever been drafted in Iceland.

ROWENA: What do you think will happen to homeopathy in this country? Do you find it worrying?

ROBERT: No, I find it cyclical.

ROWENA: So do you think it will go dormant again?

ROBERT: It will go minimal, for sure. The same people that corruptly produced the EU (hence UK) legislation to wipe out all the supplements and vitamins; the same money will essentially try to wipe out everything else. It depends on how far homeopathy abandons common law. It should never do that; it should have embraced and rejoiced in common law because that is where the freedom lies. In my opinion, it is organising itself out of its own freedom to exist. But then again if you look around the planet, who isn't? That seems to be the tone of the century - people giving up their freedom voluntarily. Selling the freedom of the individual for the rights of a slave is not 'Fairtrade'.

The elimination of anything that might obstruct the truly obscene profits of 'Big Pharma' will be eliminated and the level of sickness will be controlled downwards, to ensure sickness, so that everyone has to take drugs with no other choices available. By the way that is a 'done deal'. It is already set up and must be implemented by all countries signed up to the World Trade Organisation. What they are planning is so evil, so totally evil and unthinkable for most folks that it will be riveted into place before anyone notices, as it has always been done when totalitarian control of populations occurs.

It is insane. You get a whole country like the USA - what are these people doing? Millions of them died to get bloody freedom and now what are they doing? They are just pissing it away. You look at the USA and it has a major shortage, and the shortage is terrorism. It doesn't have terrorism; it has to have Hollywood produce it. It has to have shows on TV about it because it doesn't have any. The whole thing is a perverted fantasy; it is quite incredible. Where is the terrorism they are defending everyone against? It is, however, a politically advantageous position. The herd does that; it goes into sacrifice mode for the greater good. They will sacrifice their individual selves for the greater good, no problem. That is why men will agree to suffer and die in large numbers in armies for the good of the social totality. And politicians always exploit that in times of war or crisis. So they create the war on terror so they can exploit and get what they want.

And the USA is, now, a white van country. They can just come along in a white van, yank you off the street and dump you in the back. They don't have to tell you what you are charged with; they don't have to tell you anything else. They can just take you away and don't have to tell anyone they have taken you anywhere. They don't have to charge you. That is the state of it and it is worse than a lot of condemned countries but people are accepting it.

The sad thing is that it means that there is something wrong with the human species right now. We will have to be put into a place of extraordinary massive pain and violence with humungous quantities of dead people. At which point, maybe, we will get the point and maybe change things, evolve a little, maybe just enough to survive. It may well be done without war and projectile weapons, but that is usually the way it works. This time it may well be species extinction by pharmaceutical company or military biological or nuclear weapons. And probably also, death by Tesco.

The people with the money will then have all the money; they will all be sitting there, all these arachnoids, these spider people. They are not human beings. The people running these businesses are not human beings. There is a bit that makes a person human that they do not possess. They don't have it and as such should be put down mercilessly.

ROWENA: You mean like David Ickes' conspiracy theories?

ROBERT: You could put it that way. It is like the bit that makes them human isn't there. They will sell out of date drugs to third world countries that don't need them. As long as that type of 'opposite of empathy evil' and insanity goes on; the big picture is not pleasant. But homeopathy tends to be filled with all these optimistic tuberculars who think if we just get spiritual enough, if we just find the right remedy to change everyone, then the big mother ship from the other side of the moon, which is parked invisibly, will come and rescue us all, clean up the planet, take away all the radiation and it will be a paradise again. Then we can all live together on this planet holding hands and singing Kumbaya.

There is only so far you can go into fantasy before you die; before you self-extinguish. You cannot live in the world as if it is different to the way it actually is. Human beings happen to be the most vicious, vile, aggressive, ruthless species on the planet. That is who we are and we have to take that into account. One of the questions I ask all those nice mummies in the class is, "When would you kill somebody? When would it be alright for you to kill somebody?" "Oh my goodness" they answer, "I would never do that." "Okay" I reply, "So you are walking down the street, your baby is in the push chair and some drunk, six foot six person comes up and threatens the baby, what will you do?"

ROWENA: Kill him.

ROBERT: Instantly, the guy goes down. Absolutely. And society approves.

ROWENA: I agree that we are all capable of everything.

ROBERT: We all are. And our self-inhibition of this ruthlessness is our civilisation. Inhibition is a positive quality; it is a restriction of our violence, our selfishness and all those other things. And you can see the kids; they are so sick they have got less capability of inhibiting. The sicker you get the less able you are to inhibit the human instinct of ruthlessness.

ROWENA: I think we are all capable of psychosis too.

ROBERT: I suspect that most of us are already there. Most of us live in a complete delusion. Among this profession there is that stupid mindset that decides that homeopathy needs to be put into the mainstream; God help us. And that is what is happening. Someone who doesn't understand the established group, because he is too deep in it, and has a completely unreal viewpoint of everything, decides we are now going to have to get organised to meet that unreal viewpoint. And then the politics and manipulations begin.

ROWENA: Statutory after that?

ROBERT: Sure. The people who want that are already in place. They don't give up. There are people who have been pushing that point of view for a very long time and won't give up. It is just horrendous.

ROWENA: How do you think it will affect homeopathy?

ROBERT: We will either have to be completely university trained like clones or practise illegally. This is the control and suppress century, and it is much more violent than anything else. Previously it was done with guns and armed forces and now it is being done politically and with massive deception. Just watch the way the European Union is set up. It has an unelected set of directors who decide how parliament votes and what they vote for. And if they don't like the way the parliament votes they just ignore it. What the hell is that but dictatorship ... and it's only just beginning.

ROWENA: So what brought you to set up the Society of Homeopaths?

ROBERT: In 1977 Peter Chappell had the idea of something like the Society of Homeopaths, so a bunch of us got together and talked it through and eventually set it up. It was his idea – and a good one at the time.

ROWENA: You stayed involved for a long time though didn't you?

ROBERT: Yes, I was a Director for seven or eight years. Fortunately my natural social role is that of disruptor and I have faithfully stuck to that over the years. As such, those who have a fixed or manipulative agenda don't like me because I will disrupt it. If I were to be invited to speak at a conference, I would go there, do my thing and I would never get invited back. I remember at a Homeopathic Medical Association (HMA) conference I did a whole thing on nutrition. This was the HMA; totally 'Hahnemannian'.

You could see seventy to eighty percent of people were saying, "Why is there a need for nutrition?" and I would say, "How are you going to build new tissue if you don't have the physical materials to build it?" However this was not a problem defined in the *Organon*[4] and 'the establishment' wouldn't get it. They would have to change, learn something new and they couldn't do it. So I was rejected as a disruptor and never invited back again, of course.

ROWENA: What skills do you think homeopaths need in order to make a fruitful income from their work?

ROBERT: If you are not making a fruitful income from homeopathy, then get a real job. Homeopathy is plagued by amateurs who live on their partner's money. The kind of person who usually practises homeopathy seems to be the opposite of someone who can actually market it. It seems really hard for homeopaths to understand that all income comes from selling something. And that is what we are doing; we are selling our skill for so much per hour.

ROWENA: So we need to be able to market ourselves but what are your thoughts on personal development?

ROBERT: Your question is based on the assumption that people can develop and I have a somewhat cynical point of view on this. The only time I have ever seen people change is when they are threatened with death or there is some huge personal advantage to it. However in the case of the latter, it is usually only temporary.

ROWENA: I feel I have changed dramatically but maybe I have just compensated!

ROBERT: You have not changed; you have either become more who you are or less of who you are. At some point you were how you are now and someone crushed it, contracted you with fear and limited you in the process. What we can do with ourselves is to trust, lighten and expand. I see the incredible capacity for joy there is in my daughter. I want her to live in that joy chemistry for as long as possible before society messes her up. Schools are places where people who don't like children try to make them exactly like themselves.

If she can live in that joy chemistry long enough so that it becomes a habit and it becomes difficult for her to be sad, melancholy and depressed, then maybe she can find a way to survive the contractive repression of schools so that she is socialised but not suppressed. The challenge is to be true to oneself in a world where individuality is seen as a crime. It is why homeopathy has a continuous problem becoming popular. When people are willing to be individuals then homeopathy will be as natural to their understanding as allopathy is now. I look forward to it.

ROWENA: Well you certainly have given me food thought Robert. Thank you so much for your time, thoughts and challenges. I have lots to think about on my journey home!

CHAPTER 7:   MISHA NORLAND

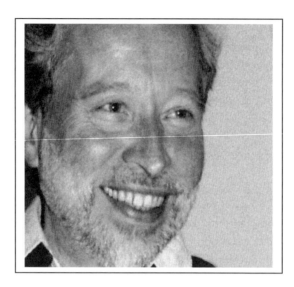

Saturday 26 February 2005 brought me to Yondercott to visit with Misha Norland, his school, his family home and his chickens. I wondered around the gardens and woodland at Yondercott prior to our half ten in the morning meeting time. The students had started their morning classes and I had some time on my hands, some space to gather my thoughts and get into the groove of the School of Homeopathy. It was a cold morning, but here in Devon they had escaped the snow that had been falling constantly all week further north where I had come from. I was already in love with this place. Misha and I found each other near the allotment, his greeting accompanied by the sound of the ducks chatting away; he was gathering eggs.

After a warm hug, we made plans to take Bear, their dog, for a walk up in the hills before conducting a more formal interview in his clinic room in the quiet of the upstairs of the house. When I say 'more formal', we did in fact sit on the floor. Misha has a wonderful way of relaxing his companion, and I felt like I had known him forever. The interview was really more of the conversation that the title of this book suggests which was inevitable as we were already familiar and relaxed with one another from our rambling around the fields. I immediately admired Misha's warm and empathetic way. Since the interview Misha has now handed down the role of principal to his son, Mani.

"I have a sort of prayer to the universe, a wish list, for homeopathy. The wish is that those who practise homeopathy should keep on looking; keep on looking at the world out there and the world inside themselves."
                                                      Misha, February 2005

CHAPTER 7: MISHA NORLAND

ROWENA: How did you get into homeopathy all those many years ago?

MISHA: There are many ways to answer that question, because there have been many steps along my journey from there to here, most of them taken unconsciously, so that only now, looking back, can I understand the sequence. I first heard about homeopathy when I was about twenty six or twenty seven while I was investigating the world of healing and healers. I was in the room of a radionic practitioner called Rosemary Russell, long deceased, a wise old lady, who had been in the field of distant healing for at least forty years.

Among the various objects and healing devices that she had were some illustrations that intrigued me. They looked like a cross between Malcolm Rae's diagrams for creating remedy potencies and astrological charts. I asked her who was the creator of these and what was their purpose. Rosemary Russell explained that they represented thought forms and that she sometimes used them in her healing work. They were created by a colleague of hers who was also a homeopath, called John Damonte.

So I received two things at the same moment, the concept of homeopathy (for she explained to me the 'like cures like' principle) and the name of the man who later became my teacher, John Damonte. I obtained his address and also her recommendation of a book about homeopathy. It was a perfect text for me, although I would not recommend it to others as an appropriate starting place unless they had a medical and scientific background. It was Clarke's *Materia Medica* [28].

I went to the Watkins bookshop, by the British Museum, because I worked within easy walking distance. They said they could order it for me. (This was in 1968. Oh, how I wished I had started all this when I was at school because here I was in my midtwenties, with so much to learn.) But I am jumping the gun - I eventually received a card from Watkins saying, "Your books have arrived." I thought I had only ordered one! They were expensive and I wasn't sure I wanted them, so I disappeared into the back of the shop and started reading, and realised pretty quickly that I loved them.

Back at home, for bedtime reading, I would pick out a remedy at random. As you know, Clarke's *Materia Medica* [28] has a 'relationship of remedies' section, and my habit was to see if I could follow the reasoning behind the relationship, which I usually couldn't. I kept on reading Clarke's *Materia Medica* [28] and was endlessly intrigued – I had got hooked into homeopathy.

I decided I definitely wanted to contact John Damonte luckily I caught him at a point when he was beginning to reach out in the world – he had started up a homeopathy class; prior to that he had just been a busy practitioner. Furthermore, and most conveniently, he lived round the corner from my parents in Hampstead, in North London. So, I could combine visiting them and my teacher. This is the short answer to how I discovered homeopathy.

For the longer answer I have to go back to my early childhood in Gower, Wales. My parents came over in 1939 from war torn central Europe. I can remember distant explosions in the night while Swansea was bombed. I lived with an ominous feeling of imminent danger. Although family life was safe and loving, there was threat on the horizon. I was not told about the holocaust and the fate of the Jews until later on, but I believe that I picked up on feelings of ambiguity about human conduct at an early age. I was fascinated about us.

I also became fascinated by war itself, and the machinery of war and how the engines of destruction worked. Once I got near chemicals, (reagents being readily available from Chemists' shops in those days) I started making bombs, the way boys do. It was dangerous. I got expelled from my first school because I got into a lot of trouble. From then on I was continuously moving schools, not that I got into trouble in every school, but the first expulsion set a pattern.

Anyway, that fascination about humans and what makes us tick (pun intended) was abiding. It has not specifically got anything to do with homeopathy, of course, but it has to do with danger, disease, and transformation - how ailing life can be fixed up and made better. Our doctor, a friend of the family, was a Viennese Jew, as was Sigmund Freud. I mention this because his views about psychology and health influenced me. Anyway, he immigrated at about the same time as my parents. When I was six years old my parents went off on holiday together and parked me with the good doctor. They explained to him that I was really no trouble at all except that I got up very early in the morning. They said that if supplied with hammer, nails and some pieces of wood I would keep myself quite happy for an hour or two. So the doctor and his long-suffering wife were woken up early in the mornings by the sounds of industrious hammering.

Being there gave me a chance to investigate the doctor's surgery. There was equipment, as doctors carried out minor surgery in those days, and many books. I remember being most interested in the books. Although I could not read them, there were illustrations and photographs of diseases. It wasn't a big stretch of imagination to see that physical disease and psychological ill health are mirrors of one another. I wouldn't have put it that way then, yet I became intrigued by both. What is it that twists people into these extraordinary distortions? I guess it is easy to be captivated by such things when you are young and half Jewish.

ROWENA: I don't think every child would make that connection.

MISHA: I am not sure I did either, consciously, but those speculations and that interest has always been there in the background. I have those same pathology and medical tomes up on my library shelf now. He wrote in his Will that I should inherit his books and bookcases.

ROWENA: What did you do workwise up until you were twenty six?

MISHA: I tried out this and that. I did A Levels in Botany, Zoology and Chemistry and got a place in Aberystwyth University to study Marine Biology, which on the face of it could have suited me, but I didn't take it up because I knew that there was a large part of me that wouldn't have been satisfied. I went off and studied English Literature, Economics and Philosophy A Levels at Westminster College with a view to another kind of university degree. I then went off to drama school auditions and got a place at LAMDA, but that didn't appeal to me either. So, as you can see I was perplexed.

This led me to sample many different jobs. Of these, the longest lasting for almost a year, was at the Medical Research Council's establishment annexed to Hammersmith Hospital. I was a Laboratory Technician, which is a lowly job, but set in an environment which attracted me. I enjoyed the detective work and the empirical spirit among these folk who, free from financial constraints, could pursue pure scientific enquiry. I attempted to interest them in researching into psychotropic substances, but the director of the team for whom I worked was dubious about finding approval amongt his colleagues. What is astonishing is that he considered my proposals! I was being heard! It was a relief to be out of school where I was treated as a nuisance at best and as a menace at worst.

Before leaving the subject of medical research, I should recount what it was that most of the other scientists were up to in the name of cancer research. This was shocking to me, and I was glad that the team I had landed with had no part in it. The subbasement of the research building, a tower block of some thirty stories, was dedicated to irradiation. It boasted a massive X-ray unit, a small cyclotron particle accelerator, a Van Der Graaf high voltage source, radioactive isotopes of cobalt and other means of producing electromagnetic rays, subatomic and accelerated particles.

The top story of the building, heady in the sky, housed a zoo. Here, ill-fated creatures such as albino rats and mice, rabbits, monkeys and pigs awaited a macabre fate. The approach to cancer research at that time was to induce growths in test animals using carcinogens. At various stages of cancerous infiltration, the animals were taken to the subbasement and subjected to one or another type of ray or accelerated particle, the object being to ascertain which mode of 'treatment' would be 'effective'.

This level of debasement, of the sanctity of life, by those very 'scientists' whose enquiry was to uncover its secrets; shocked and disillusioned me. I was nineteen at this time, impressionable and idealistic. The company of scientists was congenial to me, I liked the way their minds worked, and there were some good people there, very awake, aware and adventurous, but the work was missing a vital ingredient – the very vital, vital ingredient!

I went off travelling for quite a while and spent a year out of the country with a fair spell in Israel. I worked in a lunatic asylum there for a time. It was an eye opening experience where real healing took place. No drugs, no straight jackets. It was a unique situation, because it was set in a village in Lebanese territory that was connected by a road to the Israeli homeland. So nobody could escape. If they were to have crossed the sand bags, they would have been shot. Complete security. The director was given license to do almost whatever he liked. He was a remarkable man, dedicated to his patients and to the practise of non-violence.

ROWENA: Did he get people out of psychosis?

MISHA: He let them live out their psychosis, as long as they weren't killing anybody. It was a remarkable experience and an astonishing place. That was one of my keynote work experiences, because it demonstrated a non-invasive healing approach to the deepest levels of suffering.

I came back from Israel very saddened by the politics. I felt that the situation was hopelessly stuck; nobody had a workable solution. The policy seemed to be saying, "If you take one of our eyes, we will take two of yours!" and we all know that if we go for an eye for an eye and a tooth for a tooth policy, we end up with a blind, toothless population. That's bad, but when you raise the stakes it's horrific. I was sickeningly struck by the fact that the Jews, who had been treated so badly for many thousand years, were now treating their enemies like scum in return – that no lesson had been learnt. I realise that this is a simplistic way of evaluating an emotive and complex situation, however simplicity often highlights truth.

In England I didn't have a job to come back to, but I had somewhere to live, because my folks were still in Hampstead and had a house that was large enough to accommodate me. I had no idea where I was going or what I would like to do next. But I knew that I wanted something that involved my hands, something that was tangible. I wanted to be creative and I wanted my work to involve people. Now I must step back again and say that quite a number of my friends prior to my leaving on those travels had been interested in films, and also that we had an unusual cinema in Hampstead, called the Everyman.

ROWENA: I have been there many times but it has changed over the years. They now have great big leather seat sofas to lie on, watch an arty film and drink Jack Daniels!

MISHA: Yes, it has changed. It used to be a fleapit with hard seats; privately owned by a wealthy solicitor who ran it as a hobby. He only showed the films that he wanted to, many of which he owned. He had a garage stacked full of film cans, some on nitrate film base. this fact: he would dig them out, the old Buster Keaton and Chaplin films. The projectionist, himself quite a veteran, used to get a thrill out of living with this danger which entailed keeping a vigilant eye upon the projector at all times and cutting the ark immediately should the film fail to feed through the gate. It is dangerous because as the nitrocellulose film gets older, it becomes increasingly inflammable. Nitrocellulose is a constituent of many high explosives by the way, so the danger was very real.

Anyway, the Everyman was an inspiration, not because of these perils hidden from the public, but because of the diversity of films that were screened; the best out of the UK, Europe, USA, Japan and India. I decided it would be fun and a creative challenge to make films, and that is what I did before I became a homeopath. In order to help me, I talked to a number of filmmakers. Hampstead in the sixties was thick on the ground with them! Most said, "Try editing and learn the nuts and bolts of how films are put together." I took their advice.

The other advantage of working in the cutting rooms, apart from learning the trade, was that you could get your hands on free film and film processing. You just slipped the technician in the lab a bit of money and he would do some illegal processing for you on the end of the bigger jobs. I learnt later, interestingly, that the main laboratory that our production company used knew about this practice and secretly condoned it. This was typical of the film industry at this time. The people at the top were really encouraging to the people at the bottom because they just loved the whole ethos of filmmaking. So if someone came in and wanted to make a film on the cheap, they quietly let them get on with it and 'pretended' that it wasn't happening. I didn't know this at the time and thought I was living riskily and would get expelled from school again if they found out.

The greatest thrill was not gained through fraudulent practices however, but came after the shoot, the next day in fact, when the film was screened at guess where – the Everyman cinema! Later on in my filmmaking career the magic of cinema was gradually eroded by the necessity of earning a regular crust. You see, the industry was financially challenged during the sixties and I survived that decline by directing TV commercials, which I saw as a prostitution of the filmmakers' art because the ethos is of selling product.

ROWENA: So tell me Misha, why do you think someone should choose to learn homeopathy at the School of Homeopathy?

MISHA: It certainly is possible to vision homeopathy and homeopathic education in different ways. My approach to say, materia medica studies, is through an appreciation of how archetypal energies and signatures manifest in nature. For example, we study the spider. The spider is nothing but a representation at the physical level of an archetypal way of being. The disease, as we call it, if it is similar, is nothing other than the energy of a particular spider acting out through the afflicted person.

That person becomes its mind, its sense organs, its limbs, and acts out its essential being. See that and you see what needs to be cured. The vital being of the spider is expressed in its form and behaviour; it is its signature. So any teacher, or any book that can take me to that understanding, is where I would like to be learning. I would hope that people would come and study with me because that was what fascinated them. This in turn probably implies that not very many people are going to come to the School of Homeopathy. Not everybody is excited by an archetypal approach.

ROWENA: What do you think other people are excited by? What motivates them?

MISHA: When you go out and give talks on homeopathy, the questions you are most likely to be asked are to do with therapeutics. How would you fix the arthritis, how would you fix the bruising, tell me how you would use *Arnica* in the home, etc. It is a fix it mentality. Most people are searching for a series of formulae and methods that can help them to alleviate the pain. Generally speaking, in a group of twenty or thirty people, there may be one or two whose interest ranges beyond therapeutics.

I had a scientific education. $E = mc^2$ is a formula that has been familiar to me for a long time, and here in homeopathy we see it in action. This is another illuminating aspect to homeopathy. The potentised remedy represents a similar transformation. There is both a scientific and an artistic aspect to being homeopathic in your vision and to bringing about cure. The disease and the remedy should match at the archetypal level of signature – the art of seeing - while the potency should match the vital force – the science. My parents were artists, painters, and their vision represented a similar, archetypal way of seeing. John Damonte's vision encompassed all of that, so he was the right teacher for me.

ROWENA: Why did he die young?

MISHA: He had a heart attack. At a physical level, he suffered a congenital weakness, plus he was overweight. At an emotional level, he had a younger wife and two sons, one of who was marching into his teenage years. Like many a man of his generation, John Damonte was authoritarian while being a gentle and loving husband and father. As I understand it, both his older son and his wife were struggling to break away and gain some independence.

At a spiritual level, John Damonte was a man who primarily transmitted knowledge through devotion. This provided a gentle learning environment, because students quite naturally developed openness and trust. It is easy to learn then, because you are not threatened and you don't put barriers up. However, the family feeling within the homeopathy class was insufficient to make up for what may have felt like a shortfall in the home. At the time of his heart attack, the physical structure of his house was also under threat. The roof was under repair. Chaos in the home was the disorder of the day. As I see it, these were the salient factors.

ROWENA: Do you transmit knowledge through devotion? Do you set it up like that here?

MISHA: I don't set it up; I am it. I am like John Damonte in that respect.

ROWENA: I have to say, immediately I feel a complete trusting space with you, so if your students all feel that, then I can understand what you are saying. So other colleges that don't have those central figures, that are called gurus, how do you think it works for them?

MISHA: I don't know and I don't understand how it works. Often all I see is trouble. From my perspective, when trust breaks down things become dysfunctional. Families become dysfunctional when trust breaks down.

ROWENA: Who else was a key teacher, a guru?

MISHA: John Damonte was my major teacher, because he gave a vision of healing as well as a vision of homeopathy. He wasn't that experienced as a homeopath himself, so there was an element missing around the techniques of homeopathy. The basic philosophy was in place, but finding rubrics, repertorisation and differential analysis were not focused on. Because of the spirit of homeopathy, which John Damonte seemed to embody, we felt bereft when John died. We all knew that we needed more, so our first move was totally logical; we went to John's primary teacher, Thomas Maughan.

We sat in on Thomas Maughan's ongoing homeopathy class. This was in the early seventies. There was a wonderful crew of people including Peter Chappell, Robert Davidson, Martin Miles and Kaaren Whitney. Thomas was really hot on esoteric teachings - he felt that these underpinned homeopathy because true practise requires wisdom. If you just practise homeopathy as a technician and don't underpin it with the perennial philosophy, it is one dimensional. So he was really strong on bringing in that second dimension.

He invited the lot of us to become Druids and to follow their teachings. Not many of us stayed with it including me. My heart wasn't in it, not because they aren't valid and wonderful teachings, they are. However, within druidic practices is considerable reliance upon ritual. While this is fabulously powerful, it had been poisoned for me. If I search for a 'reason', I would have to look to the Third Reich. This was so embedded in ritual; I feel it infused it with great power and to such destructive ends.

John Damonte's other teacher was Donald Foubister, who brought our attention to *Carcinosin*. He was a fine homeopath rooted in the notion of signature, looking for the deeper picture and prescribing constitutionally.

Thomas Maughan believed that Kent was right, but he also had many ancillary methods. He said you should start most cases off with *Sulphur 10M* to clear out past drugging, but before that give *Morgan 200C* the bowel nosode, because this is like the snowplough that preclears the way. Then, when you give *Sulphur* it will do really good work and that will throw up the constitutional picture upon which you may prescribe. In the meantime, you can also use certain formulae; he liked triads, putting together three remedies and using them as specifics for this, that and the other. So you can see how the practical approach could have germinated and been nurtured in the nursery bed of Thomas Maughan's teaching.

ROWENA: Where did he get that from?

MISHA: He made most of the triads up himself; he liked to do that, his creativity went there. Hahnemann, putting his theory of *Sulphur* being the greatest antipsoric to the test, was the first to give this as a first prescription to patients, only later prescribing the homeopathically obtained specific. As for putting *Morgan* before *Sulphur* or *Gaertner* before *Calcarea carbonica* that is the work of Paterson and Bach[29], they found that there was a relationship. You will recall, they discovered that stool cultures of patients under treatment, with say *Sulphur*, showed a preponderance of the *Morgan* strain of Gram-negative staining bacteria.

I tried all those things in my practice and got terribly confused, so my next great teachers were my patients. I figured, and this comes from basic science, if you are unclear about things, you can remove as many variables as possible and simplify down to basics, to first principles. The first principle of homeopathy is the simillimum principle.

ROWENA: So is this what you call your 'salad days' of homeopathy?

MISHA: Yes, those were definitely my salad days in homeopathy. I just thought; what happens if you give a unit dose of the remedy that you think is the most appropriate on the basis of totality of symptoms? If I go back to my salad days, I would have said, "I have to recognise the patient in the remedy and the remedy in the patient." I wouldn't have used a term like 'totality of symptoms'.

ROWENA: Because you hadn't gone off to college for four years and got all that information?

MISHA: Absolutely correct. The person who supplied most of that in a big way was my next major teacher, George Vithoulkas. I had already been in practice for well over ten years and had been teaching before I went to Alonissos for the first time and was blown away by the depth of his materia medica understanding. But the main thing that his approach helped me with was the creative use of repertory. I still believe that George Vithoulkas' most original insights are to be found in the *Essence of Materia Medica* [30].

ROWENA: What is the story behind the *Essence of Materia Medica* [30]?

MISHA: We have to go to the early eighties for that. George Vithoulkas was teaching homeopathy to the doctors in California – many people we know well were there, including Bill Gray. Bill was a great note taker as well as a skilful writer. He collaborated with George in *The Science of Homeopathy* [31] but he is given small credit. One of the reasons it is so good is because of Bill, so hats off to him, he did a great job! He wrote down the lectures of George Vithoulkas and worked on them, so they do not read like raw lecture notes. They are put together as coherent and well crafted pieces.

They were not meant for publication though; they were intended for circulation among attendees of the seminars. Well, you know how things like that go! When I first had sight and a read of them they came over as the *Stolen Essences* [30], written by fairies, gnomes and elves, literally that is what they were called. It's funny, isn't it? Not funny for George Vithoulkas, he was really upset about it. But for us it was fabulous, we had got the work. George didn't get any royalties but we got the knowledge, we were hungry for it.

The next major teacher who came along my track of teachers has been Rajan Sankaran. I am so glad to say that we have cemented a firm friendship over almost twenty years now.

ROWENA: So up to date now, those are the teachers that have influenced you the most?

MISHA: Yes, they are. I don't want to sideline Jan Scholten and his fabulous contribution but in terms of personal teaching, he has not been like that for me. Teaching is a relationship between a pupil and a teacher and I don't have that relationship with Jan, although I honour him greatly. And there is one other I would like to cite, my friend Jeremy Sherr. It is not only for his wonderful teaching but also for his work on provings that I appreciate and thank him.

ROWENA: So when George Vithoulkas publicly criticised other homeopaths in *Links* [32] back in 2000, how did you react?

MISHA: I knew it was coming because he had already said those things to me in private before. We have had some disagreements in regard to certain things and we have both been in print over it.

ROWENA: So you responded to the *Links* article?

MISHA: I wrote an extended letter called *The Nature of Influence*[33], published in *Links*, which was truly the last straw for George Vithoulkas. He resigned from *Links* after the article, having made vitriolic comments about it. He wrote in the following vein, "This man who calls himself a homeopath is doing so much damage to homeopathy and you give him so much space in your magazine – I cannot go on subscribing to a magazine which publishes such views, I withdraw." So I am a bete noir in George's eyes.

ROWENA: What are your views on homeopaths making a fruitful income?

MISHA: They are very simple; it has got nothing to do with homeopathy. Some people go out there and find it easy, and others don't. People often come into homeopathy driven by idealism, which is fabulous. But idealism doesn't make you an income. You could be a wonderful homeopath and not make a very good living or a really poor homeopath and be extremely wealthy; these things are not related.

ROWENA: Do you see homeopathy becoming dormant again?

MISHA: No, I don't see it going that way again. I see it diversifying. George Vithoulkas would like to see it stay in a particular direction, but it's not doing that, it's going all over the place.

ROWENA: So how do you think that affects our profession?

MISHA: I think that is healthy. I have a clear view about the kind of homeopathy that I like to practise and model for my students. However, that doesn't mean I am not appreciative of the other camps. Dismissing what others believe in would be like saying I really don't like slugs, I wish there weren't any in the world, I wish slugs were banished. But we know that diversity is the key to success and health. Diversity in homeopathy is just wonderful. There is a slight problem I guess, keeping a term like homeopathy, if one is actually practising something that is very different from what Hahnemann wrote about. But I think most of us are guided in a fundamental way by the *Organon*[4].

I do fervently believe in empiricism; in a process of evaluating results and modifying practise according to what one finds. I also believe in Continuous Professional Development, especially at this time when homeopathy is developing rapidly and extending its therapeutic range.

Increasing numbers of students who come for interview know very little about homeopathy, quite often they have come across Andrew Lockie's book *The Family Guide to Homoeopathy*,[34] or Miranda Castro's book, *The Complete Homeopathy Handbook*,[35] and that is it. So clearly they don't come to my school because they are interested in our point of view, the overreaching philosophy, the Doctrine of Signatures or the awareness of spirit into matter. It must be the spirit that is in the school, which hopefully is described in the literature and communicated by word of mouth. People often come because they have heard that their homeopaths have studied here or maybe wished they could have done. So there is something about what the school represents beyond the outer form of the homeopathy it espouses, and I believe it is the feeling of a functional family. This family works well and teaches in depth. It provides an environment, which is safe for people; it's safe for them to be dysfunctional occasionally and not be thrown out because of that.

I have a sort of prayer to the universe, a wish list, for homeopathy. The wish is that those who practise homeopathy should keep on looking; keep on looking at the world out there and the world inside themselves. I know we are always amazed at the stories that our patients tell us, and if we get tired of that we shouldn't be practising. The looking I had in mind goes further than that: we are told the story, but the question is what is driving that story. Keep on looking. What is the thing that keeps it going; where is that coming from?

In terms of ill health, where is the vital energy being held and stopped, how is that expressing itself? Here's a simplified analogy: there is a river, this represents the energy flowing and there's a rock in the river, which the water gurgles round. This obstruction is the disease. The eddy pools are incredibly interesting. That pattern is what we are looking for and the remedy has that pattern too. We match that pattern to the remedy pattern and the obstruction dissolves.

ROWENA: How do you teach remedies?

MISHA: Through signature. It is what it is. Be with the being of that particular manifestation and you have got it.

ROWENA: I have been reading about *The Secret Life of Plants*[36] – that they have a spirit. This concept makes perfect sense to me. What do you think?

MISHA: They are manifestations of spirit, obviously.

ROWENA: I always thought then when we die our spirits would go off to the astral plane, which would be here or somewhere else. Maybe they are in the plant world as well?

MISHA: Absolutely, why would it be different, there is a different awareness and consciousness of course, but in terms of planes of existence, these 'lower' astral realms are there for all of us – through them we manifest, to them we return when our manifestation ceases.

ROWENA: Do you think we can move into plant and come back in a human form?

MISHA: Well, we do as diseases, don't we? What happens, I wonder, when creatures go out of existence, for example, the Bengal Tiger? Its days are numbered but nothing can go out of existence at an astral or spiritual level, just the physical form has gone. So the energy that represents tiger has got to live somewhere and where better than as a co-inhabitant of a human. Maybe there will be more human tigers around the place as the animals go out of incarnation. It is a speculation.

One of the things that is endlessly reinforced by patient's stories, is that we all have an unconscious theme in our lives; a theme which repeats itself. Going back to the analogy of the river and the obstruction, well it's obviously the same river, because that's life. That won't change, but the obstruction also has an unerring way of remaining fixed. The eddy pools can vary because of changing life circumstances, but basically they represent the same pattern of deviation. It is a golden thread/river that runs through. The expressions may change but the thrust is the same. This unconscious stuff is what we should focus upon because that is where the obstruction resides. The expressions, and they are usually compensations, can change, but the basic unconscious material remains the same.

If that is true then there is one basic remedy that will be appropriate for that person rather than many. So when we keep on looking, what we are doing is searching to find the nature of that unconscious, basic obstruction and the remedy that most closely matches it. One lifetime is very small and short in the evolution of human consciousness. If we think of each human as being like a cell in the body of humanity, which is itself evolving, and we know that we are a very young species, then we notice that individually we have a long way to go. One lifetime of one individual human allows the possibility to work over a particular form, shape and disturbance and that's enough!

ROWENA: Even with my classical training I was taught the concept of layers.

MISHA: I don't think that's true. I think it appears to be true and therefore it is modelled. I don't actually think that is what happens.

ROWENA: So we are this one remedy, like when you have your astrological chart made for you? The picture that is created at birth of your whole life is reflected in the chart?

MISHA: Exactly like that. Like the natal chart, it tells you everything. There is one natal chart and there is one remedy.

ROWENA: Does that mean that people don't move on? Let us say I was given *Natrum muriaticum* and it clears my disappointed love. If I kept having that remedy repeated over time is it just making me feel better and boosting my immunity?

MISHA: Yes, but let us go back to the river and the obstruction. If you are looking at the eddy pools, you note that *Natrum muriaticum* covers some of these eddies. So if these eddy pools appear and I take *Natrum muriaticum*, the river flows with less obstruction, so it's good. I don't knock it. What I am suggesting though, is that if you prescribe a remedy for somebody, even by accident, and you see the miracle of cure at the deepest level, not just some but all the eddy currents disappear.

It is the Holy Grail of homeopathy; it is the quest. It is a model that keeps us on the search for more remedies and more provings because as we develop our materia medica, we also increase our capacity to find simillima, not just partial remedies, and this in turn moves our practice away from a layer model and towards a single remedy practice.

ROWENA: So the homeopaths that come out of this college, they would go on and practise the way that ....

MISHA: What tends to happen is they walk out of this college having taken cases under supervision during which time they also learn other things and they may say, "Wow, there is a much bigger world than we were taught at the School of Homeopathy, let's try out these other methods." That often happens. They are often rebellious and experimental; it is great and wonderful.

ROWENA: George Vithoulkas wouldn't say so though. But you are very classical, so why doesn't he approve of you?

MISHA: Well, I say some 'naughty' things especially about potency and provings and he is really not into that stuff. It is also about the understanding of the remedies. He is saying that a lot of partly proven information is added to the books and he is right, too. There is speculation in there. There is insufficient clarity about what is wildly speculative, what is just slightly imaginative and what is solidly arising from the provings. I wonder what he thinks of Vermeulen's work, for instance, of *Prisma*[37]. Frans Vermeulen is very rigorous and he always gives sources. Thus you can decide whether it is reliable or not and where you would place it on the 'speculative spectrum'.

ROWENA: That is what Sheilagh Creasy got us to do. We weren't allowed to use *Synthesis*[2] at the London College of Classical Homeopathy (LCCH), but like you I am a bit of a rebel so when I brought it in and mentioned a listing of a remedy within a rubric that wasn't in Kent, she would ask who the source was. I thought this was great and really good training.

MISHA: Yes, rigour is necessary; we shouldn't loose it.

ROWENA: Tell me more about John Damonte.

MISHA: I can tell you one thing about John Damonte that is most revealing; he spent his childhood in Morocco. They lived rurally and they had chickens.

ROWENA: Interesting, so you have that in common with him. Is there a chicken remedy?

MISHA: Yes, Nuala Eising proved *Chicken*, but she did it the same time as *Fox*. She divided the class into two and gave half of them *Chicken* and the other half *Fox*; that is very unconventional. Does she like trouble or what? She is a wonderful and extraordinary woman. But to get back to the story; if you want to multiply your stock of chickens then you will want to incubate the female eggs while eating the male eggs and the ones that are infertile. The way in which this was decided upon was by use of a pendulum. John Damonte had an aptitude for it. He unerringly got it right. The eggs John dowsed to incubate turned out to be chickens, not cockerels, and they all came out of their shells, rather than turning into a smelly, rotten egg.

That gave him the confidence to be a dowser in other fields. As he said, "Caruso came with a voice, Mozart came with music and I came with an ability to dowse." John Damonte was a natural and the word got round. The local healer used to go round with a horse and cart visiting sick folk, just an ordinary man, but with healing abilities, a bit like a Shaman. He liked John and took him on these healing rounds. When John was a young adult he entered medical school, a study interrupted by the war.

ROWENA: Do you dowse?

MISHA: I am not a natural. I am only good at it if I really have no vested interest in the outcome. If it is my patient I am not so good at it. If it is someone else's patient I will be fine. So there is some weird block that I have. Another homeopath can just tell me about their patient and I can dowse for them.

ROWENA: But how do you go through three thousand remedies?

MISHA: There are several of ways of doing it, but all you need is a list really, however a book is nice because you can open it and you can halve it and then halve the half until you reach the page and the remedy. George Vithoulkas would go mad!

ROWENA: I guess he would! Thanks so much Misha.

CHAPTER 8: ANNETTE GAMBLIN

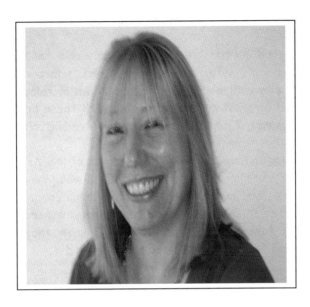

Monday 28 February 2005 took me to the University of Westminster to visit Annette Gamblin, one of the teachers who inspired me while studying at the London College of Classical Homeopathy (LCCH). Along with Sheilagh Creasy, Annette taught us most of the homeopathy philosophy. We had reconnected at the teachers' seminar in Malvern and I was eager to get to know her better and hear her story. I sat in on her class in the morning and we then found a clinic room to chat and eat sushi, soup and sandwiches; a strange mix I know!

"If you can understand homeopathy, then you can approach it authentically from your own place of truth rather than from what this or that teacher says. I think students have to find their own way of doing that."
Annette Gamblin, February 2005

"There is a lot of bickering and politics in homeopathy and I wish that people would just get over that and concentrate on the profession's future. I would love to become part of a healthcare system that works with doctors but does not compromise what it is that we do. I wouldn't want to work in an NHS clinic where somebody says, "The first consultation has to be this long" or "This patient will have to be on this drug and you just do your homeopathy around that." My vision is of working together with doctors to get a patient into a better, healthier place with a holistic approach. Doctors who are honest enough to say, "These drugs do what they do and they are helping but not healing" and who will ask, "How can we really cure this person?" And I am not just talking about homeopathy here. Let's integrate all kinds of traditional healing."
Annette Gamblin, February 2005

CHAPTER 8: ANNETTE GAMBLIN

ROWENA: So Annette, how did you get into homeopathy?

ANNETTE: That is a good question really. I think it was a 'calling', as Künzli said in his translation of the *Organon*[38]. When I was a little girl, somebody gave me lots of tiny bottles as a present to play with, and I filled them with water colours. They were medicines to me, and I proceeded to treat my autistic sister with these bottles. I didn't make her drink any of them but already I had a sense that the material itself was not necessary.

It is a cliché, but wanting to help has always been a part of me. As a child I lived in various countries and in one of the many schools I attended, I was in a class with about fifteen other kids with no more than two students from the same country. So I was exposed to different cultures, different countries, and people's varying perceptions of things. From very early on I didn't take anything for granted. I knew that how I might perceive something could well be different from how somebody else did.

When I left school I was involved in music. I did various jobs to earn money but I very much wanted to be a musician. I was in all sorts of bands and travelled with one as well.

ROWENA: Singing?

ANNETTE: Singing and playing saxophone. I had lots of adventures and at that time also developed an interest in astrology. I was living in Munich at the time and there was an astrologer there called Wolfgang Döbereiner. He had this little school that I attended. He taught a combination of astrology and homeopathy. I had never heard of homeopathy before and I thought that it was very interesting. So then when I was ill, the first thing I did was to seek help from a homeopath. At that time in Germany homeopaths mainly prescribed combinations or complex homeopathy. I ended up seeing someone called Braunger, an incredible spiritual teacher who unfortunately is no longer with us.

ROWENA: How long ago was this?

ANNETTE: Twenty five years ago. I came to England because I met an English man and got married to him. He was a musician, too. Again, when I wasn't well in the UK I saw a classical homeopath, a lovely lady called Jackie Smart, and through treatment with her the idea of homeopathy grew on me and I thought, "This is what I want to do with my life."

So I am one of those people whom it took a long time and quite a journey to get to the point of finding out what it was that I wanted to really do. At the time, colleges were just starting up and so I was able to go. I was part of the third generation of the London

College of Classical Homeopathy (LCCH). I graduated in 1991. I still love homeopathy to this day and I also love teaching it as a subject.

ROWENA: Why LCCH?

ANNETTE: It was very much on intuition. I didn't go to this place and that place to check them all out. It just felt the right choice to make.

ROWENA: Did you start your teaching career at LCCH?

ANNETTE: No, I started teaching at Barbara Harwood's College of Homeopathy (COH) and I am very grateful to her for the opportunity. When I was little I actually wanted to become a teacher. With a few colleagues, I started attending philosophy tutorials run by a chap called Yair Shemmer who was from the first intake at LCCH and soon I was absolutely hooked. We were into really reading the *Organon*[4] [38] and the classics. I feel so sad that some students don't read these great books anymore. We spent hours going through the *Organon*[4] [38] really examining each aphorism, questioning its meaning and working it all out. I just had a passion for the philosophy straight away so my colleagues and I expanded on a curriculum, with references for further reading, which Yair had developed and Barbara took it on board at COH. At that time they were looking for people to increase the philosophy input there, so straight after graduation I started teaching.

For me the philosophy really creates the foundations for understanding homeopathy and this is reflected in how I approach a case. If you can understand homeopathy, then you can approach it authentically from your own place of truth rather than from what this or that teacher says. I think students have to find their own way of doing that. All we can do in an undergraduate course is to teach the basics, and once you have the basic tools you develop your own style and make use of the methodologies that you feel resonate and work for you.

ROWENA: From my experience of LCCH, there was a strong focus on repertorisation.

ANNETTE: You have to teach the repertory as one of the basic tools. It is ridiculous to say to students in year one, "Throw out those repertories, you don't need them anymore." You can throw them out once you graduate if you find that you don't need them anymore, but not when you are learning your basic tools and it is part of the craft to know how to use a repertory. One has to remember that the repertory is not an absolute, it is a tool, and just because you have chosen certain rubrics doesn't mean that the best remedy for the particular case will just automatically pop out as a result of it; it just doesn't. I think if you work with repertorisation, a good practice to adopt would be to repertorise the case in several ways and observe what remedies come through.

ROWENA: So tell me more about the experience of studying at the University of Westminster.

ANNETTE: We have a core team of teachers here. The Pathway Leaders are the people that carry the responsibility for the management of the course, that doesn't mean that we are told what to teach or how to teach it. The homeopathy course is part of the School of Integrated Health in which there are other therapies, for example, acupuncture, herbal medicine, nutrition and naturopathy. We have a Polyclinic that is multidisciplinary and it is where all the students have their teaching clinics. When a punter comes in off the street they come into reception and they can have a session from any of these various therapies. The idea is that, if necessary, we can cross-refer and also learn from each other. There is, for example, some interdisciplinary supervision and some research that takes place, which is very interesting. The Polyclinic is a set up that really works well for us.

ROWENA: Do you ever get a shortage of patients?

ANNETTE: No, not really. I think that the only thing, and you probably find this in any low cost teaching clinic, that there is sometimes a lack of commitment from the patients. However there is an extraordinary range of cases and we do get patients with some very heavy mental pathology. The cases that come here seem to be different from those in private practice for some reason. There is obviously the added dynamic that patients are observed by students here and observation changes everything.

Students take part in the clinic from year one by initially just observing. We run it two full days a week, which I think is quite a lot. Our course is weekday full-time and for three years. We have a university modular system giving us a part-time option for students to study over five years with a tailor-made timetable.

ROWENA: Is that a popular option?

ANNETTE: We do get a fair percentage of people doing that but not too many. They are not here all the time as they obviously spread their modules out. The university structure means that they do a really good homeopathy course but they also have to complete additional modules, which belong to the structure of the University of Westminster, so the academic side of it is also quite challenging for some students.

I think the big difference between a diploma and a degree is probably in the amount of hours of attendance and study. They have this basic degree with philosophy, materia medica and clinical practise and then they do practitioner development with students on the other courses as well as the anatomy, physiology and pathology. A module that I think is very important is 'setting up in practice', which is again for all students across the courses. I think that is what a lot of people struggle with when they graduate - how to actually be a professional homeopath and make a living.

ROWENA: What do you think are the ingredients that make a successful homeopath?

ANNETTE: There are so many skills that make a good homeopath; it is so multifaceted. They should have a good philosophical understanding, be proficient in communication and listening and a good prescriber. I think it is also important to have some kind of business sense as well.

ROWENA: Can you tell in the classroom who is going to be a successful homeopath?

ANNETTE: You can never tell. Over the years I have seen practitioners become 'successful' when I thought they were actually terrible students and didn't have a clue. It also depends on what you mean by 'successful.' If you equate being successful with making money, which to me is just one element of it, then of course anybody can be successful if they have got the mind for that, but for me it is a combination of several things.

ROWENA: So are you saying that some homeopaths make a lot of money but they won't necessarily be good homeopaths?

ANNETTE: It is possible, for sure. You can make money in so many ways. You can hook people onto a machine and whiz them in and out in ten minutes and give them a quick fix. Now you are getting me into my pet hate!

ROWENA: Good, let's talk about that then!

ANNETTE: For me, classical homeopathy is not about what Hahnemann or Kent did, it is actually about an incredible depth of approach; the deeper you can address something, the bigger the shift. Now that doesn't happen overnight. It is a process and that is what I enjoy most in practice; to see the shift over a period of time. I dislike the attitude, "I have got this complaint and I just want it to be treated". Having said that, there is also this tendency for some homeopaths to ignore the physical complaints and only look at the mental and emotional picture, but that is not actually what I am talking about. I am looking for a shift in wellbeing through a process - mentally, emotionally and physically. It is not a question of expecting a very chronic complaint to just disappear overnight. Some symptoms will sometimes do that, but we shouldn't have that expectations and we should be open to a process because within that process lots of things happen.

ROWENA: How do you get your patients to understand that involvement?

ANNETTE: By educating them about the process. I make a formal agreement with them from the start so they understand.

ROWENA: So if they want a quick fix?

ANNETTE: I would recommend that they try something or somebody else.

ROWENA: So if I go to see this other person, what would that quick fix be? How would that be different from how you are prescribing?

ANNETTE: It is a non holistic approach. They might treat one aspect and give a remedy for a physical complaint while losing the bigger picture of where that particular complaint relates. It might be that this way of treating is curative but it might not. Just because a complaint disappears doesn't mean a cure has taken place.

ROWENA: So for example, a thirteen year old girl with rheumatoid arthritis came to me and she had been prescribed *Rhus toxicodendron* at the Royal London Homeopathic Hospital. She came with her mother, by recommendation, to see me soon after, and I advised against the prescription and explained that I could see a deeper and obvious constitutional picture of *Lycopodium*. She took the *Lycopodium* in an LM potency and the remedy made a huge difference to her on all levels. Is that the kind of thing you are talking about?

ANNETTE: Absolutely. The depth that we need to go in the case is where the vital force is disturbed. We are looking for the expression of the disease and then we deal with those expressions. We need to ask what the experience of that physical complaint is for that particular patient. At the end of the day what we are addressing is the disturbed vital force. There is this energy that has got a certain quality of disturbance and that is what we are dealing with and we cannot access that directly so we need to understand its expressions.

Dynamic means not static, so whatever the state is, it moves all the time and within that it has various expressions. Whether that boils down to the fact that we all have this one state that just needs this one remedy - for me that is still open for discussion. There are people doing wonderful work who seem to say that paradigm is working for them.

ROWENA: And that is how Massimo Mangialavori would see it, wouldn't he – that you need that one remedy and it works for acutes and constitutionally?

ANNETTE: But there is something about acute and chronic that is different. So for me, the whole idea of acute and chronic is like people sharing a flat. The chronic complaint or picture is that one person is really tidy and the other one is completely disorganised and untidy, and the tidy person is just getting so annoyed and frustrated. This carries on for months and months and needs to be addressed. Then one day - as has happened many times before – the untidy one is in a complete panic and goes into hysterics looking for the car keys because they need to get to the station on time. They need to get to work because they have been late so often that if they don't get there promptly they are going to lose their job and they have already had a warning.

The tidy flatmate wanted to have a chat with the untidy but if they choose this point occasion to address the chronic picture while an acute is happening, what is going to happen? Nothing, because it is completely consumed with the energy of the acute and the acute needs addressing. So the best solution to this is for the tidy flatmate to let the chronic go for now and say, "Ok, forget your keys, I will take you to the station", and when they come back in the evening to say, "There is something I have been wanting to talk to you about." That is the whole idea.

ROWENA: I remember you teaching us that analogy at college and it really stayed with me.

ANNETTE: But I think that sometimes the acute can really lift out of the chronic and get its own identity, but it also can still be mingled in with the chronic and then possibly a chronic remedy will also deal with the acute - but I am still thinking about it all.

ROWENA: Yes, me too. I was listening to you saying that and I was thinking about how I was trained and it makes a lot of sense, but how is it that Massimo Mangialavori can use the same remedy for acute and chronic? There are just so many different ways homeopaths look at a case and they get good results but with different methods and different remedies. Why do you think that is?

ANNETTE: I can see that in terms of the way Hahnemann in the *Organon*[4] [38] talks about what seems acute, is in reality, the transient explosion of the latent psora.

ROWENA: That would fit in with Massimo Mangialavori's way of thinking, I guess.

ANNETTE: So basically the idea would be that by addressing the chronic susceptibility that produces the acute, you are incorporating the acute at the same time.

ROWENA: And, I guess, I just seem to attract a lot of chronic cases so Massimo Mangialavori's paradigm works for me.

ANNETTE: And I do too, and it works sometimes but also sometimes it doesn't, and whether that means I haven't got the simillimum, I just don't know.

ROWENA: I know you have worked with people with AIDS. Can you tell me more about that?

ANNETTE: I worked for two years in a charity clinic where they had all kinds of alternative practitioners and the patients chose which treatments they wanted. I learned a lot, and it is a strange thing to say but I really enjoyed it. It did, however, take up a lot of my time and energy.

ROWENA: What do you think is the best way of prescribing for patients with AIDS – one constitutional remedy, zigzagging with the different remedies according to what is uppermost or something else?

ANNETTE: The remedy has to work with the vitality that is there, so curability for me means a vital force that can bounce back. AIDS is a syndrome, it is not a disease per se, so all kinds of disease expressions happen on the way, so it depends at what stage the patient is at; whether they have only just been diagnosed HIV positive and have never had any symptoms of any kind or whether they have been through many years on their journey and are on a combination of drugs treating all kinds of episodes of AIDS related illnesses. Your results are only as good as what you are working with at the time.

ROWENA: Ok, sure, and then the methodology would change. So at first when they just find out, in a way it is like treating cancer. The diagnosis can cause an emotional layer of shock. After you treat that, which may just involve talking and the therapeutic relationship or could be with a remedy, you are then working back to the layer of susceptibility which you could see more clearly when the diagnosis is just HIV positive. Obviously further down the line when they are on a lot of drugs, would you think of using tautopathy or something else?

ANNETTE: I have tried that, of course. When you get out into the world having studied you do try things but I just found that tautopathy didn't work for me at all.

ROWENA: Would you treat the specific 'opportunistic' issue they have at the time?

ANNETTE: You have to deal with what you are being presented. If somebody has got such bad diarrhoea that they cannot even get out of the house because they just never know when it is going to happen and they don't want to soil themselves on the bus, that symptom has to be uppermost.

ROWENA: That symptom is limiting them the most at that time.

ANNETTE: I would use the symptom as a signpost. We should always be looking at what is the urgency and are they in a lot of pain. I wouldn't dream of saying to somebody in pain, "Wait a couple of days until I work out your remedy because this one is not working."

ROWENA: It is interesting that you mention waiting because that is the reputation the classicist has when you speak to people from the Practical Colleges.

ANNETTE: I think there are lots of misunderstandings about classical homeopathy. You get the fundamentalists, the people who say, "This is how it is and there is no other way". You get that in all kinds of homeopathy.

ROWENA: You get that in all walks of life.

ANNETTE: Exactly. Like I said, to me 'classical' is about the depth of treatment and has not just been inherited from Hahnemann. For example, the way we use the miasm theory is not simply according to what Hahnemann said. Therefore is our use of that theory classical? Where are we with that concept now? For me it just relates back to the idea that everything is an expression of the disturbed vital force.

ROWENA: And there are a lot of elements to homeopathy.

ANNETTE: Yes.

ROWENA: I can see that homeopathy fits into that broader picture, especially at the University of Westminster where we have a Polyclinic that treats so many conditions with different modalities and people are mixing and matching. I know you taught the subject of methodology this morning - so is one methodology encouraged? I know in philosophy classes a lot of methodologies are discussed, but when and how is that translated into the clinic situation? Is one methodology used more than others?

ANNETTE: I think it is about teaching students the basics so they have tools, and I would never say to any student, "In order to be effective, you need to work from my understanding." It is no use me imposing my understanding as it will never their own', but they have got to have the basic tools in order to learn. In the clinic I think we do have our individual styles as well, but on the whole we do have to keep it simple so that it is reproducible for the student, otherwise they are not learning anything. I think they have to be able to observe something, learn something from it and then use it, so how I take cases would be slightly different here from how I do it elsewhere when I am not teaching or being observed.

ROWENA: Do you get to the same remedy, do you think?

ANNETTE: I cannot split myself like that; I don't know.

ROWENA: It is a different dynamic here as the patient is being observed. Do you think this stops you going deeper?

ANNETTE: I remember having talked to Jeremy Sherr about this once, as obviously he does a lot of teaching clinics. We agreed that when you are being observed taking the case you are so involved with that patient at that point in time that observation just really increases the potency.

ROWENA: Yes, I can understand that. I really liked the expression 'freefalling'; you used it this morning in class. So in the clinic here when you take a case and you are freefalling, do you sometimes have a remedy at the end of the case taking and then when it is discussed among the students your ideas change?

ANNETTE: Obviously you come to a prescription much quicker at the Polyclinic. I am not sure what to say to that really, because in my practice maybe twenty percent of the time I will prescribe immediately. I know some people do so all the time but I don't. I like to go away and think and look at different possibilities and remedies I have never heard of before.

ROWENA: Otherwise if you prescribe remedies immediately and never research you will not have the opportunity to learn about new remedies?

ANNETTE: If you prescribe on the spot you are only ever going to use what you already know about. Obviously, if you are not open to something new, you are not going to be able to use remedies that are unfamiliar to you.

ROWENA: I love the learning, especially the fact that it is just endless.

ANNETTE: When you sit down and have a consultation it is all about getting beneath the surface, really getting deeper and deeper into it, and once we get there, it is just an adventure and the landscape is so different every time. It is amazing to look at and just be. I have always felt so honoured to be there with that person at that point in time when they show me their landscape, and from day one, that has never changed for me.

ROWENA: I thank my patients because I see it as a privilege. I know you have to go back and teach in a minute Annette. Thank you so much for sharing your lunch break and stories with me today. Is there anything you want to add as your parting comment?

ANNETTE: There is a lot of bickering and politics in homeopathy and I wish that people would just get over that and concentrate on the profession's future. I would love to become part of a healthcare system that works with doctors but does not compromise what it is that we do. I wouldn't want to work in an NHS clinic where somebody says, "The first consultation has to be this long" or "This patient will have to be on this drug and you just do your homeopathy around that." My vision is of working together with doctors to get a patient into a better, healthier place with a holistic approach. Doctors who are honest enough to say, "These drugs do what they do and they are helping but not healing" and who will ask, "How can we really cure this person?" And I am not just talking about homeopathy here. Let's integrate all kinds of traditional healing."

ROWENA: Thank you Annette. It is always a pleasure to see you.

CHAPTER 9: FRANCIS TREUHERZ

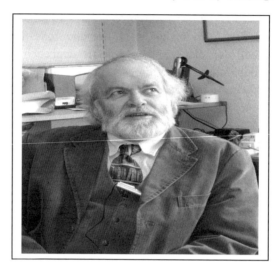

Thursday 3 March 2005 found me in Kilburn visiting the fountain of knowledge that is Francis Treuherz, a fellow of the Society of Homeopaths. He swept me upstairs to the library in his high ceilinged Victorian house, and as I relaxed in his patients' worn velvet throne, I was immersed in the sights, sounds and smells of our heritage. Nearly every book written about homeopathy adorns the many shelves of Francis' clinic room. Exciting trinkets once owned by our renowned forefathers and mothers are displayed for his patients and fellow scholars of homeopathy to view. For the several hours that I was with him I felt that I had stepped back in time.

"I don't like labels and I am only interested in finding the right way of treating any individual patient, whatever that right way may be. I have very, very rarely found that right way to involve the use of more than one remedy at a time and cannot understand how people who are creating the principles for a single register seem to be allowing that in."
Francis Treuherz, March 2005

"George Vithoulkas once talked about prescribing for people on his Greek island (Alonissos). Decades ago the patients were simple to prescribe for and they were on one remedy all their life. But now, there is so much Western influence – antibiotics, divorce, drugs and all the rest of it. Life is more complicated and it is harder to be certain of that remedy for all their life."
Francis Treuherz, March 2005

"Many homeopaths undersell and undervalue themselves. Some are unknowing of how to deal with money and how to present and publicise themselves." *Francis Treuherz, March 2005*

CHAPTER 9:   FRANCIS TREUHERZ

ROWENA: What got you into homeopathy in the beginning Francis?

FRANCIS: I was a successful patient actually. I went to see my dentist one day and made some joke about a dirty needle, because I had had hepatitis years before, and he said, "You have made that joke before – go and see my brother, he is a homeopath". I had no awareness of the word, although there was a Manchester Homeopathic Clinic at that point in an old building right next to the university. I must have driven, walked, or been on the bus past it countless times, with no conscious knowledge of it. This was in the early 1970s. I had had hepatitis in 1966, seriously.

So I went to see his brother. At the time, I was drinking coffee intravenously and the first remedy he gave me was *Nux vomica*, but that really was because of the coffee. Then I got another remedy and I remember, very, very quickly, feeling well. I used to ride a bicycle everywhere and I could no longer really ride; I just didn't have enough energy, and after the remedies I was back on my bike.

The homeopath's name was Jack Lozdan. He was also a dentist and trained with Margery Blackie, and then he went off to live in France for a while. The first book I got was Boericke[39], it looked like a bible. Then I picked up two volumes of Clarke's *Materia Medica*[28], signed by the author, without the third, for a fiver, and that began the hunt. I did eventually find the third volume.

I heard about a couple of homeopathic study groups. One was taught by John Damonte in North London, which Misha Norland was attending, and the other was taught by Thomas Maughan in South London. I was holding down full-time and part-time jobs, at the Open University and London University at the time, so I didn't have much time other than that for private reading. I decided to try and register for a PhD because I felt this was a subject worthy of study and I was interested in the history of homeopathy and in particular, as I was a social scientist, the reactions to successful homeopathic treatment of the cholera epidemics in the nineteenth century.

There had been a cholera epidemic and the then secretary of the Board of Health made a report to Parliament. He added that if he got sick he would go to the homeopaths despite his initial prejudice. He stated their mortality rate was about sixteen percent compared to the general London hospital mortality rate, which was about sixty percent. It could have been that the patients were brought in at an earlier stage of their illness; the homeopathic hospital could have been more hygienic and perhaps the patients could have been better nourished as they were from a higher economic class. The reaction from Parliament was that "This was against all reason, truth and science" and the figures were suppressed.

So I called my proposed thesis 'The Social Construction of a Rejected Science' and my idea for a PhD was rejected. The Open University said that homeopathy was not a proper subject to study. However, it was prevailed upon the London University to accept me because, after all, I had been teaching there for eleven years and I was an examiner. I wrote long chapters on Kent's philosophy and the origins of Kent's thought and on Rudolph Steiner and the apparent confusion between homeopathy and anthroposophy among homeopathic practitioners. I was trying to look at what the boundaries were of homeopathic science. I began to look at the work of Bach[29] and got as far as the bibliography, which was actually published, but I never got round to writing that chapter because I discovered that a college had emerged where homeopaths were actually being taught.

So I went to see the principal of the College of Homeopathy (COH), Robert Davidson, and asked if I could find out what he was teaching. He replied that the only way I could enter his classes was if I enrolled as a student. I appreciated the way an observer changes the subject under observation and that it would be less of a problem if I was one of the students so I agreed, although, I thought, the notes I would be taking might be different. I wrote down everything the teacher said and before long I became so fascinated that I ended up carrying on seriously studying and the PhD was abandoned along the way.

Back then I borrowed a book, Hahnemann's *Lesser Writings*[40], from the British Homeopathic Association (BHA) library. I was on my bicycle waiting at a traffic light and somebody came by on a motorbike and whipped my bag and the book was in it. So I started haunting the second hand bookshops – it took me eight years, but I found another copy. Then I found another that summer, so I kept one and the BHA library got one back. But by that time I had bought everything I could see because they weren't so expensive, and I became a collector.

ROWENA: Were you in the first year intake?

FRANCIS: No, I was in the second with Stephen Gordon, Robert Nichols, Barbara Harwood, Tony Hurley, Jeremy Sherr, Peter Adams, Susan Curtis, Stella Berg, Lesley Gregerson, John Morgan, Robin Logan, Sylvia Treacher and some others were. It was a very big year and a good one too. There are still quite a few of us around. Janet Snowdon and the late Stan Tibbs were already there.

I had contact with George Vithoulkas and his colleagues very early on. At the first ever annual conference of the Society of Homeopaths - it wasn't annual then but started off as being every year and a half for the first two or three - I was asked to give my lecture on Kent and I was still a student. Our first foreign guest was Vassilis Ghegas, a close colleague and friend of George. I had family in Greece so they asked me to be his minder. I didn't really know what to say to him as I was still new to all this and he was an apparently eminent Greek physician. He was accompanied by Roger Morrison, because it was the first time Vassilis has ever lectured in English and he knew he would need help occasionally.

I told him that I had been to Greece a few times and I bought him a whisky because I was told that was what he liked. He asked me what I did when I went to Greece and I told him I went to visit my uncle. I told him who my uncle was and he nearly choked on his whisky. He is dead now, but he was the Dean of the Medical School at the University of Athens and physician in charge of the largest hospital. He was a very modest man and I wasn't trying to drop names, but Vassilis Ghegas did nearly choke. He told me that my uncle had referred patients to him but he did not admit to it. He taught Vassilis Ghegas and the first wave of Greek homeopaths allopathy – a very weird connection.

Later on I went to Athens and my uncle gave me a book, *The Science of Homeopathy* [31] and it was by George Vithoulkas. It was first published in English in Greece and George had given it to my uncle as a present because he wanted him to adopt homeopathy. He said that he was not interested and gave the book to me. So I showed it to George and his jaw dropped. He asked me where I had got it. So I told him, and so he sent my uncle another copy because he wanted him to have it. My uncle said he would put it on the shelf in his office where he had the sort of books that furnish the room.

My uncle was regarded in Greek medicine as a great clinician, a great diagnostician and a sort of human being polymath. He could talk about Greek poetry with one voice and then write a play for a patient who is an actor the next day. He was one of those renaissance men who we don't get any more.

ROWENA: So who were your teachers at COH?

FRANCIS: Robert Davidson, Misha Norland, David Mundy, John Ball, David Curtin and Sheilagh Creasy. There were one or two lectures through which I slept, but that is my pathology. It took a while until somebody figured what remedy to give me to stop me falling asleep, as many years later I fell asleep at a Board Meeting for the Society of Homeopaths. A fellow board member, Robin Logan, gave me *Opium*. It sorted it out to some extent but it is a family trait. I am useless being taken to the Albert Hall for example. I always fall asleep at a concert.

I felt that sometimes I learnt homeopathy because of COH and sometimes despite COH, as it was terribly organised. Having come from a university background, including teaching and examining, it was a shambles. So I made a long and detailed suggestion for a revised assessment system and gave it to Robert Davidson as a gift, you might say, but I don't think he understood what to do with it. I remember saying to a friend in our first year that wherever I went it seemed quite hard to adopt a low profile and we both resolved to do just that, but it didn't work for either of us.

What happened during those early years - the very late 1970s and the early 80s - was that Vassilis Ghegas, who had been invited to our Conference, came back and did a series of eight long weekend seminars. A lot of students and homeopaths came, both medical and non-medical, and that is what gave modern homeopathy a secure foundation in the UK. Although we had the teachings by the students of Thomas Maughan and John Damonte, they didn't have their feet in the classics and in the philosophical structure in the way that we needed.

ROWENA: Was that part of the course?

FRANCIS: No, this was extra and they were not consecutive. They were a series of eight seminars known as the Greek Seminars and then George also came and gave some seminars. But those eight were elementary in a way, looking back now, but it is what we needed at the time. They were the foundations that put us on a thorough footing, back into the mainstream of homeopathic thought.

We had about thirty students in the year and we began at the YWCA in Great Russell Street and moved to Imperial College.

ROWENA: Who had the biggest influence on you?

FRANCIS: I don't think there was a 'biggest' influence. George Vithoulkas' ideas certainly had a big influence. Hahnemann and Kent have always had the biggest influences and Burnett and Clarke - reading the old masters from this side of the Atlantic. The first really good grasp I had of the history of homeopathy was a French book by someone called Denis Demarque, *Homeopathy, the Medicine of Experience*[41], which looked at the whole gamut of the history of homeopathy, and Harris Coulter's *Divided Legacy*[56]. I read that very early on before I was studying to be a homeopath. One of the reasons for choosing a project on the ideas of Kent and the influence of Swedenborg was that that was something that Harris had avoided.

I sent that early chapter of my PhD to the American Institute of Homeopathy, for publication in the *American Journal of Homeopathic Medicine*[42] and they sent it to Harris Coulter for peer review. I never heard. So I wrote to Harris asking for his advice, not knowing that he had been sent it for peer review, and he thought "Oh no, not an article on Swedenborg – I cannot stand that!" Then he realised I had got inside it in some way and said it was okay to publish, and we became firm friends and he has been one of the biggest influences ever since. Harris is steeped in the history of homeopathy and homeopathy philosophy, without being a practitioner. His former wife was a practitioner – Catherine Coulter – she practised in Washington DC. Harris' understanding of how and why homeopathy rose and fell in the nineteenth and then early twentieth century, the rise of the drug companies and so on, is really important to understanding homeopathy. He wrote *Divided Legacy*[56] and a lot of people only read one volume but it is in four volumes.

A digression, one day I was in my bedroom and I heard the answer phone going, and it was Harris Coulter saying he was going to Moscow and his plane was going to come to London for a stopover later that day. I rushed to pick up the phone, he was in Washington at the time, and luckily I was free and I picked him up from the local station. We sat and talked about homeopathy and got books from the shelves. I had this big pot of mushroom soup, we drank red wine and I had the most marvellous day. Later he went to Moscow and then to Paris and the next thing I got was a phone call saying that he had had a stroke.

He was due in Ireland, a month after that meeting of ours, to talk at the Irish Conference. I simply packed an enormous briefcase with every book he had ever written and took it over there and we lit a candle at the beginning of the Conference when he was due to speak, as I didn't know whether he was alive or not. I fished out of my bag one book after another, and talked about his work and explained what he had done.

When I returned home, I received a phone call from one of his sons asking me if I would go to Paris where he was in hospital to see him. I just dropped everything and went by Eurostar. I walked in there early in the morning, and there he was with a tube in his face, lying there in a stupor. "Hello Harry", I said. "Hello Fran" he said. They wanted someone whose voice he might recognise.

It was the only time in my life I have pretended to be a doctor. The nurse came in and I asked her what medicine he was going to be given. She replied, "Opium" and I requested that it wasn't given to him. But she came in an hour later, and again I asked her not to give it to him. As the day wore on he began to sit up and we had a conversation. He wasn't really always there, his mind kept drifting off, but by the end of the day he was sitting up, and by the end of the second day he was drinking from a cup instead of from a tube. He had told me a lot of names and addresses of people to write to tell them where he was. I was testing his memory, but he couldn't remember his own address. So it wasn't quite right. He had been proving opium, the remedy he needed, as it was given too often.

Unfortunately he has remained partially paralysed and disabled. The last thing he wrote was the introduction to Julian Winston's book *The Faces of Homeopathy*[43]. This was a few years ago now. It is possible that Harry took too much *Arnica*. He used to travel a lot and use an enormous amount for jet lag. So yes, Harry was a big influence.

ROWENA: Who influences you the most nowadays?

FRANCIS: In the winter of 1985–86, I spent a fortnight in New Delhi. From there I spent a long time in Calcutta and then over to Bombay. Someone who had a very, very big influence was S P Dey. He was taught by Donald Foubister (who has also had a big influence on me), and he gave really practical information but also a lot of ideas about miasms, single remedy classic prescribing and how it works in the most dire of pathology that you can imagine in Calcutta – and it would make your hair stand on end. Literally, walking in, seeing a woman patient dressed in shawls rather than closed garments in hospital with a breast cancer lesion pouring rubbish out. In England they would have cut it out and been horrified but he gave her a dose of *Staphysagria 1M*. The reaction was that stuff poured out, and gradually it poured out less and less and it healed. We have neither the experience nor the courage to do that here.

ROWENA: Do you do that?

FRANCIS: I don't have the opportunity unfortunately, but see my article on *Matters of Life and Death* in the *Homeopath*[44], summer 2005. On my last day in India, I got a phone call from someone from the Society of Homeopaths in England asking if I could find Rajan Sankaran and invite him to come and speak in England. It was my last day and it was a miracle the phone worked and I was still in my hotel room at the time – and that they had actually found me. I apologised and said that I had a dinner date with the most beautiful homeopath in Bombay. Coincidentally she said when we met that she had a surprise for me, and it was dinner with Rajan. So I invited him to come to England and I have a photograph of that moment. He was eating something with his hand – his mouth open, nearly choking on it. So Rajan has been a big influence, and I am happy to say that I am responsible for inviting him for the first time to come to England to our Conference in 1986.

ROWENA: Tell me more about your journey – your career within homeopathy.

FRANCIS: I have a tendency to get involved with things. "If I am not for myself who will be for me? And if I am only for myself, who am I? And if not now, when?" This quote is from a Talmudic book known as *The Ethics of the Fathers*[45]. It is a Jewish ethical statement, which I learnt early on. When I was growing up, my father spent a lot of his spare time helping to manage and run, in a practical sense, a Jewish old peoples' home in Manchester. So I learnt to get involved with things. I was secretary of a youth club attached to my synagogue, of which I was a member. So I got involved with the Society of Homeopaths, and the first thing I did was edit *The Homeopath*[46], then I was on the Board at the same time as doing that. At that time there wasn't a time limit for being on the Board so I was on it for about ten years. Then I had a gap, and I have now been on it again for five years. I will withdraw in 2006 because six years is the end of the term you can have. This time it will be the end of my term as Secretary.

ROWENA: How come you got to be Honorary Secretary?

FRANCIS: Because I have a background in public administration and because it is the sort of work which a lot of people find boring. In the early days our work was much less differentiated. I was involved with planning, running and organising seminars; with setting up a proper disciplinary procedure because although we had a *Code of Ethics*[47] at the Society of Homeopaths, nobody actually knew what to do when somebody did something naughty – how to actually organise it. I got involved in everything, but all Board members did at one time or another. We initially didn't have staff, then we had Mary Clarke, and then things gradually grew, but we were hands-on when really in a legal sense, a Board ought to do solely governance. But there was no other alternative.

I got involved with computing fairly early on. *MacRepertory* was invented and I took to it like duck to water. I got involved with David Warkentin who started *Homeonet*, a very primitive e-mail service. He and I virtually met when I found a remedy for him the first time I logged on. He was living in California and after that he began to pick my brains about literary things – why the remedy abbreviations in Boericke[39] didn't match those in Kent's *Repertory*[16] and stuff like that, very basic. He was a big influence and has become one of my best friends.

There are books on these shelves that went into that repertory because no one else had got them. So my obsession, my pathology, is collecting books. I got involved with *MacRepertory* and ended up helping to develop it, helping to sell it and most importantly, helping to teach people how to use it because it is both intuitive and simple but very deep and rich. There is an enormous amount there that people don't use because they never think to click in every one of the possible click boxes.

Because of my involvement I started going to lots of seminars. The idea was that I would only go to a seminar if it would pay for itself. I went to loads and I learnt loads. I started teaching in Helsinki; I went four times a year for about five years. Five years later when Helsinki had its tenth anniversary I was invited back to teach a seminar. I went to teach in Prague; I went to teach in Sweden, but I very much preferred to teach within a programme rather than coming on as guru teaching without responsibility – turning up, teaching, and disappearing again. I didn't like that as much.

ROWENA: So where have you taught in the UK?

FRANCIS: I have taught at COH in London; bizarrely they kept asking me to teach when I lived in Manchester, less so when I got back to London. The London College of Classical Homeopathy (LCCH), as it was known before it merged with COH; I taught quite a lot for the British School of Homeopathy when it began in Swindon. I taught for the Yorkshire School of Homeopathy in York and Leeds. I teach regularly but not frequently for one or two colleges where I go along for a day only and talk about the history of our literature. I taught in Manchester for the longest, whether I lived in Manchester or in London – ten years of regular teaching at the North West College of Homoeopathy (NWCH) where I also ran their bookshop. I have given odd lectures at the Northern College in Newcastle and the South Downs School of Homeopathy in Chichester ..... and who knows where else.

I literally get scholars from all over the world coming here. I have been to the USA three times and done some lecturing there and individual seminars. Very early on I got to know Dana Ullman who runs Homeopathic Education Services in California[48], a big publisher and publicist for homeopathy. I met him and helped him run his stall at a conference in Lyon, France in 1985. I met a lot of people that way. So I have been to quite a lot of conferences to try and hear all different viewpoints about homeopathy.

ROWENA: Where do you stand now having listened to all these people?

FRANCES: I don't like labels and I am only interested in finding the right way of treating any individual patient, whatever that right way may be. I have very, very rarely found that right way to involve the use of more than one remedy at a time and cannot understand how people who are creating the principles for a single register seem to be allowing that in. There is a vast library here and the only books about mixed remedies are a handful and published by pharmacy companies who make them. There isn't a book about the philosophy of it, so I am not sure there are any principles for this type of prescribing except expediency.

Approximately fifteen years ago the Faculty decided to hold an intellectual debate in the old British style of debating for and against the motion. The person organising it came to chat with me to ask what the motion should be. They knew what the subject was but wanted to know how it should be phrased, and I suggested, "The single remedy is the medicine of experience" – that was one of Hahnemann's titles from his early essay *The Medicine of Experience*[40]. The event was open to medical and non-medical (professional) homeopaths. David Curtin and I spoke for the motion, the late June Burger and George Lewith against it. The motion was overwhelmingly carried. I spoke seriously but with some jokes about what Hahnemann called 'half homeopaths', and crabs, scientists who walk backwards! The debate was published in *The Homeopath*[46] and the *British Homeopathic Journal*[49] in 1993.

Before I became a student of homeopathy, when I was only a patient, I gave a child the *Nelsons' Travel Combination remedy* for travel sickness and it really did the job as an acute prescription. It contains *Cocculus indicus, Theridion curassavicum, Tabacum, Nux vomica, Apomorphine* and *Staphysagria*. That is the only sort of combination remedy I have used. I have got a seven year old now where *Cocculus indicus* alone never does it whereas the combination does. Within forty minutes of a journey in our car he will be sick if he doesn't get some relief. I have never used a combination remedy on any other patient.

I do prescribe single remedies in a variety of potencies and LM remedies, but every now and again I will also give mother tinctures of plant based remedies, and I have given those at the same time as a potentised remedy. I had a case where I gave somebody *Carduus marianus* in a 6C potency. He had left-sided liver pain and haemoptysis – he was coughing blood. It wasn't a question of organ support, it was the remedy that came through the repertorisation; I gave it to him in the sixth potency and nothing happened. I went over the case again and gave it in the mother tincture and it worked immediately.

ROWENA: Tell me about your experience working in the NHS.

FRANCIS: When I first became a homeopath I had a nightmare; it was rather like when I first had a mortgage. Me settle down and own a house in Northwest London? Me go into private medicine? I had recognised the NHS was the National Sickness Service, not the National Health Service, but I felt it ought to be free at point of use for all. So when that phone call came from an NHS GP asking if I wanted to be interviewed to work there I phoned a very good friend, Miranda Castro, and asked her if I could come over to her house and talk about it. She replied that I could have, had she not been invited too.

Anyhow, it was me that got the job and I have written and talked about it many times. It was the most stressful work experience I have ever had in homeopathy because the clinic was stressful. Physiologically it was in a basement with skylights and a bit of natural light, and that was all.

ROWENA: Was that soon after you qualified?

FRANCIS: Well, that is a relative term. I started practising in the summer of 1984 and this was in the summer of 1990. I did an audit of my practice at the Marylebone Health Centre which showed how successful I was being; no more nor less than anyone else, seventy to eighty percent of patients were satisfied, either doing well or very well. I was the only homeopath there at the time, but there had been a homeopath previously and I was asked at my interview how I behaved in situations of conflict. I wondered what my predecessor had created so I made various placating noises and I got the job. Apparently she had not been a single remedy prescriber.

So I did very well, and when my audit came through they didn't believe it. They said that it must be because I was so nice to the patients – and I was sacked! In the book about Marylebone Health Centre it was as if I was never there. I was airbrushed out of the place – it was very, very weird. However, I contacted a friend who was a GP and told him my predicament and he asked me to come over and sign on the dotted line immediately. So I never looked back. I happily worked in the Fitzrovia Medical Centre for ten years.

I spent thirteen years in that area, and during that time I was invited to do a research project for the Faculty, which was to create a drug dictionary for the NHS computer service so that you can go 'click click' and print a homeopathic remedy into their automatic prescription printing service. It was a few years on before it was actually used, but that was quite interesting, so that filled up the gap of declining NHS patient numbers.

And then quite separately I started at a GP group practice in North London. I had seen a patient there, a baby who was vomiting after every feed. I discovered that the mother had been given castor oil to help the birth. The idea was if you open your bowels, a purgative, the baby will come out, too, because the muscles will all get going. She didn't tell me initially because, of course, it was something 'natural', so my first prescription didn't work. We made up *Ricinus communis* (castor bean) into the sixth potency there and then, and gave her some. The baby stopped vomiting.

I did it as a presentation at a Society Cases Conference where I gave a series of short cases of small remedies. *Ricinus communis* increases the quantity of milk in nursing women and is a purgative, so she was getting more milk than the baby needed and there was all this digestive stuff – and he stopped vomiting. The baby's father was a GP. I was there for six years and it was well paid in NHS terms. I carried out a practice audit with help from a grant from the Faculty there, which the Society of Homeopaths published and I presented it at a Faculty Conference – it was very, very satisfying. One of the GPs from there set up a practice on his own and asked if I would come and join him before he had even got a practice nurse. I was still seeing private patients from his neighbourhood.

I wept when I gradually got the sack from those practices - thirteen years of working part time with the NHS and it was over. The way I practise and what I did with patients clinically was never questioned; I was allowed to practise how I wanted. The doctors had to sign the NHS prescriptions, but clinically I could have as much time as I needed. I saw pathology that you wouldn't see anywhere else and which I wouldn't have been able to cope with if I hadn't been in India before working for the NHS.

ROWENA: How did the *Homeopathic Helpline*[18] come about?

FRANCIS: Once upon a time I worked above a pharmacy for many years in East Finchley. I was already working there when I got recruited for NHS work and I stayed working there as well. The pharmacist, David Needleman, had studied homeopathy. He didn't own the shop and the owner said that now he was doing homeopathy all these people were coming along for free advice and ringing him up and blocking the shop line. The owner asked David to get his own phone line. David thought of getting a pay line but obviously he couldn't do it seven days a week, so when he had a day off I was his first reserve and I still am.

I suddenly realised when I was on duty on the first working day after Christmas, the day when everyone nowadays goes shopping – every homeopath in the land was still on holiday. Everybody who had suppressed their flu or cough over Christmas now rang the *Homeopathic Helpline*[18] and I got over one hundred calls a day – and this winter it has been like that almost throughout December and January. It is very, very busy and routinely homeopaths now put the number on their answer phones and patient literature.

We receive calls on everything you can imagine, but we also get people who have never used homeopathy before but they have been recommended to call us by a friend. And of course, they don't have remedies so we have to have a mental map of where the people can get remedies from all over the UK. Neal's Yard Remedies, a small chain, is actually very, very useful.

We have to be very careful. For example we might say, "It is possible, and I am just saying this as a routine question, I think you have got pneumonia, but I don't know at this distance away. Why not go and see your GP; you will then have a prescription of antibiotics as a safety net. Then don't let them frighten you. If your GP says that you have, then you are welcome to ring up and tell us, and this will give me an idea as to which remedy to give." I know in these circumstances that they have got the safety net in their prescription. I haven't said to them to do anything other than a citizen would say. It may be pneumonia, it may be something else, but I suggest they go and see their doctor, get the diagnosis and ring back. We don't need the diagnosis to prescribe. We need the symptom picture. But the doctor can listen or observe or say which lung is affected, which will help chose the remedy. For example, I cannot see what sort of rash a person has, on the telephone.

ROWENA: Do you often recommend they go to the doctor?

FRANCIS: Or Accident and Emergency, yes. I am going to suggest a remedy – a child has got a bump to the head and has been unconscious and may need more than *Arnica*. I say that if there is any disturbance to vision; if a squint develops or there is vomiting, I tell them to go to hospital. I may have said take *Natrum sulphuricum* but they don't have it or they might not obtain it fast enough. Or they may not improve from the remedy and I am not there to observe and prescribe again. That is where these little kits are so wonderful, because you can always tell people, if you have got a kit the *Homeopathic Helpline*[18] is so much more useful, because there is a chance that you have got the right remedy.

ROWENA: And your experience to draw on?

FRANCIS: Experience I didn't realise I had, but yes, I could be cooking a meal or changing a nappy but I have got a headphone on and I can turn round and get on with it. You have seen me do it, haven't you? There is a strangely disproportionate use of the *Homeopathic Helpline*[18] in terms of the population in this country. There are many orthodox Jewish communities – Northwest London, North London, Salford and Gateshead are where the main concentrations are.

ROWENA: Do you think it is because they find out that you and David Needleman are Jewish?

FRANCIS: No, it cannot be only that. With so many children in the family they get loads and loads of acutes. What is funny is maybe two or three will get an acute and the others won't. I think they have a distrust of the authorities and so they distrust vaccinations. We saw a measles epidemic run through that community and we dealt with all of it. We even had a doctor who was Jewish, from Gateshead, ring us, discussed the campaign and the epidemic and then he sent people to the *Homeopathic Helpline*[18].

One of the things that I have enjoyed doing is not only collecting books but reading them and writing book reviews. I have seen a lot of mediocre books and obviously read some interesting ones as well. There seems to be an enormous concentration on trying to understand what Hahnemann really said, or what he meant by what he said, and it is a lot more complicated even than reading *the Bible*[27]. There are many ways of being right and the problem is that numerous teachers and writers insist that theirs' is the only way of being right. Hahnemann, Kent, Clarke and Burnett, they were in different centuries, different cultures and had different sources from which they learned. Clarke gathered his information from all over the place. Burnett was unusual for an Englishman in that he understood and spoke German and French and then studied in continental Europe so he knew the writings of Rademacher.

ROWENA: How do you feel about the philosophy that there is one remedy that a patient resonates with all their life?

FRANCIS: This is an ideal state. George Vithoulkas once talked about prescribing for people on his Greek island (Alonissos). Decades ago the patients were simple to prescribe for and they were on one remedy all their life. But now, there is so much Western influence – antibiotics, divorce, drugs and all the rest of it. Life is more complicated and it is harder to be certain of that remedy for all their life. I also think that when an epidemic turns up the 'remedy for all their life' is not going to help them when they have got mumps or if they have got septicaemia. They might need *Jaborandi* or *Pyrogenium*. Quite often when they turn up with a more chronic complaint, arthritis or anxiety, the 'remedy for all their life' might help them. And you might think that it should help their sepsis, too, but often it doesn't and then you are in trouble if you don't have other tools up your sleeve.

The question is what to do when the philosophy doesn't fit the patient. As long as you are prepared for the exceptions, philosophical approaches are very useful; they are heuristic devices, ways of understanding the world and the patients within it.

There have always been innovators and seekers after a new truth. Eizayaga from Buenos Aires was a medical doctor and fitted his way of prescribing with his view of pathology. I think his best work wasn't his attempt to explain the philosophy but his way of looking at the repertory, which is less well known. If you are new to medicine, although you have a grasp of homeopathy, and a patient comes to see you with multiple sclerosis, do you know how to look for diplopia - visual disturbances or whatever else they have got?

So Eizayaga extracted all the rubrics, which apply to MS from the repertory and created a series of books called his Algorithms (now available on computer as part of *MacRepertory*). So I read through the repertory to see the pathology, not to ignore the individualistic aspects, but to help differentiate. Eizayaga's way is not to ignore the mentals but to look for the pathology to guide the way through the repertory. Kent's *Repertory*[16] is full of pathology and not only the mentals. Swedenborg talks about the mind ruling the body, and that is true, but the pathology is still there.

ROWENA: Tell me what you know of Swedenborg.

FRANCIS: Well, Swedenborg had a big influence over Kent. Once upon a time, a long, long time ago, there was an Englishman by the name of J J Garth Wilkinson. Wilkinson set off on a holiday to Iceland and he observed the sheep on this volcanic mountain called Hekla. They had got bony growths on their jaws and legs. Due to his homeopathic imagination he thought that it was because of the water, the grass and the lava – the sheep have got 'hekla'. So he had a lump of Hekla mountain brought back to England and made it into a remedy and behold it was good for bony growths. I looked up Wilkinson and what I found was he was a doctor like Hahnemann, who gave it all up and became a translator. We have heard that before haven't we? Hahnemann was also a translator.

But what he did was to translate Swedenborg's mid-eighteenth century Latin into mid-nineteenth century English. Who wanted to read these translations? People like Ralph Waldo Emerson, and other transcendentalists on the Eastern seaboard of the USA. Henry James senior, the father of the novelist, and William James, the psychologist, ran a magazine called *The Harbinger*[50]. Through Henry James, J J Garth Wilkinson's translations of Swedenborg became known to the intelligentsia in North America and many of these intelligentsia were homeopaths, and so Swedenborg's ideas filtered into the homeopathic community, not only to Kent, but to all of them. This started in the 1840s and for the next couple of decades.

Swedenborg was a Swede and he was a mining engineer, philosopher, Christian and a hallucinationist. People afterwards founded what became known as the New Church of Jerusalem of Emmanuel Swedenborg, a nonconformist sect, but that is about as much as I know. They have got a reading room and library in Bloomsbury. So that is the short version of how Swedenborg came into homeopathy. We believe that it is possible that Hahnemann knew about Swedenborg but he never admitted it. Kent absorbed it in a more wholesale fashion than a lot of the other Swedenborgian homeopaths, and quotes him.

ROWENA: So what influence does Swedenborg have on homeopathy?

FRANCIS: The idea of the 6C, 30C, 200C, 1M 10M series of potencies. Levels of energy in the universe have this harmonic scale, this series of degrees, for example. The idea of the mind as an influence on the body is a Swedenborgian concept – forward thinking then, taken for granted by us now. *Oeconomia Regnum Animalis – The Economy of the Animal Kingdom*[51], he wrote it in the mid-eighteenth century, the body (economia) is ruled by the mind, (anima).

ROWENA: On another subject Francis, do you think it was easier to be a homeopath when you first studied, because there were so few?

FRANCIS: Intellectually, morally, emotionally, it is always as difficult or easy as you make it. Did you mean economically?

ROWENA: What has made you financially successful at being a homeopath?

FRANCIS: Dogged persistence and a positive attitude, I suppose. Many homeopaths undersell and undervalue themselves. Some are unknowing of how to deal with money and how to present and publicise themselves. There are a lot of homeopaths who have other sources of income in their families; their husbands or wives are the main breadwinners. I don't know how many homeopaths are financially independent, but obviously some are and it is their main source of income.

There are a lot of unsuccessful clinic businesses, too. People set up half-baked health centres in an unprofessional, unbusinesslike way, where there are a number of different disciplines working together in an ill thought-out way. And they neither know how to relate the different practitioners together nor how to run a business in a community, either. So generally a lack of business sense is the problem. Middle class people who have come at it from only ever having been in public employment might find it difficult. I had only ever been in public employment and somehow or other, that wasn't a handicap for me. If you have only ever been a schoolteacher, it is very, very different from earning your own money by being self-employed.

We are talking about issues of so-called poverty consciousness and prosperity consciousness and the culture that blames patients for being ill and blames practitioners for earning money from them. It isn't that stuff. I have not found it difficult, although I know that patient numbers have ebbed and flowed. It takes dedication, persistence and being good at it – and marketing is part of that, too.

Of all of the things about long-term practise I would like to say, never bullshit patients about the possibility of curing them. If I have seen a patient three times but I haven't found the remedy, I stop and I say that I think that we are really getting on fine in relation to each other, but I haven't grasped their remedy, so I don't feel I should be taking their fee anymore and that I regret I haven't been able to help them. I suggest that they go and see my colleague, and I have a short list of homeopaths that I refer to. Sometimes I actually say to a female patient, that maybe they would be better off with a female homeopath. They may never go, but I don't feel I can carry on if I think I haven't cracked it.

ROWENA: Homeopathy has obviously gone through a renaissance these last thirty to forty years – do you see it becoming dormant again?

FRANCIS: No, it is too successful for that. I am an optimist. I hope it has learned its lessons for keeping its head above water. I just think it has grown too much.

ROWENA: What, do you think, has contributed to its growth this time?

FRANCIS: The world is beginning to realise that allopaths are busy inventing medicines and then withdrawing them because they are dangerous. There are these things like Methicillin resistant Staphylococcus aureus (MRSA) and flu epidemics. If only we could get in there with our foot in the door, that would make a huge difference.

ROWENA: From your experience, do you think we have remedies to combat MRSA?

FRANCIS: It will depend on the remedy epidemicus. It is likely to be a snake venom like *Crotalus horridus* or *Pyrogenium*, but it depends on how it presents in any hospital or region at any one time. There is an *essay by Pierre Schmidt*[52], which is only in French, on the epidemic remedy. It has never been translated but it would be very useful at this time. It boils down to the economics of publishing; nobody wants to do translations because they cost a lot.

ROWENA: And finally, Francis, what do you think makes a good homeopath long-term?

FRANCIS: You have to be a fanatic. I don't mean that you go around converting everybody! I just mean you have to be fairly single-minded about the intellectual and emotional demands of the job – and keep at it. And be a member of a team, that is to say whether it is with a supervisor or a colleague – you cannot be a loner. If you are alone a lot you have to find ways of relating to teams so if your Continuous Professional Development, like mine, is devoted to reading books and you are alone, you actually have to go out and meet people and go to seminars as well and learn from other people.

ROWENA: That is good advice Francis. I know that is why some homeopaths want to leave our profession, because they feel unsupported and alone. Many thanks for your time and stories today Francis. What would we do without you!!

CHAPTER 10:   CHARLES WANSBROUGH

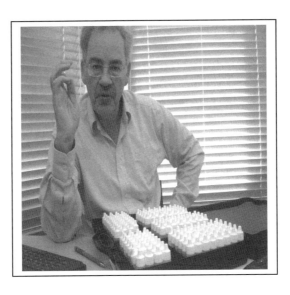

Saturday 19 March 2005 took me to the work place of Charles Wansbrough, the man, money and mind behind the New College of Homeopathy (New College) established in 2003. I had not listed him as an interviewee prior to a couple of weeks before we met, but several homeopaths, when they heard I was having conversations with teachers for my book, pointed me in his direction as a must to include. His clinic space was impressive, a wooden floored through room filled with crystals, and a mantelpiece adorned with before and after photographs of his patients, a beautiful bowing Buddha statuette in the middle of one room and a large rather curious black box standing to attention in the far left corner of the other – his unique machine. Charles sat behind a big table and I perched opposite him on his patient's chair, taking it all in. Since the interview the New College has unfortunately had to close.

"I was determined to prove whether classical homeopathy worked and found, using my machine, that it does work up to about fifty to sixty percent of the time."

Charles Wansbrough, March 2005

"Generally homeopaths don't realise that everything is shifting. That is why we are in a crisis, because cyberspace, in my opinion, is not dissimilar to homeopathic space. Cyberspace has actually created an extraordinary degree of subtle energy. If everything is intention, basically we as individuals are actually creating what we see. We create our reality. The New College is an exercise in establishing a particular vision that may work. I don't know if it will work; it depends on the people we pull along with us."

Charles Wansbrough, March 2005

CHAPTER 10:   CHARLES WANSBROUGH

ROWENA: How did you get into homeopathy?

CHARLES: I was trained as a dentist, qualifying in 1977, and worked for four or five years developing appalling back and various other problems. In short, my health plummeted. In those days they did not really know what was wrong with me, but I had developed a neurodegenerative disorder. No one could basically pinpoint what it was and no one understood it. I had only ever wanted to do dentistry, but had to give it up and didn't know what to do next. At twenty nine years of age I left for India and spent a year and half there being a hippie, but unfortunately my system collapsed again, so I came back and within three years I was virtually crippled.

I studied Sanskrit during this time at the School of Oriental Studies and completed the first year. It was hard work – twenty five of us started and only two got through. At that point I was getting so bad and so crippled, and then luckily someone told me about homeopathy. Being from a medical background I just thought it was all mumbo jumbo, but I started to pick up and I thought, "Well this is more interesting than being a monk in India", which had been my plan.

From then on I trained at the College of Homeopathy (COH) with Barbara Harwood and Robert Davidson. It seemed okay, but because I was from a dental and medical background I seemed rather like a fly in the ointment.

ROWENA: Who was in your year?

CHARLES: Gordon Sambidge, Ian Watson, Sue Josling – all the people who ended up starting colleges. It was rather experimental to put it mildly. After that I started practising and common to other homeopaths, it was not easy to get patients at first. Then I joined the Martin Miles group about eight or ten years ago - the Guild of Homeopaths (Guild). That is when meditative provings came into existence and various other exercises. We spent about eight years, once a month, going down and spending the whole day, from about nine in the morning until three in the afternoon, sitting in a circle meditating and commenting. At that time there were a number of people in it. Janice Micallef was the main homeopath, who ironically enough had been told to teach because she is an extremely busy homeopath and she has psychic powers. She and Martin Miles were both Druids but I don't know anything about that, it is not my area. Colin Griffith was also part of the Guild.

One exercise we did was to potentise sound which was very interesting. When you potentise sound you are basically creating a remedy but it decays after a few days. A colleague and I spent about five years messing around with these parameters, a bit like the work Benveniste did. Finally we managed to find a way to lock the sound into the solution, in other words we created electromagnetic remedies – we could actually potentise any sound to any frequency to any level. The frequency generator, which was especially adapted, could potentise electromagnetic frequencies to six decimal places.

When we actually potentised sound we had no way of applying it, no way of knowing how you read someone and work out what sound they needed. But I have developed this work since then because I went off to the USA and met a woman called Sharry Edwards who is the founder of Bioacoustics, who basically had the ability to be able to sing sound waves. This is absolutely extraordinary, because normally you can only sing in harmonics, but she had a peculiar quality and that is when her ability started. She reverse engineered how to give someone the right sound by taking their voice and then breaking it down to the notes to see where there were holes in the voice chart.

I was using very low frequencies – alpha, beta, delta - going from 10hz to 30hz, which is the beta alpha wave. If you prescribe very low sounds, what you are really doing is re-engaging with the orchestra in the brain. So, a bit like homeopathy, if you superimpose a different coherence on the brain it will snap back and throw out the correct signals. This is the field of Bioacoustics - we are made up of millions of sounds; the heart giving off one, the brain giving off another.

During my days with the Guild I started to develop the use of crystals, which is something similar to homeopathy but seems to work on another level. I was at the HIV Clinic some ten years ago and I was prescribing them left, right and centre which lead me on to develop a double tier system of treatment. When homeopathy didn't work I would use crystals at a higher level and these seemed to work perfectly, but I couldn't understand what was going on.

ROWENA: How did you choose the crystals?

CHARLES: This is the complexity and it is highly intuitive. That was another development. I am endlessly continuing to develop my styles of prescribing. What seemed to happen with the HIV, when the homeopathy didn't work the crystals worked perfectly, so I was left rather stunned. I used 10MM - very high potencies.

ROWENA: So you potentised the crystals?

CHARLES: Yes, to 10MM and I started to realise that you could create what I call orchestral manoeuvres. Because lots of sensitive patients come to see me, I started to pick up which crystals move where, and some of them go up and some go down. So I started to divide them up and then I went back scientifically to see the structures and to see if I could understand any coloration between them. In the end, I abandoned the whole thing because it was chaotic and I couldn't come up with anything firm, unfortunately. I still use them now every so often. The more sensitive you are the more appropriate crystals are, that is the only comment I can make. There are downers, uppers and neutralisers and you can shift someone's energy very quickly all the way through these particular variations.

ROWENA: So what happens with amethyst?

CHARLES: Upwards probably. After the crystal phase I decided to abandon everything, as I had never been that impressed with homeopathy. Like everybody I was getting good and bad results. My type of mentality allows my interests to spread right across from consciousness studies to music and magic, and my thoughts in these areas started influencing me. I went to visit a lady who was using liquids, but they weren't homeopathy. She told me the man who invented them called them chelates. He was basically modifying subtle energy in some way, so I wondered if it was the same or different from what I was doing.

So I went for a couple of treatments and nothing worked, but she was a very powerful lady, so I thought either the whole thing is a load of rubbish or she is creating an incredible force with this technology. I wanted to get back to the source - Patrick Richards, who had created the machine she was using - but I was suspicious that the machine was rubbish. For about a year I couldn't get anywhere, then one day I was sitting in bed ill. I had done my back in as usual and she said she was going off to the USA to see Patrick Richards – he was at a conference. So I got one of those corsets that hold your back together and off I went with her.

So that is when the next phase in my colourful career started – I came home with one of his machines. I wanted to prove to myself that the black box was not a viable exercise, though Patrick Richards the inventor swore it worked well. I was intrigued by the challenge and by the technology he had invented. You can read more on the website *www.biolumanetics.net/tantalus*[53].

Having taken the machine on, I had to decide whether it did or did not work. That has been rather an awesome exercise and I have no idea still, as it behaves in the most peculiar fashion. Patrick Richards had established a protocol when taking a case to first photograph a baseline. One explanation is that your energetic field is interfering with the energetic field of this generator and it is being caught in the Polaroid photo. There have to be certain factors, which allow this to be done, and from Patrick's point of view this occurred purely by chance. We do not understand this technology and I can give you certain comments on it but I really have no idea. But what basically happens is that your energy and the machine's energy snap together. Normally you get very, very fuzzy photos.

ROWENA: So this machine is on all the time?

139

CHARLES: It cannot be turned off. The protocol is that I take a case for an hour, after which I decide what remedy you need. You hold the remedy in your hand and you take another photograph and the image will change. It sounds extraordinary, I know. My first challenge was to work out if this was viable and it was rather complicated, as you can well imagine.

ROWENA: When it comes back into focus you know the remedy is a good choice?

CHARLES: Yes, so what we are dealing with is coherence on an orchestral level. What the energy of the remedy is doing is to snap the person's energy field back into coherence. Firstly I have to decide what the correct remedy/simillimum, is, and then what we are dealing with and whether it is valid. My first observation was that something seemed to be going on.

It doesn't operate like normal machines, as you are really operating on the subquantum levels where the entanglement of people has just as much to do with it as you and me. I realised I needed to learn the whole materia medica fast because I had no way of scanning it and I didn't know the parameters I was dealing with here.

My problem and challenge was to find out whether the technology worked with homeopathy, because Patrick Richard's own experience with homeopathy was not particularly informative, neither had he managed to get any homeopaths to use the technology properly. So the real challenge was deciding whether the photos taken in this peculiar field generated by the black box were genuine, or whether it was all in the intention of the practitioner. Patrick had already established from clinical experience and practise that when a patient went clear holding the chelates, then that patient experienced an improvement in their health.

So I had to decide whether a clear or coherent photo that the patient created when they held a good remedy was equivalent to the simillimum. It turned out to be more complex than that, but in essence a clear photo holding a good remedy would lead to an enormous improvement in the health of the individual being treated at that time. The homeopathic principles of similarity together with its emphasis on the unique qualities of each individual suddenly meant that I had to learn remedies very fast, including many small remedies I had never even heard of.

So I basically set it up as in the kingdom approach. I set up these taxonomic aid books, then I processed twenty years of journals, put them in the computer, read the lot, created a networked web for myself and for two years I went to Kew Gardens and looked at all the plants. Slowly I evolved. I was determined to prove whether classical homeopathy worked and found, using my machine, that it does work up to about fifty to sixty percent of the time. After that it doesn't, and you are moving into an entirely new area of engagement, for want of a better word. I have to stand back from myself sometimes, because I know I can be completely wrong.

When I first started practising homeopathy with the machine, one of the most difficult exercises for me was the nightmare scenario that I was wrong the whole time. In other words, most of the remedies I would try did not go clear and it turned out to be a very steep learning curve. The first two or three years were very hard to take. My ego was constantly pummelled. Also, I had another homeopath with me, a colleague I trained with, and we would take about ten to fifteen photos in any one session until we found clarity. So in some way it was like always searching for the best remedy in one session, and as I have gained more experience it has become easier to find the simillimum at the first session if it is present.

Homeopaths may search for the correct remedy, but in essence the placebo effect is used until they find the right remedy. But for me the first two or three years were so hard. Every time I thought, "Oh yes! This is a *Lycopodium*" for example, and then the photos showed up incoherent, I had to think very fast to know or have some intuitive feeling where to go next - or just feel utterly exhausted in the session.

Basically, I set up kingdom domains in my own head, which were subdivided. Now I just snatch through the whole thing and go, "This is a snake domain" or "This is a spider domain"; you learn to move very fast. You need to develop some feedback mechanism. My greatest strength is my level of uncertainty. If I don't know, that is fine by me. But the first two or three years were very hard work because I kept telling myself that I was crap. Nowadays it just doesn't disturb me. Sometimes I just give up and say I cannot do it, but in those days I had to try and prove myself.

I want to develop further than that now and create a universal model to pull everybody else's models in. We have a problem with epistemology, for want of a better word - what holds true and what is right. So I have differentiated between linear and nonlinear cases – that is the first step. Linear cases that are classical - you stay the same core but you will move up and down that particular core without any particular problems; you will move in and out of that state – that is a linear case.

They have discovered in the past fifteen years that there are now no linear cases; they don't exist. But within those parameters people will still stay within the linear. When you get to nonlinear you are treating different states and my suspicions are that your identity is in question. If you have a very strong identity then you stay linear, if you have a weak identity you have a different number of states that you will basically merge into or out of. These are my own observations. So you will actually move around these states. You will never be a state because these are all states. That is as far as I can make it out so far.

My interest in the technology and its relationship to homeopathy is what has fuelled my research, and the most interesting area is that of the relationship between consciousness and homeopathy. For example, I have not used the miasmatic theory to get me out of even hard cases. I have found the whole conceptual domain of miasms to be clinically useless in my practice. Not only do I never use them unless they come up as a remedy, but the whole miasmatic theory has never proved of any value in my own prescribing style. I prescribe on states; any state should and can be matched by a remedy.

I have a protocol, which is that I treat a patient three times classically. After three visits I should have found the simillimum but if I haven't then I search elsewhere and use Patrick Richard's chelate solutions, which in essence is using polypharmacy since you can mix a number of these chelate remedies. In essence we have about six thousand remedies available to us, but we are searching for a remedy that matches a state - a frequency - and one can mix polypharmacy to produce an even larger set of frequencies. After nine years of using this technology, I tend not to use the chelates very often, as my homeopathy is good enough to find the remedy nowadays.

However, if the case is intractable and has not responded to homeopathy, and I need to see someone only for three visits before deciding whether they will respond to homeopathy rapidly, then I move to sound therapy or Bioacoustics, which is an entirely different exercise. I very rarely use potentised sound. It is interesting but I have found very little use for it. With myalgic encephalomyelitis (ME) patients, if you find the right frequency that they need, they can put it on a mini disc player and carry it about. They do not have to hear it because the frequency being generated is enough to put the orchestra back in balance. If they play it for six to eight hours, after about two or three months they begin to centre and feel their energy coming back. Then you go in with homeopathy because it is at a higher level, and that is basically what I have been doing recently.

ROWENA: What do you teach at the New College?

CHARLES: I teach what I call neoclassical homeopathy, for example, the works of Massimo Mangialavori and Jan Scholten. I basically teach the themes, for example, I teach the social insects and give a lecture on them with handouts. My teaching is all done in mind maps. Students see two videos then we discuss the variations on the themes. If you cannot make links between themes, you don't know where to go when searching for and understanding remedies. If you split up the learning of materia medica into tiny bits, you cannot make links.

We have a memory theatre so that we can learn to hold all the information in our heads. In the same way that Scholten has developed the periodic table, which is also a memory theatre. Each map is like a room at home and it becomes embedded in your mind. You can then basically hook things in those rooms, and that is the way you accumulate vast amounts of knowledge. This is the art of the memory. Shakespeare's The Globe is based on these concepts, so it is quite fascinating.

The New College was my idea but I stay in the background. I cannot stand for more than ten minutes with my condition so I have to be very careful.

ROWENA: Which teachers of homeopathy have you been influenced by?

CHARLES: No one. I am a complete outsider.

ROWENA: Even when you were at college?

CHARLES: I just thought most of it was bullshit, to be entirely honest.

ROWENA: And now?

CHARLES: I have deep respect for Rajan Sankaran. He used a particular taxonomy in plants created by Arthur Cronquist, which is the main one, but there are six. What is interesting is if I change the taxonomy, some of the plants get shifted around all over the place. So who is to say it is solid, but it is clever. Unlike myself, who is a solitary person, Rajan Sankaran is surrounded by an enormous amount of people. Massimo Mangialavori is very clear on his cases. To get to that level you need to use a recognition model and this is what experts do.

ROWENA: Do you feel Hahnemann should be taught in homeopathy schools?

CHARLES: I am dividing The New College's teaching into the historical perspective and the contemporary. The contemporary perspective is a matrix - the secret life of puppets, are we in control? The placebo effect, what is it? There is a whole series of lectures on Renaissance magic so that they have contemporary as well as historical. People tend to not read outside, because once you take on a particular model that is it. It all closes in and that is what you know, which is fine. The matrix changes; it is not solid.

ROWENA: How did the New College come about?

CHARLES: Well basically the New College is run by Valerie Probert and Linda Razzell. Before that they helped to run Barbara's college, COH, which was taken over by Gordon Sambidge, who as you know was a colleague of mine. I think he is very clever and he is a good businessman. I am basically not interested in business at all. I am only interested in research. No one would let me lecture anywhere - what I teach is too unconventional. So I put in a bit of money and asked Linda and Valerie if they wanted to start up. I would basically be the ideas man, but I don't know how to run a college and it doesn't interest me.

Generally homeopaths don't realise that everything is shifting. That is why we are in a crisis, because cyberspace, in my opinion, is not dissimilar to homeopathic space. Cyberspace has actually created an extraordinary degree of subtle energy. If everything is intention, basically we as individuals are actually creating what we see. We create our reality. The New College is an exercise in establishing a particular vision that may work. I don't know if it will work; it depends on the people we pull along with us.

I have dumped the classical; not because there is anything wrong with it, but because you cannot keep increasing the amount of information without a new way of looking at it. Data is ten a penny, we can download ten provings; so what are you going to do, read them? No. It is all about how we process the data to make useful information. You have to teach the taxonomy at the beginning so that you categorise. I can read a proving in ten minutes, so I go okay, where does it go? Okay, I know which tree it is, which family it is under, which order it is, so you can actually snap in quite quickly. It is the art of memory and it can be learned.

ROWENA: Do you see homeopathy becoming dormant again?

CHARLES: No, I don't think so. There is far, far too much activity. There are far too many good minds out there developing methodologies. Rajan Sankaran has done very interesting work. In my opinion what he is doing is actually creating a higher level metaphor and he is able to construct and sometimes it will work brilliantly. What he has managed to do is break this appalling tie between learning the pattern, the narrative, and then not being able to find the remedy, and that he has done brilliantly. One of my problems is learning all this information. How was I going to keep absorbing it? So that is why I have evolved in this particular way.

ROWENA: What about homeopaths making a living?

CHARLES: It is difficult to know. One of my problems is that there are lots and lots of homeopaths and it is a pity because people do homeopathy as an inspirational vocation and in a way it is psychotherapeutic; it moves them into an entirely different realm. There are too any homeopaths and not enough patients, in my opinion, and even if you do become a homeopath, the amount of experience you need to acquire is so vast.

ROWENA: Vast like the ocean; it takes a lifetime to learn. Thank you for sharing your fascinating perspective Charles.

CHAPTER 11: JEROME WHITNEY

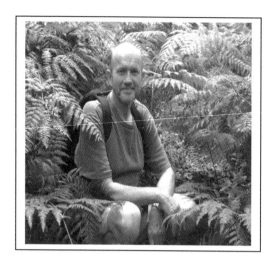

Jerome Whitney was one of the first to go on my list of 'must interview'. My introductory session with him at college back in 1998 made me really sit back and listen! I had found someone that was really going to change my life and my thinking and I attended his esoteric classes with my eyes wide open, totally engrossed and hungry to learn. Personally he also really helped me. My youngest son Theo at the time was just turning six years old and suffered from repeated nightmares about wolves. *Stramonium* had done something for him but the wolves kept tormenting him.

I discussed his fears with Jerome one lunch break and he suggested young Theo befriend the wolves in his dreams. Before bedtime that night I suggested this novel concept to Theo who listened, questioned and then went to bed. The following morning he woke to say that he did indeed chat to the wolves in his dreams and from that day his fear was dispelled and his nightmares ceased. You can see why I am in gratitude to the wise old owl that is Jerome. We met in the very noisy but most beautiful Green Park on Monday 11 April 2005 and we chatted away for hours.

"Even Thomas Maughan said, "If it isn't the 'simillimum', it isn't homeopathy.""
Jerome Whitney, April 2005

"The profession is growing, and the idea of the various professional registers, after years of arguing, getting together to understand each other and realise that we have the same goals and the same willingness to allow diversity; that kind of openness has really been healthy for the profession. So even though we are slowly moving towards a single register, it is healthy, because while there are limits, there is also openness, so the balance between limits and openness is being acknowledged and recognised." *Jerome Whitney, April 2005*

145

CHAPTER 11: JEROME WHITNEY

ROWENA: How did you become involved with homeopathy?

JEROME: Well, back in 1970 I was doing graduate work at New York University.

ROWENA: Is that where you are from?

JEROME: I grew up in western New York State, actually, halfway between Buffalo, New York and Cleveland Ohio, almost five hundred miles from New York City. Anyway, by 1970, I was at that time married to Kaaren and living in Connecticut, seventy miles from New York City, and we decided to come on holiday for a few weeks to London. At that time, as well as doing graduate work, I was also searching for gurus. And on the night before we came we were given the name of Thomas Maughan, who was the chief Druid. In the meantime, we arrived here and went and heard Jiddu Krishnamurti.

ROWENA: Lucky you!

JEROME: We saw Jiddu Krishnamurti live and also Sangarachita, who is British, and the leader of the Friends of the Western Buddha Order. We went to see Thomas Maughan and I was very impressed with him and with the way he expressed the Druid teaching and the role of Druids in society. In the meantime we discovered he was also a homeopath, which was of great interest to Kaaren, who was on prescribed medications.

ROWENA: Not homeopathic medications?

JEROME: Not homeopathy; very heavy conventional medicine. And as a consequence of the interaction with Thomas Maughan, she decided to stop using them and proceeded to switch over to homeopathy and then had what we might call a miraculous cure. And out of that came the idea that we would come to England to study homeopathy and the Druid teachings as well.

ROWENA: So what had you been studying in the USA?

JEROME: I was studying social history, race and ethnic minorities.

ROWENA: And what about Kaaren?

JEROME: She was at that time a children's librarian and running a very active library in Connecticut.

ROWENA: How old were you at the time?

JEROME: It was 1970 and I would have been thirty six and that was the start of it. We flitted back and forth during 1970 and 1971, and then in the autumn of 1971 we got everything arranged and shifted to living here, and have been living here as permanent residents ever since. That was the beginning of the study of homeopathy and active involvement in the Druid Order and of course, that lead into becoming part of the homeopathy classes that were being taught by Thomas Maughan. At that time, he ran a number of classes; one was for the public and one for members of the Druid Order. After 1972, when he became ill, he combined the two classes and so there was a whole range of people at different levels of homeopathy altogether in one room being taught simultaneously. That group became known as the South London group.

ROWENA: Who were the members then?

JEROME: Members of that class included Robert Davidson, Martin Miles, Peter Chappell, Kaaren Whitney, Peter Firebrace, Jennifer Maughan and I, and there were many others who were not members of the Order including several doctors who are now members of the Faculty. There were also people that we knew who were going to classes in North London lead by John Damonte, who was a good friend of Thomas Maughan's. He was also a very fine homeopath in his own right. As a consequence there was a great deal of interaction between us all, and when Thomas had to be away, John would come and teach his class in South London. And because John was active in the Order, I got to know him quite well and went directly to a few of his classes in North London too. In October 1975, John died of a heart attack, and then in June 1976 Thomas Maughan died. The two classes combined in 1976 and in 1977 many of its members began the discussions that lead to the formation of the Society of Homeopaths in 1978.

Robert Davidson had taken over the teaching of Thomas' class after he had become too ill in early February 1976, and later on Martin Miles also taught the class. The two of them founded the College of Homeopathy (COH) in the autumn of 1978. In the meantime, I was teaching physics and chemistry in American International Schools to earn a living while Kaaren and I were studying homeopathy, first with Thomas and then with Robert and Martin Miles. Kaaren went on and began actively practising while I was working and teaching and also I was very involved in the Druid Order's organisational structure after Thomas' death.

In about 1983, John Hocking, a person of a varied and interesting background in law and teaching in Africa became the bursar for COH. He felt that the students needed grounding in the background and evolution of homeopathy and that its context needed to be developed. John then asked me if I would present a series of lectures for COH on the history of our discipline. My approach was to draw on the past and see how it informs the present giving us deeper insights into how we practise now. This provides us with a broader understanding of homeopathy in terms of its philosophy and principles.

It was not just about looking at the history of homeopathy, but at vitalism, the vital force and how these concepts are ignored in conventional medicine. I focussed on the struggle between the materialistic biochemical paradigm and that of homeopathic vitalism. I began researching how different homeopaths practised, in particularly Constantine Hering and other contributors to homeopathy philosophy; Paracelsus, Rademacher who took on Paracelsus' organopathy and Compton Burnett who used organopathy and became, simultaneously with Kent, one of the two great figures of homeopathy in the late nineteenth century.

ROWENA: You wrote a book on it, didn't you?

JEROME: Yes, I wrote *Vitalistic Medicine from Ancient Egypt to the 21st Century*[54]. My research lead me to look into the Cooper Club of which Compton Burnett was a member as well as John Clarke, who was responsible for writing books to assist non-doctor 'lay homeopaths' or professional homeopaths, as they are known today. He wrote many books to help them prescribe, making him very important to the evolution of today's homeopathy. I also researched Thomas Cooper, who was a very intuitive homeopath, and Swedenborg, who inspired Kent into developing the concept of what became known as constitutional prescribing.

ROWENA: How did that happen?

JEROME: Kent married in his twenties, but his wife died shortly thereafter. Meanwhile he trained as a naturopath at the Eclectic Institute of Cincinnati, Ohio. Even though he was one of the top in his class, he was unable to do much for his second wife, who had a terminal illness. Luckily a friend of his, who was a homeopath, was able to make the end of her life much more peaceful and pain free. As a consequence, Kent then took on board the study of homeopathy, and that is how he became a homeopath. When he married for a third time, his wife, who was also a homeopath, introduced him to Swedenborg's spiritual teachings. Interestingly, if you look into the lives of homeopaths of the nineteenth century one finds that many other American homeopaths, along with Constantine Hering, were followers of Swedenborg. Kent went on to apply Swedenborg's spiritual concepts, in a practical way, and developed a powerful method of prescribing that became known as constitutional prescribing.

My research led me into asking, "If all these people were involved in Swedenborg's teaching, what were they getting out of it?" The answer was that Swedenborg kept diary accounts of his lucid dreaming state and in them, he recorded how he had been taught by ethereal beings about a model of the Universe where people are born free, rather than with original sin, and that they have choice. He was also being taught that there was nothing in heaven that did not have its correspondence on earth; in other words, for everything that was on the different levels of being, all the way from here to abstract spirit or God, there was a correspondence.

Swedenborg wrote that there is nothing here in the physical realm that isn't in the spiritual, but just in a different and denser form. Kent took on board that idea and related it to homeopathy, showing that mental symptoms can be found in another form in the emotional and physical symptoms, reflecting an exact correspondence on each level. This is consistent with Hahnemann's model of illness in that outer symptoms are an external expression of the inner malfunctioning vital force.

Kent then went on to elaborate the concept of constitutional prescribing, which is a very powerful tool. Up until Kent, one had to be very knowledgeable in pathology, anatomy and physiology. With Kent, we now had the potential for a system that allowed us to use the symptoms crosschecked against the remedy, without having to be that knowledgeable in basic body function and pathology. The result was that a person could now, with Kent's constitutional approach, find the mental and emotional symptoms and check to see if the physicals agreed. If they had two or three potential remedies, they could then have two areas that they could check. As an example, they could identify the mentals and the physicals, and they could check them against the emotionals. What it amounts to is that you take any two of the three categories and find a potential remedy and check to see if corresponds with the other. In this way, the person could literally have almost no knowledge of anatomy and physiology and would still be able to prescribe the simillimum very effectively and that was the basis of constitutional prescribing.

Kent's contribution added power to homeopathy, and that is why his constitutional prescribing was taken on board so rapidly by very serious homeopaths in England, the USA, Europe, India, and in other countries around the world. While Swedenborg inspired Kent, homeopaths such as Hering and Compton Burnett were inspired by Paracelsus. Compton Burnett, who became inspired by the writings of German physician Rademacher, came in contact with the Paracelsian idea of treating organs. Burnett had patients coming to him with morbidity so great that the average homeopath, and even the average doctor, couldn't even prescribe for it effectively. He was able to obtain results with tumours and cancers utilising organ prescribing that both of those groups failed to achieve and this all happened back in the 1880s and 90s. Introduced by Kent in the USA and Compton Burnett in England, we had two incredibly powerful approaches for prescribing remedies added to the homeopathic tool kit.

As we moved through the twentieth century, Kentian prescribing became very dominant in the practice of the profession. However, from the late nineteenth century alternative therapies progressively lost favour with the public and the number of practitioners fell. Homeopathy declined from 1885 until 1960 when it and the other alternative therapies experienced a resurgence then. Homeopaths such as George Vithoulkas began to come forward. By the late 1970s, he was one of the most well known homeopaths in the world, and a strong advocate of Kentian prescribing.

With George Vithoulkas and others of like mind, the profession experienced the emergence of what I call 'Capital C' Classical Homeopathy, which is a method of prescribing focused primarily on the early work of Hahnemann and Kent. Gradually 'Classical Homeopathy' became popular in many countries around the world. especially, in India. The South and North London Groups, practised homeopathy that utilised a synthesis of the later Hahnemann works, and those of Kent and Compton Burnett who I would call, along with Hering, the four great lights of the nineteenth century.

By 1960, the Faculty that represents the doctor homeopaths in England collaborated with the American Institute of Homeopathy and performed a survey of homeopaths in England and the USA. Out of that study, which was published in the *Journal of the Faculty*[55], they found that homeopathy was in what they called the terminal phase. This was because in 1960 it looked like not just homeopathy, but all alternative medicine was on its way out and had been superseded by 'scientific medicine'. But in their study, they also noted that more than half of the homeopathic doctors here in England and in the USA subscribed to some type of spiritual philosophy. They were either Swedenborgians or those who followed teaching of Rudolph Steiner and anthroposophy or those who believed in reincarnation. Some were even fundamentalist Christians.

ROWENA: Was Swedenborg a Christian then?

JEROME: His father was one of the bishops of the church of Sweden and at the age of seven he would often have an intellectual discussion about the sermon when they walked out of church. Swedenborg later became an esoteric Christian and like Hahnemann and Hering; he was a genius from the very beginning.

ROWENA: Are there still Swedenborg followers?

JEROME: There are. Swedenborganism became very popular. Its three most popular places were London, the area between Preston and Leeds in England, and Philadelphia, Boston, and New York. Hering was a member of the Swedenborgian church of Philadelphia, and he was a very close personal friend of the minister of the Swedenborgian church in New York. The New York Swedenborgian minister officiated at Hering's funeral. When he died Hering also had the largest private collection of Paracelsian writing in the USA.

Swedenborg knew that his writings were too revolutionary so he never published them in Sweden. They were published in London for friends and groups of people that he knew would be interested in reading them. His writings were so profound that a following developed and they gathered together into discussion groups. These study groups were the seed from which the Swedenborgian Church got started; he wasn't out to start a religious institution.

A mile down the road from where I live there was a Swedenborgian Church. I attended a service there back in the late 1970s, but it was basically what I would call an ordinary Protestant type of modern twentieth century service. It has now been renamed Swedenborg Court, and provides apartment space for retired people. But there remains Swedenborg House very close to the British Museum so there are still residual elements active today. What has happened is that the teachings of Swedenborg were never reinterpreted into a modern language; his books are quite intricate to read but nevertheless are full of amazing ideas. Many of Swedenborg's ideas have now become accepted and taken on board; he was just ahead of his time.

ROWENA: You were talking about the survey before I interrupted you?

JEROME: Yes, the survey showed that there was a tendency for doctor homeopaths to be interested in spiritual philosophies, which were much broader in context than traditional Christian philosophy. Or they were interested in Christian religious teaching that was more compatible with the idea of the vital force and that each person isn't condemned by original sin but has the power of choice. This idea was very appealing to thinking homeopaths in the nineteenth century. The same is true of the other spiritual philosophies that have appealed to homeopaths in the twentieth century.

The context, in which I was being taught homeopathy, by Thomas Maughan, was from a model of the universe in which you learn about the inner processes of life and humanity from observation of nature, of natural processes, from signs, signatures, and all these different concepts which are reflected and resonate within each one of us. In other words 'what is within is reflected in what is without'. This is what Hahnemann was saying in that you don't need to be clairvoyant, clairaudient or have any psychic powers; the whole inner story of the vital force is in the external symptom picture, which is, again, the same principle that Kent worked from using Swedenborg's influence.

In my case, I was treated to a very rich experience of homeopathic education. As an example, Thomas Maughan, in the way he was teaching about the cell salts, was pointing in the direction of the work that Jan Scholten was later to take up. Scholten, of course, had no contact with Maughan but he took an idea forward that was in the ethers. It was a very logical progression when Jan started working with the minerals and the periodic chart and was no surprise to those of us who had studied with the South London Group in the 1970's.

Basically we had a taster – a finger being pointed in different directions by Thomas, which was later taken up independently by different homeopaths around the world. One of the rewarding things for me is to see how this person, who was literally ahead of his time, pointed possible future directions and said, "This is an area that could be of interest", and influenced people to carry on in these areas and add to them. Remember that when an institution is dying, which was the case in the period 1885 to 1960 for homeopathy and alternative medicine, there is no surplus energy to innovate and explore.

One can only preserve the past and learn and make suggestions for the future. Unfortunately, all the books that were available at the time, not that I want to put down *Boericke*[39], were very basic. At that point not that much new material was around. As an example we can now see from the compilations of Vermeulen and the homeopathy computer programmes how the bringing together of the work of the past and the present produced a new base for homeopathic research, understanding and innovation. This in turn provides avenues for a constructive liberation of energy for investigation as more and more people are drawn into homeopathy and alternative medicine.

ROWENA: Why do you think the energy was right for it to then have this big resurgence?

JEROME: Well, several things were happening here in England. The resurgence came about because people were beginning to become concerned about the use of penicillin, and the miracle drugs, which were starting to show serious problems. By 1970 even the Pill was revealing many drastic side effects. Homeopathic and alternative practitioners were beginning to have women, who had been on the Pill, seeking them out with problems that needed to be dealt with; not being able to conceive, having blood clots and things like this. There was a whole symptom picture, which was emerging from people who were on the Pill that was not being addressed by conventional medicine. Meanwhile in the 1960s the hippies were also responsible for a trend towards more natural cures for ailments and vaccine induced illness.

ROWENA: Other than Thomas Maughan, who had the biggest influence on you and has the biggest influence on you now?

JEROME: Probably the biggest influence on me after Thomas was Martin Miles, when he told me to look into Compton Burnett. I took the ball and ran and that opened up a whole area of understanding about how Thomas prescribed because it is from Compton Burnett that we have organopathy and innovative ways of prescribing the vitally important remedy categories of nosodes and sarcodes. In that sense, Martin was a major stimulus. At the same time, there are many, many people who have inspired me and to whom I am also indebted.

ROWENA: So do you think that homeopathy will become dormant again?

JEROME: It could. In a breakfast that I had at one of the homeopathic conferences with Harris Coulter, who wrote *Divided Legacy*[56], Harris and I discovered that we had independently come to the same conclusion that somewhere around 2040/2050, we might see the decline of alternative medicine. We both felt that as conventional medicine tries to adopt certain aspects of alternative medicine into mainstream treatment, without actually including the concept of vitalism, the consequence may contribute to its dumbing down and decline.

ROWENA: Do you not think that is happening already?

JEROME: Yes, it is, but fortunately at this point, there are still many people in homeopathy who are not pro integration. You see, consciousness is not equal; some people have a larger field of understanding than others. No matter how many facts you bring to bear, you cannot convey principles or concepts to someone that are beyond their range of understanding or capacity for subtle abstraction because you cannot make them understand it.

It is impossible for homeopathy to be accepted or understood by conventional culture. By 'conventional' I mean people who want to believe only in a materialist, biochemical structure and who refuse to accept the idea of vitalism. As a high school physics teacher of twenty years, I had no difficulty in accepting the model of homeopathy even though materialistic science does not yet have instrumentation to measure the energy of homeopathic dilutions. Does one trust two hundred years of results or does one trust only crude instruments of measurement?

The difficulty is if you try to reduce, say acupuncture, to being something that just deals with pain as you have then dumbed down acupuncture. So to be true to acupuncture, to be true to its paradigm and its guiding model, you cannot sell your soul in order to be accepted by the greater culture. This was done in the late nineteenth century by Richard Hughes who was a very famous English homeopath, who was the leader of the majority of British homeopaths in the latter part of the nineteenth century. Hughes expressed the view that the only way to look at symptoms was with pathology. So he threw out all of Boenninghausen and Hering, all of the things that Hering had put into *The Guiding Symptoms*[57], because they weren't objectively observable pathological symptoms. I doubt that you ever heard of Hughes' *Cyclopedia of Drug Pathogenesy*[58] a testimony to the 'pathology level' of prescribing.

As a consequence, the average homeopath of the late nineteenth century was a very superficial practitioner. Whereas a very small number, perhaps only five in one hundred homeopaths, were practising at a level of the way that students are being taught in their first and second years at the colleges of homeopathy in England and around the world today.

ROWENA: Do you think there are less classical homeopaths today? There are less classical colleges, aren't there?

JEROME: There are several types of homeopath - classical, eclectic, and as I said before capital 'C' Classical. I wasn't trained as a capital 'C' Classical homeopath; I was an eclectic homeopath in a Classical college. Of the three founders of the London College of Classical Homeopathy (LCCH), the person that was the leader, Anne Larkin, was by birth a Libran. I mention this because Librans like balance so although she ran a Classical college, she wanted students to be aware of a broader context. For me, I saw that classical training was about fundamentals, and those fundamentals are important and need to be taught and are taught in most courses in England and the rest of the world.

The problem is that if you teach primarily Kent, or a particular version of homeopathy, as THE only version of homeopathy, then you are in trouble. This is where the Classicalists posed problems, because they began to claim that if your interpretation of Hahnemann's works didn't agree with their interpretation, then you weren't classical. You then have an internecine political war going on, which is not helpful to the profession.

However, it needs to be kept in mind from a developmental standpoint, many things crept into homeopathy over the declining years and many principles and practices were simplified or misunderstood, and people no longer understood why they were doing what they were doing. The role of Classical homeopathy, as a movement, was to take homeopathy back to basics, look at fundamentals and get a good grounding. And then a person could take on board organopathy, intercurrents and drainage remedies. In other words, the first step was to learn some homeopathy, the fundamentals and the principles, and then you can begin to manipulate how it works.

The first part of the *Organon*[4] is so beautifully philosophical and so naturally true; many people began to believe that the methods described by Hahnemann in later chapters were also principles. Because the Classicalists mixed up methods and principles, that then introduced a problem, which lasted through the 1980s and 1990s and out of which we are now only emerging. There are many ways and routes to reaching a goal or following a principle. To put it another way, 'there are many roads to heaven.' In politics there is a tendency for each political party to say "Our method is the only way" and it turns into a simplistic yes/no, yes/no debate. Then we have the problem that in this fruitless argument, both sides forget the goal. By the same token, it doesn't mean that everything that is done in the name of homeopathy is homeopathy. Even Thomas Maughan said, "If it isn't the 'simillimum', it isn't homeopathy."

Let us say, if I fall down and hit my head on the corner of the desk really hard, and somebody says, "Here, take an *Arnica*", and I take it; that is not a homeopathic prescription. Although it is homeopathically prepared *Arnica*, it is an allopathic prescription of a homeopathic remedy. If I have the same fall, the same serious banging of my head, and someone says, "Would you like an *Arnica?*" and I say, "No, I'm ok", then I have now exhibited a mental symptom of *Arnica* – the denial that I need help. If I take the *Arnica*, it is a homeopathic prescription. Homeopathy has to do with the basis of the prescription. This is a type of prescribing which differentiates label prescribing from simillimum prescribing.

I think one of the problems we have as a profession was created from circumstances back in the 1980s. In 1980 George Vithoulkas came to England and at that time most of the people that were studying homeopathy had been doing so only for a short time. They were still impressionable and were immensely influenced by him. John Damonte and Thomas Maughan had died, Phyllis Speight was still alive but was no longer teaching, and various others of the famous old timers, who had taught through the 1930s, 40s and 50s were now very old, or had also passed on.

The newer generation were really turned on by George Vithoulkas. As a result a whole bunch of them went off to Alonissos, the Greek island on which he lives, and spent a few weeks there with him learning and as a result they wanted George to come here four times a year to teach regularly in the UK. They planned to set up a homeopathic institute; however it really never got off the ground because he just wanted to talk to doctors and saw the others as impressionistic vague hippies.

The problem was that there was a misunderstanding of the concept of 'single remedy'. Vassilis Ghegas, George Vithoulkas' disciple, who came to England to lecture, made it look as if George only gave one remedy, but when people began passing around tapes of George's lectures, I heard otherwise. George would say, "I gave a certain remedy, it didn't do badly but not enough, I gave something else and it didn't do anything, I gave another remedy and it did a little bit, and then I gave such and such a remedy and it worked and I didn't give another remedy for a year." How many remedies did George give? Four. Vassilis made it sound as if George only gave one, which lasted for a year! Thus we have then the introduction of the idea of the single remedy, which lasts for a very long time and that it was the only remedy that had been prescribed. It is this misinterpretation of George's teaching, which created a problem within our profession.

I remember back in 2000 I was suddenly awakened by a phone call at two in the morning from a student who had graduated in the top of the full-time course at LCCH. He was saying, "My wife is in a hospital in Glasgow and they think that she is coming down with meningitis." And I replied, "*Belladonna* 200C." But he carried on giving me her case and I repeated, "*Belladonna* 200C" but he still carried on being a good classical constitutional prescriber trying to give me her full case. What we had was an acute situation, and I said, "*Belladonna* 200C", but I had to finally say, "Listen, stop and just listen! Give *Belladonna* 200C and take the case again in the morning." And I have had other phone calls from former students whose Classical training, as such, did not prepare them for what is going on out in the world in terms of day-to-day immediate prescribing needs.

It wasn't until graduates did Jeremy Sherr's course that they really became confident homeopaths. This wasn't only true of LCCH but of other colleges too. One of the needs for student homeopaths is to develop the confidence to prescribe and not be afraid of not selecting THE right remedy. As the years have passed their confidence level has improved with the growing maturity and eclecticism that has evolved within the colleges.

ROWENA: You were involved in writing the BSc course at the University of Westminster, weren't you?

JEROME: Yes.

ROWENA: So how did you get involved in that? I assumed you worked at COH and then at LCCH.

JEROME: In 1988 I started teaching for LCCH

ROWENA: How did that come about?

JEROME: John Hocking had retired from COH after five or six years of working as registrar there. Because of his experience, he was hired as a consultant by Anne Larkin for LCCH. At that time Liz Danciger, a very fine homeopath and a very inspiring person had become seriously ill and Anne needed someone to fill in for her to teach the history and background of homeopathy. John Hocking recommended me, and that is how I began teaching.

ROWENA: When did Anne set up LCCH?

JEROME: LCCH was set up in 1986 as a full time course and I taught the Evolution of Medicine and Evolution of Homeopathy there from the spring of 1988. After I had been there several years, Anne Larkin started teaching students who wanted to do a fourth year, to support them in their practice and to do additional graduate work. Anne introduced and taught the first class session of a teacher training module and asked me to come in on the second week to take the class as she had to attend a meeting. She then found she was so busy that she asked me to teach and develop the teacher training module.

During August 1991, I received a call from Anne saying she wanted me to help write a module for South Bank University. We then began writing and rewriting more and more modules from 1991 through to 1993, at which time we received tentative acceptance for validation at South Bank. At this point, the head of science at South Bank discovered the education department was on track to validate our course in homeopathy, and he went berserk and wrote a letter to Anne Larkin, saying that "Homeopathy is not science" and "It would be a discredit to South Bank's reputation to validate a course that has no scientific basis." He also sent a memo to the heads of the other university departments and the Vice Chancellor. Up to that time we were on the validation schedule and the South Bank had set the date of 14 July for formal validation session. However, we were taken off the calendar and no validation session was ever held.

In response Anne Larkin then approached the University of Westminster for BSc validation and from late 1994, for the next two years, we worked with the University of Westminster writing and rewriting modules. During the process Anne died, her daughter, Mandy, carried on, and the University of Westminster went ahead with its Pathways for Complementary Therapies programme. For the next five years I taught the Comparative Medicine module I had written for the BSc programme. I still go as a visiting lecturer from time to time to the University of Westminster.

In the meantime the LCCH course combined with COH, while remaining a separate curriculum entity within the Combined Colleges of Homeopathy (CCH). The purpose was to reduce costs by sharing the same physical facility. However the cost to maintain it eventually brought the system down after the University of Westminster broke its contract and went its own way. And the sad thing was that, at that time, these two colleges had, academically, one of the most organised structures complete with comprehensive module guides and now the two most structured colleges, no longer exist.

ROWENA: So what are you doing nowadays?

JEROME: I teach at Kathy Pitt's college, the South Downs School of Homeopathy in Chichester. It has a lovely atmosphere and sits in beautiful grounds; it provides a very friendly environment to study in. I also teach at the College of Practical Homeopathy in the Midlands (CPH Midlands), now renamed the Homeopathy College, and also for the College of Practical Homeopathy (CPH) in London, the School of Shamanic Homoeopathy , and in Helsinki for the Institute for Homeopathy. I have been teaching for Thames Valley University and occasionally for the University of Westminster I also still teach numerology on the Lewisham Adult Further Education. For the past five years I have been the Council for Homeopathic Colleges (CHC) representative on the Council of Organisations Registering Homeopaths (CORH) single register Accreditation Working Group.

ROWENA: Are you enjoying it all?

JEROME: Yes, very much.

ROWENA: And do you practise?

JEROME: I have a very small practice. My recent patients have been graduate homeopaths or practising homeopaths, but I don't solicit patients.

ROWENA: So what do you think makes a good homeopath? I ask because so many train yet so few go on to practise.

JEROME: Well, first, there are many good homeopaths who don't necessarily practise formally. I think the first skill you need in order to be a good homeopath is to be a good listener. So it isn't even about knowing homeopathy; the first thing is to really listen and understand your patient. You don't have to agree with your patient, you need to understand them. You know, people don't have to agree with us for us to respect them. If they know that we understand them, then we can have good relationships with people we don't agree with. If you agree with your patient, they will never get well because you won't prescribe non-judgementally.

In homeopathy you have to translate the patient's language into a new language, which can then be linked to the repertory and materia medica. You need three things to be a healer and it doesn't matter whether it is within conventional or alternative medicine; you need to know the patient, you need to know the illness and you need to know the remedy. It is as important to get to know your patient and any propensities that bring on illness, as it is to get the feel for remedies, understand and learn them and not just know their rubrics.

Then the last stage, of course, is the remedy selection, which causes great stress in homeopathy because there are remedies that are very close to one another, as you know. And that is where knowing your patient and relating to them comes in. Homeopathy is an art and a science. But the first thing the homeopath needs to be is a good listener. Even if they are not the best homeopath, they can consult with other homeopaths and if they are willing to do so, they will get the remedy.

To be a really successful homeopath, you have to be able to market yourself, you have to be able to be willing to stand up for yourself out in the world and really look around and find ways to show other people why you are of value to them as a homeopath. To be a homeopath, you basically have to learn to be independent. The current Labour government took away individual funding of GP surgeries and that was very sad. This meant that some of our well-known British homeopaths, such as Francis Treuherz, were no longer able to continue in many of their previous places of GP employment. The Conservatives had set up the system whereby an individual fund holder could apply the money as they saw fit. The more regional mode of control, set up by Labour, has meant that individual GPs have in many regions, been prevented from authorising funds for specific therapies which sometimes includes homeopathy.

ROWENA: So we should be voting for the Conservatives?

JEROME: Well, vote to reduce the Labour majority; that is what I say. Because the basic rule is that you should never trust the party in government. In fact it is good to change every few years, because usually the other party won't do any worse. You wouldn't want a dictatorship, would you?

Anyway, so what is a good homeopath? You see, if a person attracts the right patients for them, they put effort into it. They don't have to be what is considered by their college, by academics or by their peers as a good homeopath. If you attract the person that is right for you to treat, then if you are doing your best for them, that is the right remedy. It doesn't matter if everyone else disagrees with what you do. It is true in any therapy; acupuncturists can needle in many places to treat the same condition.

ROWENA: So you think the answer is not just one remedy?

JEROME: No. In classical homeopathy it is called the centre of the case. But in actual fact, what state you or I perceive a patient to be in is likely to be different because we all have different criteria and powers of perception. This affects what we see and sense needs to be cured. It is true that you may need one specific remedy if you have an immediate acute, don't get me wrong. But when you are talking about something which is deeply embedded, it is, to some degree, what you see a human being to be that will determine how you centre the problem. That means that different people will prescribe a different remedy.

As I said, my analogy for that is in acupuncture. When I have had acupuncture treatment from time to time, my acupuncturist who is also a good friend, would be saying, "Well, I could do these points or I could do those points". He is not asking me, he is just carrying on an internal dialogue out loud with me. What I am trying to convey is that if I had gone to another acupuncturist, I might have been needled in other places, and it is the same way with remedies. At what level one engages in curative intervention is a judgemental decision.

ROWENA: Do you think homeopaths can make a fruitful income?

JEROME: One of the problems in relation to this is that many of the people in homeopathy started from the old three pounds for a whole day of yoga in the 1970s. Unfortunately, homeopaths started out not charging enough for the amount of effort that they were putting in. There has been reluctance, interestingly enough, for practitioners to really want to charge their value. And even today, you will find nationally and internationally known British homeopaths who charge no more than students who have just graduated. The problem isn't with the new graduates; it is the fact that among experienced older homeopaths, there is still this reluctance to really charge what they are worth.

ROWENA: So what do you think experienced older homeopaths should charge?

JEROME: Some experienced homeopaths are still charging forty five to fifty pounds for a one and a half to two hour extended first consultation; they should be charging probably seventy five pounds. Also, I have never personally heard of a homeopath that doesn't give concessions in some way. There are also people who may not give concessions in their practice, but will do work in various clinics for free. I would say that they have been doing very well in giving back to the profession and in sharing with people. In other words, homeopaths have tithed well. It doesn't mean that other professions haven't either, but homeopaths have, to some degree, undervalued themselves.

On another area of evolving professionalism, in 1960 Thomas Maughan and others founded the first society of homeopaths and he became the first chairman, but it did not last very long. They wrote a constitution, and when the discussions in 1977 started with a view to form a Society again, I gave Robert Davidson a copy of that original 1960 constitution. It became the discussion document around which the Society of Homeopaths was founded. Currently there are ten registers and for the past few years they have been working to create a single register.

Where the profession is at now is that the various, different forms of homeopathy are beginning to come together and blend. And there is a greater understanding among homeopaths than there was in the 1980s and 1990s. There isn't any one of the educational programmes now that doesn't give some extended time to various methodologies of drainage and organ therapy and the like of that. They all have their own ethos, and there is now recognition of different ways of achieving the goal and that homeopathy can be utilised in many ways. There is a greater understanding, and this is very welcome and very, very good.

Homeopathy has been very powerfully influenced by the work of many different people. Frans Vermeulen's eclectic compendium *Prisma*[37] is an example of bringing together information about remedies, their source and myth which gives a deeper understanding encouraging us to extend our knowledge and their use. There is the ongoing work of meditative provings, which was quite controversial ten years ago. The idea of meditative provings may not be everybody's cup of tea, but more and more people are using them with positive results.

ROWENA: Were you involved in the Guild of Homeopaths (Guild)?

JEROME: I taught for the Guild and also participated in a number of meditative provings. Once a remedy becomes used clinically and has results, it doesn't matter how it was introduced, because homeopathy has always had new remedies coming through from several directions. They come through poisonings, through clinical experience, from provings, and the idea of the signature has also been a strong source of remedies. People like Hahnemann were prescribing remedies long before they proved them; Hering was drawing on the folk tradition and the Doctrine of Signatures. But once you begin to collect clinical results, you then begin to have a solid basis for prescribing.

I have found that people, who were laughing at *Berlin Wall* as a remedy ten years ago, are now recommending and using it, following positive responses in their own practice. The Guild's publishing of case histories in their journal, *Prometheus*[59] served to demonstrate the effectiveness of such remedies as *Berlin Wall*. There is nothing like results, and if it is results that are causing homeopathy to evolve, that is because results are reality.

ROWENA: Did they make a remedy from the Twin Towers after September 11?

JEROME: I assume someone has; they must have. Innovation is part of our culture. Remedies were being made from sun, moonlight, and the blue ray of the spectrum in the 1860s. We can see from studying the nineteenth century literature that they were just as innovative in that era as we are now. It too was an era of growth, and that is what is so exciting about now. The earlier eras of arguing are giving way to getting together to understand each other and realise that we have the same goals. There is now a larger mindedness that accepts diversity of methods.

The profession is growing, and the idea of the various professional registers, after years of arguing, getting together to understand each other and realise that we have the same goals and the same willingness to allow diversity; that kind of openness has really been healthy for the profession. So even though we are slowly moving towards a single register, it is healthy, because while there are limits, there is also openness, so the balance between limits and openness is being acknowledged and recognised.

ROWENA: Thank you so much for your time and insights Jerome; it has been an education and a pleasure.

CHAPTER 12:   MIKE BRIDGER & DION TABRETT

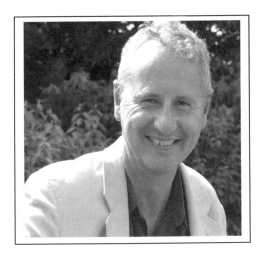
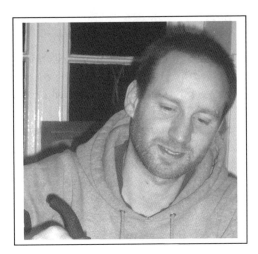

Friday the 15 April 2005 took me to Nelsons Homeopathic Pharmacy in Duke Street, London to sit in on an Orion class, which was very interesting, and later chat with Mike Bridger in a local pub. Dion Tabrett, his partner in crime, joined us for a drink initially and answered some questions about his story too. In Malvern, at the teachers' seminar in November 2004, I had shared several meals with Mike, Bill Rumble, Kate Chatfield, Jean Duckworth and some colleagues from Germany so I was very familiar with Mike's energy – perhaps a little too familiar now I look back on it – my questions were a little cheeky – but hopefully the time we shared that Friday evening will make for an interesting read. He is such a charismatic personality; one cannot help but be inspired by him. Since then Mike has moved his practice to Ainsworths in London and Dion continues to practise from Nelsons.

"I am classical but I am also contemporary. 'Classical' became a misused term, a kind of false fundamentalism which was neither Hahnemannian nor Kentian. Kent would have turned in his proverbial if he had heard his name being used to justify some of the nonsense spoken about him. Kent became synonymous with prescribing only on mentals and emotionals because to prescribe on physicals would be suppressive. These misconceptions were responsible for a trend of amateur psychotherapy in the profession. My 'practical homeopathy' is basic Hahnemannian and Kentian homeopathy. It does me very well and it is contemporary."   *Mike Bridger, April 2005*

"If you think back to your college days, how many of Hahnemann's cases were you instructed in? Probably none and there is a good reason for that; he contradicts most philosophical tendencies of today. He completely breaks all the rules altogether."
Dion Tabrett, April 2005

CHAPTER 12: MIKE BRIDGER & DION TABRETT

ROWENA: How did you discover homeopathy Dion?

DION: Well that is quite an interesting story and involves an old friend. He wanted to have children with his wife but she was diagnosed with polycystic ovaries and couldn't conceive. So they went to see a herbalist who said that she needed to have watercress soup every day. They thought it was a bit wacky and so she rang you (speaking to Mike) and you took the symptoms and said *Magnesia phosphorica*. They didn't take that either but eventually the husband decided to plant a vegetable garden and he thought he would grow some watercress as their herbal book said that it is rich in magnesium phosphate. Consequently, she took the remedy, drank watercress soup, became pregnant and had two daughters as a result. He went on to study homeopathy, saw me puffing on an inhaler and said that he needed patients for college and asked if he could treat me. So he treated my asthma and I discovered homeopathy.

ROWENA: And where did you study?

DION: The College of Homeopathy (COH) in the period 1989 to 1992. I practise in Nelsons in London and Newbury in Berkshire.

ROWENA: Tell me about your teaching. Where do you teach?

DION: At Mike's Contemporary College of Homeopathy (Contemporary College); I run the clinic with him and at the Orion Postgraduate Course here at Nelsons . I also teach fairly regularly at the Centre for Homeopathic Education (CHE) and occasionally other places. I don't like working too many weekends so I have had to whittle it down.

ROWENA: So what kind of homeopathy do you practise?

DION: Now this is an interesting question. I can quite happily say Hahnemannian. So in my case, George Vithoulkas is completely wrong in his assertion that we have all lost our way. He actually contradicts Hahnemann particularly in his book *The Science of Homeopathy*[31]. He thinks you should have an aggravation and that is a good thing. Hahnemann thinks otherwise quite explicitly in the *Organon*[4]. That is one of the reasons he invented the LM system.

ROWENA: What subject do you teach? Do you specialise?

DION: I teach some of the methods particularly James Compton Burnett and Eizayaga. If you think back to your college days, how many of Hahnemann's cases were you instructed in? Probably none and there is a good reason for that; he contradicts most philosophical tendencies of today. He completely breaks all the rules altogether. He gives more than one remedy, repeats remedies and prescribes on old symptoms, on return of symptoms and all sorts of things.

ROWENA: So what books do you recommend to your students Dion?

DION: I would probably recommend specifically *The Best of Burnett* [60] but also some of Clarke's books. I think we draw too heavily on the American homeopaths, especially Kent, when we have a lot of philosophical lessons to learn from the old English homeopaths. Apart from the Contemporary College, it is always a surprise when I teach them elsewhere. Students have heard a bit about Burnett – generally about *Thuja occidentalis* and vaccinosis but any of his deeper stuff just isn't taught so I think there is a whole range of books that we don't touch that are actually essential.

ROWENA: How do you think we can prevent homeopathy becoming dormant again?

DION: I think it is quite compartmentalised. Homeopathy is a predominantly white upper class and middle class domain still. It doesn't really reach across the spectrum of society. For a lot of people, paying seventy five pounds for a consultation is immediately prohibitive. So I think we price ourselves out of an entire spectrum of society. We spend thousands of pounds studying and then we go out and practise. I would like to be paid by a health authority so it doesn't matter how many people I see or how many prescriptions I give, as the service is free. That is one sure-fire way it would retain its popularity and spread. But the structure isn't there for it and the inclination isn't there either particularly because that side of things, in my opinion, is sewn up by the pharmaceutical industry.

ROWENA: Who influenced you while you were studying Dion?

DION: James Compton Burnett without a doubt and also Ellis Barker, John Clarke and Thomas Cooper. I really like Robin Murphy; I have seen him a lot and studied *his tapes* [26]. And of course, Hahnemann.

ROWENA: And the teachers at COH when you studied?

DION: I would say Mike, Robert Davidson, Tony Hurley and Ian Watson. Those are the big ones that spring to mind.

ROWENA: What do you think are the qualities that make a good homeopath these days? There are so many that don't survive. What skills do you think you have to have to be a good homeopath? Why do you think so many homeopaths don't succeed or choose not to practise?

DION: I think we are a prejudiced bunch. I think there is so much that goes on with dreams and interpretations and periodic table and kingdoms and things like that. We don't actually listen to the people sitting in front of us and fix the problem they are paying us to fix. If somebody comes to you and has on average three visits to cure what they are paying you to cure, if you don't do that then simply they will go elsewhere. So I think we too easily spiral off on our own fantasies, which may be indicated but if you don't fix that itchy skin and the kid gets an infection they will end up on antibiotics. You can only do that so many times before parents will say this it isn't working - even though we are convinced that we have hit the right remedy. We tend not to treat what is in front of us; what people pay for - and the cold harsh reality of clinic is that if you don't fix what you are paid to fix, people won't come back and won't recommend you.

ROWENA: So how do you do that? How do you treat what is in front of you? The symptoms? Would that not be suppressive? I am just playing devil's advocate here but how do you view a case?

DION: Well, at the end of each case taking, I will make a treatment plan with the patient - what are we treating here? What is the emphasis? Then what they decide on is what I work with and that is purely how I work.

ROWENA: So what happens if the symptom they come to see you for is something that they have had for a while but there is a new layer sitting above it. You cannot prescribe for what they want immediately because it is not uppermost. How will you work their case?

DION: In that scenario you reflect it back to them, explain your position and ideally come to some bargaining point where you can negotiate what you are doing. If you don't achieve what they want you will lose their trust anyway and ultimately them as a patient and then their recommendations.

ROWENA: So open, clear communication?

DION: Yes absolutely.

ROWENA: So this whole area of practitioner development and personal development. Do you think that plays a part?

DION: I think it is crucial for some people, yes. Seriously I do.

ROWENA: So knowing their stuff and knowing their prejudices?

DION: I don't think you can always get round it but you can be aware of it. We are top heavy in this country; we are mental and emotional prescribers. That is how I was trained predominantly and that is how most people are trained. Why do we shy away from pathology? In Hahnemann's cases he was strictly a pathology prescriber; miasms and pathology time and time again.

ROWENA: So Mike, you have been around our profession for a long time haven't you?

MIKE: Yes.

ROWENA: So how did you discover homeopathy or how did homeopathy discover you?

MIKE: I was in Totnes with a girlfriend. I hated anything to do with health, health food or anything like that; the only thing I liked was organic bread.

ROWENA: How old were you?

MIKE: Two and a half; I was a precocious boy. She went in to the health food shop and came out saying that she had found an advert for a homeopathic college. She would always get the bread because I wouldn't be seen in an organic shop. I didn't have a clue what homeopathy was but I sent away for this leaflet and it said you treat people with minerals and really nasty little substances. I liked that idea so I got hold of *Kent's Lectures*[61].

ROWENA: When was this?

MIKE: I would have been twenty four.

ROWENA: And this was in 1981?

MIKE: Yes. I read it overnight on a coach to Scotland. It was fantastic!

ROWENA: What were you doing before that?

MIKE: I was a playwright and I still write plays now.

ROWENA: Tell me more about play writing.

MIKE: Plays are about people and how they interact. It is all about dramatic moments and that is what you are looking for when you are talking to patients; the dramatic things that have happened to them physically, mentally or emotionally and you sit there and listen to it. People sit there and talk to you in a way they would have talked to the priest, the vicar or the doctor a hundred years ago. So I ask personal questions, which I probably wouldn't ask most people, about what they do and how they react. It is like detective work. Writing a play is like detective work too; you are working out what people do, how they interact and why things happen. This is what I do as a homeopath.

ROWENA: I appreciate that you still write plays but were you looking to come out of that profession and do something different?

MIKE: From playwriting? Yes. Theatre is a very neurotic world; you are in your own head. You have to be engaged with the outside world, with people and their stories otherwise you just write how you think people are. They can be two different things. When it comes to homeopathy you are actually applying a pill or a medication. You can test out a perception which you cannot do when you are writing plays. In some ways I am introverted otherwise I wouldn't be a writer. I am not an actor and I would never want to act. I wouldn't like to be a director either. Naturally I am a writer but there is this other part of me that is a bit more extroverted really. It enjoys the engagement, or whatever you want to call it, which you don't get writing plays except with the imaginary people in my head who talk to me all the time.

ROWENA: So you are a bit of a paradox. So what intake were you in at COH?

MIKE: I think it was about the second or third year of the original Robert Davidson college; COH.

ROWENA: So who was in your year?

MIKE: I cannot remember. Robin Logan, I think, and a few others.

ROWENA: Who taught you?

MIKE: Misha Norland, Robert Davidson, David Mundy and David Curtin. Tony Hurley I think was the year above and was doing a bit of teaching.

ROWENA: So who inspired you the most?

MIKE: I really liked Robert Davidson. Robert is a saboteur who doesn't understand why he sometimes upsets people. Actually he is much softer than he makes out. He is like a saboteur without a centre. He likes to throw everything into disarray, which I love. He is a wonderfully empowering man. I don't know anybody who empowered students as much as he did and probably still does.

ROWENA: How does he do that?

MIKE: He does it by making everything alright, and because he is so exciting in what he does. There is an awful lot of warmth in him and a great deal of charisma. He just challenges everything as he is a nonconformist. The fact is he is always reacting and then moving off. He will never sit in a comfortable place where he belongs to something so people can get disillusioned with him because he doesn't seem to commit himself to anything for very long.

ROWENA: What are you known for?

MIKE: What am I known for? By whom? By the police? I am not really sure but probably for all the wrong reasons. I don't like pretentiousness. I don't like the kind of homeopathy that invests itself in making people have psychological symptoms when they don't have them. If someone comes with rashes or hay fever, that is what I deal with. I think I am categorised as an unspiritual, atheist, practical, bread and butter homeopath with nothing really original or interesting to say except that I make people laugh a bit. But if I really thought there was nothing more to it than that, I wouldn't be happy at all. I am probably known for remedy relationships as well.

ROWENA: Tell me a bit about the remedy relationships.

MIKE: Looking at the relationship of remedies gets you away from the idea of the single remedy. We are looking at energy not at some sort of golden essence or centre. Energy moves and therefore remedies must move too. Where do they move to? Both Hahnemann and Kent talked about this. Why do people disdainfully refer to 'zigzagging'? It is important to understand the movement of the remedy and the patient from place to place. You cannot be a homeopath without understanding 'zigzagging.'

Homeopathy is about energy and not about fixed 'pictures'. We hear from homeopaths the crappiest kind of fake diagnosis and we are hearing more and more of it. The 'deep' kind of, "The patient said they feel rotten so that is a delusion that they are putrefying" or "Their favourite film is the *Wizard of Oz*[62] so they should have Rainbow 10M." This is about ego and laziness and has nothing to do with homeopathy. Ironically it is another manifestation of the worst kind of allopathy and you hear this kind of stuff at seminars sometimes. The analysis can sound brilliant, poetic and plausible, but often the patient doesn't get better.

Quite often I have heard of cases used in seminars by homeopaths where the patient didn't get better at all and the remedy and the case were presented as a cure. Now that is really sad. When we have important people teaching from that perspective then there is something seriously wrong in the profession or what the profession seems to respect. To say that the analysis of the case is actually more important than the cure of the patient is the same as saying, in allopathic terms, that the diagnosis is more important than what happens to the patient. It is ridiculous to say that the analysis of the patient, the symbolism of what the patient says, is more important than whether the patient actually gets better or not.

ROWENA: I understand what you mean. So where did you learn about the relationship of remedies?

MIKE: In practice and reading about comparative materia medica. I was always very interested in the latter from the start. I looked at remedies in relation to each other to facilitate learning them; that was very important for me. I didn't want to see them in isolation so I spent time working out the differences between remedies that seemed similar. I was interested when I read somewhere that a remedy moved to another one or that a remedy would complete the action of another one. It seemed academic when you read it in a book but then when you have got a case that isn't getting any better – somebody is haemorrhaging and you think, the symptoms are still *Calcarea carbonica* - what do you do? In that case I read in Hahnemann that Mercury (*Mercurius solubilis*) and *Nitricum acidum* will often come up as aggravations after *Calcarea carbonica*. I prescribed the *Mercury* and the bleeding stopped so I got really interested after that.

ROWENA: Those little tips....

MIKE: Kent and Hahnemann were always interested in that stuff.

ROWENA: So what do think of these new methodologies that are around these days?

MIKE: We have to be careful that they are not used in a literal way and that we end up categorising patients and putting them in boxes. I don't think that is how people come into my practice; they don't come in layers at all. They come with arms and legs and bits and pieces. I am prescribing quite often on one or two physical generals, some pathological and maybe a mental. One symptom may be from one 'layer' and another from another 'layer'. Students get terribly confused, unless the subject is taught really well; Dion teaches it really well.

If the characteristic symptoms are mental that is called the Kentian method but I don't know a case by Kent in which he prescribed on mentals! Burnett never said you just prescribe on an organ; he prescribed on the symptoms around an organ. He talked about prescribing when the vitality is so reduced and limited that all it can do is produce symptoms around an organ and then it MAY be a small remedy, but if it is *Sulphur* they need, you prescribe *Sulphur*. Allopathic medicine is about putting things in boxes; grouping symptoms in terms of diseases. Homeopaths have to be careful not to do the same thing in different ways.

DION: I think it is all down to perception really. When practitioners attach themselves to a particular model of homeopathy that they understand, they are limiting their perception. The fortunate thing about homeopathy is that it will always change and teach you something different and after ten years of practise people will still come in and surprise you. They present with something that contradicts your previous experience but then it does depend on your perception. Mike is a people person. If you go out to dinner with Mike, he is chatting with the waitress and she is telling him about her fluffy dog and she is laughing all over the place. Whereas I compartmentalise things and like treating pathology, so that is what is attracted to me.

ROWENA: Do you use timelines?

MIKE: No because I can see what is happening now to the energy. Timelines don't do anything for me. What do they say? They don't tell me where the person's energy is at the moment.

ROWENA: How does Orion work?

MIKE: How does it work? We thought we would work well together. We didn't know why. We wanted to get away from the idea of courses being run by individual personalities, or gurus. Orion is not about gurus; it is about homeopathy.

ROWENA: Do you think your charisma attracts people to study with you?

MIKE: I certainly don't try to mystify or pretend that I have something that other people don't. I want to make sure I come from a place where students feel empowered. It isn't a matter of personality. Dion and I come from different places, which stop us coming from ego. We get on with the business. People see us discussing cases and we can disagree, slag each other off and even laugh at ourselves. As a result the students or practitioners around us start to relax and drop the pretence of being holy. Holiness doesn't work with us. It is a 'No No'. We eat guru types for breakfast. We actually want to see people enjoy themselves. Being pretentious or pretending to be more important than you are is not enjoyable; it is sad and lonely. Our job as homeopaths is to be vital; to make people feel good about themselves and to give them more energy. If we cannot find that magic in ourselves then we should get another job.

ROWENA: Do you want to be associated with a university?

MIKE: Well I might do, yes, but I wouldn't sacrifice the stuff I have just talked about though. A lot of homeopaths out there are quite lost; it is an isolated job and not the most financially rewarding. Some have been trained in the oddest ways and, surprisingly, there is a lot of fear around prescribing and how homeopathy works. There is a lack of confidence too. Orion is about simplification and getting back into oneself as a practitioner as well as understanding where patients come from. We have students from all backgrounds and from all approaches. We have had people who have been practising for twenty years and others who have only just qualified but the point is; none of it matters. We give them simple and common sense strategies, and we inject them with self-belief and above all, energy! You see them blossoming as people and practitioners. You see their cases blossoming too, and they go out and their practise changes.

ROWENA: When you are prescribing, do you give one remedy at a time?

MIKE: I tend to, yes. Sometimes I use tissue salts if there is mechanical tissue damage or something like that. If I know remedies work well together I will use two remedies - one high and one low. I tend to use organ support as well. Today I have given a patient *Natrum sulphuricum*, although her mental picture is more *Natrum muriaticum*, her physical picture is more *Natrum sulphuricum*. It is not that similar to her mentally and emotionally but I don't want her to aggravate, so I am giving it in low potency and then she will have *Natrum muriaticum* once a week.

ROWENA: How do you treat cancer?

MIKE: Same as I treat anything else. It depends where the focus of the symptoms are. If there is mental and emotional stuff going on then that is what I will treat. If predominantly the energy is dealing more with the physical symptoms, then that is what I will treat.

ROWENA: So not the Murphy method of treating the cancer first?

MIKE: No. I look for where the energy is. The awful thing about cancer is that sometimes it seems the energy doesn't seem to be bothered by it; it isn't reacting to it in any way whatsoever. We rely on how the person reacts to prescribe, so we can get stuck. If there is a reaction going on, ok. If not, you have to look elsewhere in the case. If you find nothing, you best find a remedy to match the cancer and location etc. This is Burnett stuff and Robin Murphy would agree, I think. Obviously if the energy is disturbed on another level, dare I say, mentally and emotionally then you would treat the cancer through that channel. It depends where the energy is and what it is trying to tell you. That is always the issue for me.

When people started dying from AIDS, homeopaths panicked not knowing how to treat these patients. I just said it is like everything else - you treat it in exactly the same way. You treat the symptoms! People were losing their heads about it. This was the new frightening pariah of disease and this was going to be totally different. So I did a bit of work with the Terrence Higgins Trust and treated the same way I normally do. I took the symptoms - the same with cancer. Homeopaths get panicked, thinking somehow we need a different way of treating this when in fact it is the same thing. Cancer is energy, tonsillitis is energy and hay fever is energy. If we lose touch with that and start prescribing from a different place we better know what we are doing. Interestingly, from my experience, people with schizophrenia somehow lose their schizophrenia if they develop cancer. So ignoring what the rest of the energy is doing is nuts but I don't actually think Robin Murphy is saying that.

ROWENA: Well I have read his lecture notes[14] and he talks about zigzagging and honing in on what is going on now. What are your views on the *Ramakrishnan method*[21] of treating cancer?

MIKE: It still has to be specific to the symptoms. I don't know enough about that to judge really but I know he has treated a hell of a lot of cancer cases.

ROWENA: Do you think homeopathy can change people's karma?

MIKE: Karma is a word that is often misused. Karma is about where you are at now, how you got there and it suggests that you can choose to go somewhere else if you want to. People are saying that somehow karma means you are here because of consequences, like a punishment or something but it is not that at all. It is about free will; it is about choosing. If homeopathy gives you more choices then it changes your karma but I don't think there is anything deeply weird or wacky about it. We have different words in psychotherapy and homeopathy for the same thing. It is what it is, whether we use the word karma or not.

ROWENA: Do you think remedies can shift people into a completely different space?

MIKE: Yes, but they can also not. We don't like to think that some people don't want to go into a different space. Sometimes you can give them a remedy and they don't move anywhere like where I would like them to go. They still go on playing golf or stay in a relationship that sounds to me boring. I give them *Staphysagria* - they can explode or divorce or whatever but sometimes they just say, "I am much happier now with my alcoholic husband. I don't mind him beating me up so much." Homeopathy is powerful and powerless at the same time. It won't take anybody where they don't want to go. It might be someone has just got hay fever that needs curing. Homeopathy can be fantastic for someone who has got a painful joint and cannot walk their dog; if we get rid of the swollen knee, they can walk their dog. That is what makes them happy. You have done several interviews now Rowena, do you see common stuff coming through each one?

ROWENA: The common stuff is that people are very passionate about what they do and they all seem to be working with integrity.

MIKE: I would accuse you of sitting on the fence a little bit. You must have a kind of sense of where it is all going.

ROWENA: I think I have to sit on the fence. I went to the London College of Classical Homeopathy (LCCH) and had a very classical training. I approach each interview with an open, non-judgemental mind, as I do with my patients. I was with Ellen Kramer recently and I thought she was very inspiring. She taught me that she treats her patients who have had breast cancer and are now taking Tamoxifen, with *Tamoxifen* in potency first as they often come to see her with the side effects of that drug. Her approach opened my eyes and it made sense to me. She really believes in it and is getting good results. Then I speak to someone else and they are getting good results with another method. I am not an 'on the fence' kind of a person actually. I am an Aries after all!

MIKE: How do you know people are getting good results?

ROWENA: They say so...

MIKE: Good, but I have heard of people doing cancer seminars when they have only treated two cancer cases for God's sake. That is really scary. What would you like to see at the end of all this? What would you like your book to be? Can you say, in one sentence, what you would like it to achieve?

ROWENA: To shed light and to help with the confusion that exists within our profession.

MIKE: I think there is room for pointing out that there are differences and discrepancies that need to be resolved. Personally, I think that would be a very good perspective. Let us look at the differences as well; let us look at the unresolved issues. Never mind that we are all beautiful and we have got good intentions and all the rest of it. We need to sort some of these differences out so that we present a solidly united profession.

ROWENA: I don't think there is an answer. How can the profession be a united front when everyone's practising in a completely different way? I don't know how that can come about but if you can tell me how that would be great.

MIKE: In my opinion, we are not critical enough. It is a liberal middle class profession. We are too indulgent in terms of saying, "It is all OK." I don't feel it is OK. I get very angry with what I hear, what I see and what I observe students doing. I get very angry about it and that is seen as very uncool actually. In this profession people don't like that. People don't like people making a big stand about stuff and saying that is wrong and that is bad. If people are treating semi-delusions with patients that have got cancer, in my opinion we cannot sit back and say that is really beautiful. Collectively we all do that; we all kiss and cuddle at the Society of Homeopaths' Conference. It is all very nice really. But some things are serious and we have a responsibility to patients. We need to decide what we are teaching. What do you think of that, Rowena?

ROWENA: I am in agreement with you, of course, but how can that be fixed?

MIKE: By taking the ego out of it. By getting people to feel strong enough to be able to argue and stand up and answer questions. "What do you think about treating people for the complaints they come with?" Why don't we, as a profession, debate that question. How do you do it? With piles what are you looking for? Are you trying to treat the psychological issues, their karma, or the pain in their backside? The idea that everything is ok is very outmoded and old fashioned now.

ROWENA: So someone comes to you with piles; what do you do?

MIKE: I wouldn't tell them to sit down. I would stand up to keep them company.

ROWENA: And then what would you do?

MIKE: I would look at where they are disturbed and talk to them about that and say, is that right or is it wrong? Ultimately they choose. I would put it back to them and say, it seems to me there is also this other issue? Which do you think is most important?

ROWENA: I think those you criticise, whoever they might be, would argue that being speculative and judgemental is not how to practise homeopathy either. Most practitioners know that being speculative and judgemental gets in the way of seeing the case, don't they? Do you ask your patients about sex?

MIKE: You have to be careful because it can be very invasive and I am not into invasive questioning. Sex is a very personal thing. A lot of patients are women and to go to a male homeopath is a big deal. Their food cravings tell me that they are *Sepia succus*, they don't need to say they have gone off sex. I can work that out for myself, to some extent. If a patient volunteers to talk about it, that is different. It is abusive to move in when somebody is obviously uncomfortable. If somebody has trauma, I don't need to know what that trauma is about. I don't have an investment in having someone telling me something that they don't feel ready to tell me about. Most people aren't ready to talk to a stranger about sex on their first consultation.

ROWENA: In this country?

MIKE: I have only practised in this country.

ROWENA: It is more of a British taboo isn't it?

MIKE: I doubt that. I think most countries talk about it in a very superficial, anecdotal way. I don't think other nationalities are actually any more open about themselves than we are really.

I would also say as a practitioner, always question yourself and invite other people to question you too. Always be prepared to take some stick about what you think and believe and change your mind accordingly if you realise you are wrong. That is true whether we are questioning a patient, the profession or ourselves.

There are students that are leaving colleges and don't go into practice because they are totally frightened and disillusioned. The teachers who have had a negative influence on them are probably unaware of the message they gave to them. They are all lovely people; the students are lovely; the teachers are lovely and they do all the right things but somehow there is a shadow that we haven't dealt with and we need to do so as a profession.

ROWENA: Maybe some of the readers of this book will take you up on it and a debate will ensue. Do you feel you know yourself pretty well Mike? Do you feel this is a prerequisite for being a successful homeopath?

MIKE: I know myself well because I am not frightened when I discover something else about myself that I didn't know before. And I am not frightened that I didn't know it either. If I am coming up against something and learning that it is OK. It is a positive thing not to be scared of oneself. That is my answer; I am not scared of myself.

ROWENA: Do you go to a homeopath?

MIKE: I do occasionally and I have been in the past. I went to a psychotherapist and that was life changing but I know the 'system' with homeopathy so I can manipulate it.

ROWENA: So you could go to Brian Kaplan; he uses Provocative Therapy to treat homeopaths for that very reason. On another subject Mike, do you feel that we need to create new remedies?

MIKE: Well I think it is a bit of a game. If we are going to create new remedies, let us also reprove some of the old ones for which we only have small pictures. The argument that people have changed enormously so we need these new remedies, is debatable. Some of these provings read like poetry and symbolism, not sensation and observation. Meditative provings – forget them.

ROWENA: Now you sound like George Vithoulkas.

MIKE: He is a very clever man. He knows more about homeopathy than most people in the profession.

ROWENA: So why is your college called 'Contemporary'?

MIKE: Because everybody else was calling themselves 'classical'. It sounded like painting classes. I am classical but I am also contemporary. 'Classical' became a misused term, a kind of false fundamentalism which was neither Hahnemannian nor Kentian. Kent would have turned in his proverbial if he had heard his name being used to justify some of the nonsense spoken about him. Kent became synonymous with prescribing only on mentals and emotionals because to prescribe on physicals would be suppressive. These misconceptions were responsible for a trend of amateur psychotherapy in the profession. My 'practical homeopathy' is basic Hahnemannian and Kentian homeopathy. It does me very well and it is contemporary.

ROWENA: If I came to you and you were my homeopath, would you be looking for one remedy which sums me up?

MIKE: Isn't that idea awful? I am not that arrogant that I seriously believe I can sum up someone in that way, as one remedy. I would ask, "What upsets you? What disturbs you? Is your energy disturbed in that area or somewhere else you didn't know or hadn't thought about?"

ROWENA: What you say makes perfect sense. I too work with what is in front of me.

MIKE: When you take a case how do you read your patients? How much of your own experience comes in to case taking?

ROWENA: When you say my experience, could you clarify what you mean by that.

MIKE: Everything you have been through - your ideas, beliefs, emotional life; all of that.

ROWENA: Of course I draw from my own experience and I think that is when you worry as to whether your stuff is going to get in the way.

MIKE: We teach personal development in homeopathy to try to deal with that. The idea that there is a neutral place, the unprejudiced observer, is a lie; it is not true. You have to come from your own sense of things and that is the only place you can reside. How do I read *Natrum muriaticum*? Suppression. How do I read suppression? When have I suppressed? I am using my own measurement of what is suppression. I have got to use mine as I cannot use yours. There is no objective truth about it. When I am questioning a patient how do I measure *Hyoscyamus*? What boundaries do I use for *Phosphorus*? How do I measure hysteria? When have I been hysterical? When have I been out of control? I only have myself. I never block that. How else do you measure it? I am looking at patients; I am talking to patients from absolutely all my prejudices and observations. We all have to learn to be more assertive about our prejudices. Actually our prejudices are often just observations anyway.

ROWENA: When did you set up your colleges - Contemporary College and Orion and why?

MIKE: It is a long story and a tale of professionalism and ethics. Part of it also entailed a group of doctors at the medical centre where I was practising who was very encouraging and allowed us to use their rooms for our own teaching clinic. I thought, fantastic, because I wanted to work with the medical profession and I still do actually. I like some of what they do. I want to break down the idea that homeopathy is the only thing. Homeopathy is as bad or good as you make it. So is medicine, so is spiritual healing, so is religion and so is golf.

ROWENA: I watched ER last night and it was a fantastic episode. A young woman, age thirty five with three children, collapses with a stroke. In the next scene you see her in hospital and her right side is completely paralysed. You hear her voice asking, "Where am I? What am I doing?" but she is not heard by those around her. The words are inside her head because she cannot talk. So we hear all her thoughts and feelings while the nurses and doctors diagnose she has had a stroke. In the end they do an operation to clear the clot and it is unbelievable - her face reverts to normal and her speech returns. And yes, I agree with you, doctors can really do a very good job and perform miracles. It was so awesome. From your experience do you think *Arnica* could have achieved that?

MIKE: It can do but it isn't about that in a way. It is about the notions of good and evil. It is the idea that homeopathy is good, spiritual stuff and allopathy is evil. Well there are some really bad homeopath's out there and there are some good nurses, doctors and physiotherapists too. I would rather go to a good doctor than a bad homeopath. When Hess landed in Scotland he had homeopathic remedies in his pocket. The Nazis used homeopathy. Things aren't as black and white as we like to think sometimes.

ROWENA: What, in your opinion, is bad homeopathy?

MIKE: Screwing around with people's heads.

ROWENA: Do you think there is 'a truth' Mike?

MIKE: Of course there is.

ROWENA: According to whom?

MIKE: The truth is a bit like the vital force isn't it? We don't know what it is or why it is there but we know it is there. We can kid ourselves that it isn't so we can do exactly what we want. We can lie and say that this is our truth and everybody else's truth is wrong. That would be bad karma though eh? It is when we are totally congruent. When our stomachs are doing what our hearts are doing what our spirit is doing then we are content and truthful.

ROWENA: I thoroughly enjoyed this conversation Mike. Thank you so much for spending time with me. Please thank Dion when you see him later. I hope the reader will pick up on some of your questions and start some interesting debates.

CHAPTER 13:   ERNEST ROBERTS

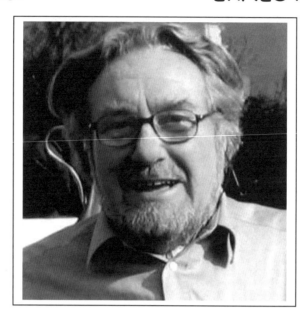

Tuesday 19 May 2005 found me at the end of the telephone to Ernest Roberts, principal of the North West College of Homoeopathy (NWCH) in Manchester. I would have loved to have met this very enthusiastic character face to face but time would not allow me the journey so a telephone conversation had to suffice. But I could feel his infectious passion through the telephone wires and was very pleased to have had this opportunity to chat with him. Since the interview Ernest is now no longer principal as he has retired and he has handed the helm over to his long trusted colleague Dave Evans.

"In my opinion, the whole issue about methodologies is ridiculous. It is breaking up homeopathy into neat compartments, which is totally false."   *Ernest Roberts, May 2005*

"Teddy Roosevelt was a patient of Kent's and when he gave money out to the medical schools he didn't give any to the homeopathic schools and Kent asked him why. He replied, "Well, it is unteachable". Well it shouldn't be, not now, not in the energetic era we live in. Most of our graduates are doing good work and are busy."   *Ernest Roberts, May 2005*

"I encourage people to charge what they are worth and if you are good your patients will pay and recommend many people. If you are good you will cure people with homeopathy and you will be busy. Years ago I put my fees up in order to get time to myself but I got busier. They thought I must be the best because I was charging the most."

Ernest Roberts, May 2005

CHAPTER 13:   ERNEST ROBERTS

ERNEST: During the last fifteen years and up until recently I have been going to Alonissos to visit George Vithoulkas every year. We always have a chat and he frequently asks me what homeopathy is like in England, but I admit I do have quite a jaundiced view. In particular, last year, we had quite a long conversation and I told him, in my opinion, I feel certain teachers have tried to destroy classical homeopathy. I really do think they have spread a kind of image of what classical homeopathy is which is totally erroneous. I think this has done a lot of harm to the British scene and even though I think there are some very good things going on, there is a great deal of antagonism towards what I consider Hahnemannian homeopathy.

ROWENA: How would you say they portray classical homeopathy?

ERNEST: They say that classical homeopaths give a high potency and then they wait and wait and wait; this is a parody. You have got to know what you are waiting for. Kent says it quite clearly, you are waiting for a return of old symptoms; you are waiting to see the direction of cure in correspondence with the order the symptoms came in the first place. It is a scientific process but they caricature it and there are several other things all along those lines. So it puts people off and causes them to question the validity of the *Organon*[4]; of Hahnemann in this day and age. Homeopathy is going through such transformations at the moment. I have just finished reading Rajan Sankaran's new book, *The Sensation in Homeopathy*[63], have you read it yet?

ROWENA: I have got it here but I haven't read it yet.

ERNEST: It is a hell of a book. I think what Rajan Sankaran has done is rewritten the *Organon*[4]. It is absolutely amazing how he has just gone back to the original meanings.

ROWENA: So rewritten it in a good way?

ERNEST: Oh yes, it is absolutely fantastic; the man is a genius. I have known Rajan Sankaran for many years. He visited the NWCH and stayed a few days and I have attended his seminars and sat in with him in Bombay for a period. I know the man very well and am full of admiration for him.

ROWENA: Do you think colleges will now be teaching Rajan Sankaran's new system?

ERNEST: No, not all colleges.

ROWENA: Will you?

ERNEST: Oh, we do already. We give lectures on his methods and have done so for the past two years with the fourth and fifth year and also as a Continuous Professional Development programme for our graduates and students from other colleges.

ROWENA: And is it seen as a 'methodology' or is it just an extension of classical homeopathy?

ERNEST: I am not sure what you mean by methodology. I recommend Ian Watson's *A Guide to the Methodologies of Homoeopathy* [64] to my students, and then I will tell them to read it critically and to compare it with my own book *Homoeopathy; Principles and Practice* [65], so as to put it into perspective. In my opinion, the whole issue about methodologies is ridiculous. It is breaking up homeopathy into neat compartments, which is totally false. He says about 'classical homeopathy' that it only takes into account the emotional and mental symptoms and not many remedies are known to that extent and therefore it has a very limited application. This is the absolute opposite to what homeopathy is about. I have shared my views with George Vithoulkas so maybe he has a slightly jaundiced view of homeopathy in England because of listening to me.

Janet Snowdon said to me the other day that she thinks that the best homeopaths are now the medical homeopaths. In my early days, I think they were the worst. There is an article by Margaret Tyler called *How Not to Do It* [66]. She explains her experience of changing from being a doctor using homeopathic medicines to being a classical homeopath after having trained with Kent. She just writes down all the terrible things that I heard about when I started practising in 1983. In those first ten years I came across many patients who had been prescribed by medical homeopaths, many different remedies all in high potencies as if they were dolly mixtures. When they came to see me some had confused pictures as a result of their homeopathic treatment.

That was always my impression of medical homeopaths because the Faculty had been cut down so badly in the 1940s. But then I met two or three doctors working in the Royal London Homeopathic Hospital. One of them was Philip Bailey, the author of *Homeopathic Psychology* [67]. David Curtin began his training of doctors properly and they are very good, very professional and quite classical. They all mostly trained to some extent with George Vithoulkas. There is Dietmar Payrhuber who is an old friend of mine who lives in Salzburg, Austria who also trained with George. His book, *Dimensions of Homeopathic Medicine* [68] shows how to cure very advanced cancers using Scholten's method with great success.

I believe there is a lot of hope within homeopathy but it is hard to put your finger on it. In my book [65], I give this anecdote, which I got from Michael Haggiag. Michael is from the USA who studied with Misha Norland at the same time as me and he went back to the USA. He said that Teddy Roosevelt was a patient of Kent's and when he gave money out to the medical schools he didn't give any to the homeopathic schools and Kent asked him why. He replied, "Well, it is unteachable". Well it shouldn't be, not now, not in the energetic era we live in. Most of our graduates are doing good work and are busy.

ROWENA: So how do you get that over to them; how do you get them to earn a good living?

ERNEST: We always say charge what you will; look around at other people's fees, look at the medical doctor homeopaths' fees and value yourself fully. We always say that right through the course. It is very important. I charge ninety five pounds for a first consultation and forty five pounds for follow ups. I encourage people to charge what they are worth and if you are good your patients will pay and recommend many people. If you are good you will cure people with homeopathy and you will be busy. Years ago I put my fees up in order to get time to myself but I got busier. They thought I must be the best because I was charging the most.

There is this new way of prescribing called 'sequential' and what I have seen is that it is like working with formulas but you cannot work with a formula in homeopathy; it has got to be individualised. It is only by chance that you will get a result if you work with formulas.

ROWENA: So what do you think of the *Ramakrishnan method*[21] of prescribing for cancer then?

ERNEST: I think it is excellent; I think it is classical homeopathy. It is what Hahnemann and Kent say, when you have got serious pathology like cancer. Kent says to treat the pathology paying sufficient attention to the nature of the patient. If the prescription doesn't have some connection to the patient's nature then you are palliating but palliation is within classical homeopathy. It is a valid part of treating incurable cases and you have got to know when a case is incurable and when it isn't.

Dave Evans mainly teaches the medical side here at the NWCH but he does bring in therapeutics as well. I think there is a place for therapeutics but organ support is not part of homeopathy; it is not part of classical homeopathy at all. If you are palliating then it is useful. If you are treating a person curatively and you need an organ remedy you are going to have to work with what Kent says; you have got to fit judiciously to the nature of the person or else it is not homeopathy. It is naturopathy and there is nothing wrong with that and I admire naturopathy. What I have done is taken some of the common organ remedies like *Digitalis* and one or two others, and found some excellent mental and emotional symptoms and modalities - totality of symptoms of the remedy - and written them up including the remedy's organ affinities. I always teach affinities as they are very important. You cannot ignore affinities and regions when you are taking a case. The onus is not purely on the mental and emotional level.

We know you can get one-sided cases on any level, not just difficult ones. It is very important to be able to recognise the kind of case you are dealing with and that is what I teach. I ascertained most of my information about organ remedies from George Vithoulkas. Kent says of *Magnesia muriatica* that it is one of our prime liver remedies and you will find that in George Vithoulkas' *Materia Medica Viva*[69].

I use George Vithoulkas' *Twelve Levels of Health*[70]. If you have them in mind you know what you are treating and what to expect. If you start taking the case and you have got the history of the patient's illness, you know whether you can just find a polycrest and then sit back and watch the patient getting better and better on repeated doses of that one remedy. These are simple cases of healthy people with just one or two layers. When you get patients who are further down thet *Twelve Levels of Health*[70] framework; then you know you are working with more complicated cases.

George Vithoulkas isn't popular in England, in other countries and in Greece you get hundreds of homeopaths enrolled on his video courses. I have a very close friend who did the original one and she benefited from it tremendously. The *Twelve Levels of Health*[70] is quite simple. There are four groups and the first group has a history of very few acutes. They don't have lots of treatments, they get over acutes fairly quickly or with very little treatment and they have very healthy constitutions.

Then the next level has lots of acutes; this is the group we get most of really. They have a history of cystitis or headaches and migraine every so often and therefore they have had to have lots of treatment. And in this second group you will find there are probably two or three remedies or two or three layers. I relate this to when I am teaching how to handle people on allopathic drugs because there is a crossover. There is a relationship between the *Twelve Levels of Health*[70] and taking allopathic drugs. At this level you have got to look for a top layer. You have got to spend a lot more time, very carefully, finding what the first remedy is because there is no such thing as a constitutional remedy in groups three and four. There is only a series of remedies prescribed in the correct sequence; can you say that the constitutional one is the first one - the one that opened up the case - or the last one that actually finished the cure? There isn't a single constitutional in complex cases, so we teach people to know what to look for, what to treat. If you get the first remedy correct you begin a process of deep cure and then you have to get the best remedies in the correct order.

The third group is where there is very serious advanced systemic pathology and the same thing applies as the second group, although it is not so easy and you cannot see the remedy so clearly. This is where you need a lot of experience to get the right remedies and this is where Rajan Sankaran is working. He gives you a terrific insight and an inroad and key into these difficult multilayered cases. He says that to find the remedy you have got to know the substance. It is fascinating.

ROWENA: I want to know how you got into homeopathy in the beginning Ernest.

ERNEST: Well, it was through a horse really.

ROWENA: Well that is unique!

ERNEST: I was lecturing at polytechnics and I gave my job up and then my first wife and I ended up in a commune in Norfolk. This was when the kids were tiny and we built gypsy caravans and repaired horse drawn vehicles. Then I got this horse. I bought him on the cheap because he had rheumatism and a friend of mine turned up and gave him a homeopathic remedy, which improved his rheumatism, so he was then able to pull the cart better and be quite active. My friend told us all about homeopathy and my wife and I decided to enrol on Thomas Maughan's homeopathy classes. We used to go to London every fortnight to sell bread. We made bread, which was one way for the commune to make money, and took it to health food shops and stayed with friends. We went to Thomas' homeopathy classes on Fridays and Saturdays up until he died in 1976. And then the College of Homeopathy (COH) started and I joined the second intake. Janet Snowdon was in the first intake and David Mundy and Misha Norland were two of our teachers.

ROWENA: Who else was in your intake?

ERNEST: I sat between Jeremy Sherr and Murray Feldman and Jeremy and I argued the whole time!

ROWENA: What did you argue about?

ERNEST: Anything! When we came back to London from the commune and we lived in Blackheath I did go for homeopathy myself. I started teaching yoga and healing and I went to Martin Miles for something and it cleared up quite quickly.

ROWENA: So what was Martin Miles like in those days?

ERNEST: He was the same man he is now. He was my teacher and friend and I used to go to his class, which used to be Thomas' medical class every other Saturday. I used to go to Kaaren Whitney's class every fortnight, too, and to Misha Norland's class every Monday and that is how I learned homeopathy. When I started going to COH I didn't learn as much as in these classes, which I continued to attend.

ROWENA: Why?

ERNEST: Well, the teaching was just so erratic. We had one project that was never marked or given back to us. They had a few clinics run by students who had just graduated and, to be quite honest, by that time I knew more than they did, because I had been attending classes with all these wonderful teachers for two years.

ROWENA: Who inspired you most in those days?

ERNEST: David Mundy. He is one of my great teachers, even now. As you know, he teaches at the NWCH on our course. He teaches every month for twelve hours and lives in Manchester now so we get his brains regularly, but to be honest we always have done. And Misha Norland was good too.

ROWENA: So what is it that David Mundy does that is so special?

ERNEST: He is just absolutely devoted and dedicated. He works so hard and reads everything. He goes to every seminar and he is always learning. Years ago George Vithoulkas asked all the teachers around the world to a big teachers' conference in Alonissos. David Mundy and his wife Tasha were there. Rajan Sankaran and Jayesh Shah attended as did the big names from the USA and it was a great conference. When it finished we had a few days before we got our flights back home and I went fishing with Tasha while David went around the islands with Rajan and Jayesh. I asked Tasha what he was doing and why he wasn't relaxing, and she said that he had to learn and he wanted to make the most of being with Rajan all the time.

ROWENA: So when did your wife study?

ERNEST: My second wife is one of our graduates and has been practising for twelve years. I am divorced from the wife who is the mother of my children and she didn't go into homeopathy. She went into counselling and does very well.

ROWENA: Other than David Mundy and Misha Norland, who inspired you at your time of study?

ERNEST: David Curtin was very good. He taught us medical sciences. He was the first person we knew who went to Alonissos with other doctors and he came back with teachings on the materia medicas which he had learned from George Vithoulkas. That was the first time we had come across George's teachings; it was just wonderful. David is a very good homeopath. Sheilagh Creasy taught at COH and I was very impressed with her because she is a good classical homeopath and I got her to come and teach at the NWCH.

ROWENA: So tell me more about your relationship with George Vithoulkas?

ERNEST: Yes, well, he has been my greatest friend always. He started these seminars in London and they were held every three months for two years but they were planned to go on indefinitely. I went to them all and this was about the time I met a lot of those medics like Brian Kaplan and a few others. We always got on really well and shared our experience of homeopathy. I took a case to a seminar of a high-pressured businessman with a peptic ulcer. Before I was under the influence of George Vithoulkas' teachings, I had been giving him *Kali carbonicum* because he was so rigid. He had a Japanese garden and he was very closed and uptight and to my mind he was a *Kali carbonicum*. In the intervening period when he got the abdominal pain I was giving him remedies like *Robinia pseudacacia.*

I had learned at COH about organ support and remedies for the immediate acute condition and that is how I was prescribing for this case. That is what is great about the *Twelve Levels of Health*[70]; you know when to do that and when not to and I was doing it wrong. So I took the case to George Vithoulkas. It was crowded and there were eminent doctors from Germany, the UK and the USA there as well as leading non-doctor homeopaths including David Mundy. And it was obviously a simple and clear *Natrum muriaticum* case and everyone looked at me quizzically. George was so good; he really looked after me and ever since then George and I have got on really well.

ROWENA: I found him very warm, kind and inviting last summer when I interviewed him. So tell me what would you say are the most important qualities for a successful homeopath?

ERNEST: I don't know. You have either got it or you haven't.

ROWENA: Do you think you can tell early on if someone is going to be a success or not?

ERNEST: By halfway through the course you can tell, I think.

ROWENA: So what is it?

ERNEST: The ones that have it understand the more subtle. They are not always looking on the outside and on the outer; they understand the inner. You see, I once had a patient complain about the fact I hadn't addressed their physical symptoms and that I hadn't examined them clinically. Afterwards I said to the students who were sitting in, the patient will never benefit from homeopathy because they are only concerned with the outer flow; they are not concerned with anything inner. Obviously we get a tremendous input of skills and experience and professional ability at the NWCH, the students are fantastic and make a big contribution. We attract very good students and it is only very occasionally when we realise we have got someone who is not. They usually leave because they realise they are not suited to this work. It is not very often, because our interview techniques have improved tremendously so we don't need to lose many students.

ROWENA: How many students do you have in the NWCH?

ERNEST: We take between twenty five and thirty five and we don't lose many. A few leave but they often come back. We failed one student who just did not do the work to the required standard.

ROWENA: How do you feel about the new remedies? Do you ever prescribe them?

ERNEST: Rarely. I have seen David Mundy prescribe them and sometimes they work and sometimes they don't. But did you read an article, *Dogmatism in Homeopathy*[71] by Scholten? Briefly, he said if you take Hahnemann's proving of *Arsenicum album* you won't find any *Arsenicum album* symptoms that you prescribe on. The picture of the remedy is ascertained from years of clinical experience. There is another article by Vassilis Ghegas[72] on the same lines. I think the idea of dream provings is not very healthy and I think most modern provings are not very good, but on the other hand I have seen a few excellent ones.

ROWENA: I cannot imagine that someone like Martin Miles, who uses his own remedies, isn't getting results from them; otherwise why would people be going to him? You know what I mean?

ERNEST: It depends on their level of health. What I have found is that people use these methods for advanced pathology. Ordinary patients at better levels of health who are prescribed remedies in that way can consequently have their 'all picture' destroyed and become incurable thereafter.

ROWENA: Realistically, Ernest, how long do you think it takes to set up a busy practice?

ERNEST: Seven years. I didn't start teaching until I had built my practice up but I do remember spending two days a week for a month struggling, writing up all the homeopathic remedies for rheumatism using Herbert Roberts' book *The Rheumatic Remedies and Repertory to the Rheumatic Remedies*[73] as a base, and blow me the next two months I began to get busy with rheumatism patients. You keep working and you tell people what you do. You treat them properly and charge them what is fair for you, and you cannot but succeed.

ROWENA: What lessons do you think are crucial for a homeopath to learn?

ERNEST: Not to want quick results, to wait and be patient and follow the principles.

ROWENA: Do you think there is no such thing as a quick result?

ERNEST: Well, it depends on which of the *Twelve Levels of Health*[70] you are at. It depends on the patient and how good the picture is.

ROWENA: How long have you followed the *Twelve Levels of Health*[70] then?

ERNEST: Well, George Vithoulkas taught this to me in a different form many years ago when it was not quite so simple and clear. I went to Alonissos first in 1984, and even in his early days he used to talk about layers and prescribing within a layer. Prescribing so you get a profound change in health and how patients would then jump onto a layer, which is healthier. So he always had this concept, but with these *Twelve Levels of Health*[70] he has refined it and made it much clearer and simpler to understand and much easier to use and that is in the last five or six years. He has always taught the importance of knowing what level of health your patient is in when they sit in front of you and not to prescribe inappropriately; what to prescribe for first and for which layer. He has always told us that in all his casework and all his teachings.

ROWENA: Do you see homeopathy becoming dormant again?

ERNEST: No, I don't think so. Obviously it depends on the kind of opinion among the people and you cannot predict that and it is said that things go in cycles. But I don't think so. The NWCH is pretty vibrant and I think other good colleges are too.

ROWENA: So why do you think students should come to the NWCH?

ERNEST: Well, we get the best teachers and we have such good fun.

ROWENA: It sounds like it from speaking to you! You have such enthusiasm!

ERNEST: We have got some great people who make good contributions. We are extremely thorough and we have very close supervision. We spend a lot of our income on supervision so the students are constantly looked after. I think that is very important. We have recently just discovered that some students are having difficulty with their contracts - how often they can see their supervisor - so we are working to improve it. We are constantly working on improving things all the time.

ROWENA: I have found that classical homeopathy training is accused of leaving graduates fearful. What do you think of this opinion?

ERNEST: I think it is the opposite. That is what happened at COH. We left there confused and we hadn't been taught classical homeopathy properly. Now our students are very confident. We have got some very good graduates practising in the area and they are all busy.

ROWENA: Thank you very much for your time Ernest. I am sorry we couldn't have met in person but hopefully our paths will cross at some point in the future.

CHAPTER 14: GORDON SAMBIDGE

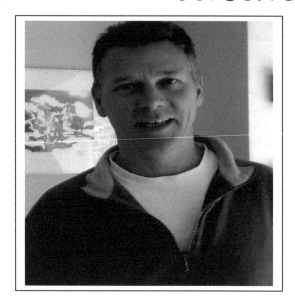

Gordon Sambidge, the principal of the Centre for Homeopathic Education (CHE), the biggest school of homeopathy in Europe and based in Regent's College) in London, kindly invited me to his house not far from my home in Hertfordshire on a beautiful, sunny spring day – Wednesday, 20 April 2005. He greeted me at the door and showed me through to his garden where I met his chickens and all of a sudden I got a sense of de ja vous. It had only been a few weeks since I had visited Misha Norland and his chickens. I wondered if this was prerequisite for being an inspiring teacher of homeopathy.

Relaxing in his sitting room we chatted away for a couple of hours having already met when I was working as an education adviser for the Society of Homeopaths the year before. It was easy to feel comfortable with Gordon, but it wasn't only that. He has a lovely, soft-spoken and rather alluring quality about him; I could have listened all day.

"Homeopathy finds you, you don't find homeopathy."　　　　*Gordon Sambidge, April 2005*

"If I stop practising, I will still be a homeopath and I say that to my students too. I say to them that even if they study homeopathy for one year they will always be a homeopath because every question is then loaded."　　　　*Gordon Sambidge, April 2005*

" To learn homeopathy was so liberating for me, that I want others to have that experience. People start at one point and they transform their belief structures and their spirituality. It is not so much about the homeopathy but taking people through transformation."

Gordon Sambidge, April 2005

CHAPTER 14: GORDON SAMBIDGE

GORDON: I want to set up a Fellowship of Homeopaths and I have spoken to a few of the homeopaths that I would like to join – Tony Hurley, Melissa Assilem, Colin Griffith, Martin Miles, Mike Bridger and Hilery Dorrian. I just want to see what happens with us spending time together debating - even our differences.

ROWENA: What a fabulous idea, and a good name, too.

GORDON: Hopefully something will come out of it and I think everyone will be willing. We are just going to sit around the table and see what comes out.

ROWENA: I think that would be great. Actually, that is part of my agenda with this book. I think what is going on with homeopathy right now is very confusing and hopefully the interviews will provide some clarity. So I wanted to start by asking you how you got into homeopathy in the beginning.

GORDON: Homeopathy finds you, you don't find homeopathy. And in all honesty, it is something that I feel that I was always kind of doing. I went to university and I studied Botany, which is along the same lines as homeopathy but I didn't go to many lectures. I ended up sitting in the coffee bar talking to everyone, gossiping and finding out about their problems. So at university I was already doing it! And then I didn't want to go straight into a career so I just travelled for about five years to lots and lots of different countries. I kind of dropped out and I did every job I could do while travelling. I was a taxi driver for three years in Sydney, Australia. Then I came back and I delivered flowers and then during my last two years before I studied homeopathy, I made my living as a bus conductor. My time spent as a taxi driver and bus conductor was all about people.

And I thought, "Well, I could be a bus conductor all my life if that is what life has planned for me and I will be a good bus conductor or even the best bus conductor." But then I thought that I better go and study because that was not really what I wanted to do! So I contemplated herbalism because I had studied it before in evening classes but I didn't actually want to be a herbalist. I didn't want to be an osteopath either or an acupuncturist. So there was this other one - homeopathy. Coincidentally I had won a book on homeopathy in a raffle, and I thought I should check it out. It was early September 1985 and I phoned up and asked about places to study and was told that the first full-time course in homeopathy was just starting at the College of Homeopathy (COH). The part-time course had already begun. And so I went along for an interview with Barbara Harwood and I was basically told that I could join if I had the money. So I enrolled and sat for the first few weeks with my eyes popping out of my head, realising how right homeopathy was for me.

I think I was always meant to be a homeopath. Even when I was a taxi driver, I was interviewing people about their lives. I very much feel that it is an expression of who I am. If I stop practising, I will still be a homeopath and I say that to my students too. I say to them that even if they study homeopathy for one year they will always be a homeopath because every question is then loaded.

So back to your question, I found homeopathy accidentally but it was always meant to be. I was always meant to be a homeopath. It was the right thing at the right time. I wasn't ready to do it any earlier but I was ready when I sat down in that classroom.

ROWENA: So who inspired you back then Gordon?

GORDON: Oh God, everybody! They all did! Robert Davidson was incredibly inspirational as he had a revolutionary way of seeing things. Because I was a bit of an anarchist myself, I loved Robert's rebellion, disdain and anger. I liked his humour too. So he was very inspirational as was Robin Murphy. He came along and put homeopathy in a different framework. A lot of the classical homeopaths really didn't like him and what he was saying and he just disappeared to the USA.

A few years later in 1992, when I was travelling around the USA I decided to search him out and found him in the middle of nowhere right up in the mountains in Colorado. He didn't know me as I had been just one of his many students. I assured him that we in England did not all hate him and persuaded him to come back and teach us. I told him he was the best teacher I had ever had. He was just writing the repertory when I saw him then. Tony Hurley, Roger Dyson, David Mundy and Murray Feldman also taught and inspired me. Credit to them, they were all fantastic. I just soaked it up like a sponge.

ROWENA: And now some of your teachers are teaching with you at CHE.

GORDON: Yes, I like to offer different ways of practising homeopathy. So we have David Mundy who is quite classical, Colin Griffith who is very eclectic and Melissa Assilem who has taken part in a lot of provings. I like to offer the range. A person practises and teaches as an expression of who they are. Some people like to prescribe therapeutically and not look at inner process work whereas others process all the time. Perhaps people who only practise therapeutically have got issues around looking at inner process work and people who are very rigid and only practise one way maybe have issues around being too inflexible.

ROWENA: So what was your practice like before you set up CHE? Did you teach in other places?

GORDON: Yes, I taught at the College of Practical Homeopathy in the Midlands (CPH Midlands) and the College of Practical Homeopathy (CPH) with David Howell and Robert Davidson. They – God love them – gave me the opportunity to teach. And then they made me vice principal of CPH in London.

ROWENA: So why did you set up a college?

GORDON: I like teaching homeopathy and empowering people. To learn homeopathy was so liberating for me, that I want others to have that experience. People start at one point and they transform their belief structures and their spirituality. It is not so much about the homeopathy but taking people through transformation and that is why I love doing it. 1998 was our first year and we got twelve students, which isn't bad. The next year we recruited forty two new students - bigger than any intake around the country.

ROWENA: How did you manage that?

GORDON: Because the homeopaths in the community liked us and what we were doing; the fact that we are not rigid, structured or dogmatic.

ROWENA: Do you think the big numbers then attract more big numbers because it looks like it is a very successful college?

GORDON: Yes, possibly.

ROWENA: How many do you have now in your first year?

GORDON: It is about sixty or something like that. And we have got the degree now as well.

ROWENA: Have you got a full-time course, part-time course and a Masters?

GORDON: No, we haven't developed the Masters yet but we will do. What we want to do in about a year's time is to set up a course which will allow people who have graduated from any college in the country to do a degree and get a BSc in homeopathy in one and a half years. I think that will be quite fun and useful too. There are lots of things I would like to do; it is just a question of finding the time, you know. I am not a workaholic so it is about creating a balance between work and life.

ROWENA: Do you have a busy practice too?

GORDON: I used to have a busy practice. Now I only practise one day a week but I used to see patients four days a week. I work in St John's Wood, on the High Street, where I was born so I haven't moved an inch!

ROWENA: I am interested to know what happened when Barbara closed her college, COH, because you got quite a lot of her students, didn't you?

GORDON: The story is she took over the lease of the Russian Embassy when she bought the London College of Classical Homeopathy (LCCH) from Mary Hood in 1999 and combined it with COH to form the Combined Colleges of Homeopathy (CCH). Basically a bill for one hundred and fifty thousand pounds came in to repair the building and Barbara didn't have the money so she went into liquidation. She asked me if I wanted to take over COH before the Christmas of 2002. I was reluctant but I wanted to facilitate the students to finish their studies so Marcus Fernandez (the vice principal of CHE) and I took a big gamble.

She offered it to us if we ran the course for the last six months of the year without any money. So she kept all the students' fees, including two years' fees for some people, and we contracted to run it for six months in the hope that the students would come back to us at the end of that time and not go to other colleges. If you interview every last one of them now they say that they were really pleased that they did stay but we could have lost fifty thousand pounds easily. The reason I wanted to do it was basically to honour the tradition that had come through COH. From Thomas Maughan, Martin Miles, Robert Davidson and Barbara Harwood who taught Misha Norland, Jeremy Sherr and Tony Hurley – I wanted to honour that tradition and that is why I decided to take the gamble and it was a big one.

ROWENA: So how many students came over to you?

GORDON: Forty five, so not that many. We got the old druid symbol from COH too - the trees, the acorn and the snake going around them.

ROWENA: So tell me who was in your year group at COH?

GORDON: Ian Watson, Sue Josling and Charles Wansbrough who set up the New College of Homeopathy (New College). Charles is a dear friend of mine; we get on like a house on fire. Twenty nine students started the first year and only nine graduated. We were a very revolutionary year with some huge personalities in it. I feel there is something to learn from everyone, always. If you don't resonate with the information, just watch the teacher and you will learn.

ROWENA: So CHE is marketed as a college that teaches both classical and practical homeopathy?

GORDON: Yes, but the reality is that it is not about homeopathy at all. It is about taking people through transformation so that they can sit with another human being in compassion and understanding. Then if you can teach them to have a conversation with someone and then crystallize it into a pill - that is homeopathy. It is like the Steiner school we send our kids to; they don't learn anything about Rudolph Steiner but they are in the system. So it is not about homeopathy; you will learn that if you have got a brain. It is about the process that goes on.

ROWENA: Do you see classical homeopathy as a methodology?

GORDON: Yes, definitely. I would like to give any one of those classicists a difficult case. What do they do when someone is on loads of drugs? What do they do?

ROWENA: What do you do?

GORDON: Well, basically I support the system that is in pathology and then eventually try and get them off the drugs and then deal with the emotional aetiology. But you cannot first do an emotional aetiology, I don't think, because the energy will go up, hit the drugs, hit the pathology, and they will get a huge aggravation and never come back again. It is almost naïve, you know. I think all illness and disease comes from a spiritual, mental and emotional dis-ease. Something is going on and that is the thing that needs to be addressed. That is the problem that goes into the system. You cannot deal with chronic rheumatism with the classical totality remedy on their central state; it doesn't work unless I was a crap classical prescriber.

ROWENA: But you have got classical homeopaths teaching at CHE – so how do they approach those cases?

GORDON: I don't know. I haven't sat down in discussion with other homeopaths. Homeopaths don't sit and discuss what they do very often.

ROWENA: So do you think you will do that within your Fellowship?

GORDON: It is not about discussing cases; it is about discussing where homeopathy is going and the spirit of homeopathy. And it is about also having another voice that isn't a registering body. Registering bodies have too much power. We need another voice.

ROWENA: So within this Fellowship, will you only have people in it that you....

GORDON: Like, yes, exactly. Exactly.

ROWENA: That would make sense.

GORDON: People who deserve to sit around that table. But I haven't done it yet; I haven't organised it.

ROWENA: What makes someone deserve it?

GORDON: I don't know - that I like them and feel easy with them! But I haven't organised it and it's quite a long way from happening but I keep thinking about it. But what I might do is expand it as an organisation so that anyone can join. It is just a question of getting it together. It is not for me; it is for homeopathy. I will tell you why I started the idea of the Fellowship. There is a rose garden outside Regent's College, where I used to play as a child and where CHE is based. One day I was walking with my wife and she noticed a variety of rose called 'Gordon's College.' We couldn't believe it. Months later I showed it to Robin Murphy and he noted the coincidence and asked me if I had set it up but I told him that from my research it had been a variety of rose that had been growing for forty years! Strange isn't it?

ROWENA: Yes. Unbelievable but at the same time, not...

GORDON: Robin Murphy suggested I read it like a sentence including the rose beds to its left and right. So left to right it read 'Rising Star', 'Gordon's College' and 'Fellowship.' So I thought that I would try and set up a fellowship and that is my reason for doing it.

ROWENA: So tell me Gordon, do you ever fail students?

GORDON: Yes, and of course they don't like it very much. But we give them opportunities to improve.

ROWENA: Do they see it coming?

GORDON: Hopefully they do because we interview each student each year, especially the ones that aren't doing well.

ROWENA: What do they usually fail on?

GORDON: The main difficulty I have is their inability to sit with patients. It is their clinical skills - inappropriate case taking, poor rapport skills, no understanding of the case. It is the way they are with another person.

ROWENA: And those are the kind of issues you cover in practitioner development, aren't they?

GORDON: Yes and clinical development. Some students just haven't got the self-awareness to sit with another. People do struggle, and sometimes we don't have the resources to individually support them. Homeopathy should be an apprenticeship where we give students as much as they need but sometimes I feel that we give them too much gold.

ROWENA: What do you mean?

GORDON: We give them great, wise teachers with twenty or thirty years of experience; Mike Bridger, Hilery Dorrian and Tony Hurley and they are getting gold, lecture after lecture. It is just always there but maybe we are giving them too much that they are not autonomously digging themselves. We are spoon-feeding them. We need to have a look at that – that is the latest flavour at the moment.

ROWENA: Do you think that can be disempowering sometimes as well?

GORDON: Yes, totally, but we don't try and set it up that you can only practise homeopathy 'this well' after twenty years. We do try and make it very simple as we are 'training' homeopaths. The only way homeopathy will ever expand is by homeopaths working out there in the public and being successful.

ROWENA: So how do you build that confidence?

GORDON: Letting them do it, and not judge them by their mistakes.

ROWENA: So they start practicing early on in their studies?

GORDON: Yes, by the second or third year. They realise that homeopathy is safe and the only way you learn is by experience.

ROWENA: Do you think it is always safe?

GORDON: Yes, more or less, unless it is in the hands of a complete idiot who gives someone with eczema *Sulphur 10M*. Most of the time it is very, very safe. I don't think there are situations that can be too damaging and if you get a balanced practitioner then they won't do the stupid things. If you get someone who is not balanced, they are capable of making ego based decisions like for example, prescribing *Plutonium nitricum* in order to blow a closed patient open. This is perhaps a projection of ones own sense of needing to be blown open. But generally it is very safe and students are confident. After four years part time they are itching to get out and practise.

The main teachers of homeopathy are your patients. I can write a certificate with your name on it and say you have completed training in homeopathy for three or four years but that isn't what makes you a homeopath. It is your patients that make you a homeopath. You start to feel you are a homeopath when people come back to you and give you money. It is not the certificate on the wall but your community that makes you a homeopath. The patients are your greatest teachers by far. No one teaches you homeopathy like they do.

196

I practise homeopathy because it helps me grow. I sit with other people and I grow, expand and look at myself. I sit with students and I get reflected back. In this work you can think you are an important person but really you are just a servant.

ROWENA: Do you think that homeopathy will become dormant again?

GORDON: I don't know and I don't really care. It is like once upon a time, there was a castle and it stood in a beautiful garden. I don't know what future generations have for themselves but I was allowed to practise homeopathy. I was allowed to teach homeopathy. And maybe, when I die, I will go to that place where there is homeopathy all the time. But I don't know what the karma is of future generations.

It is now that there is homeopathy like this. It is what it is now and it will move on. There is a wonderful Rumi poem called *The Drunkards*[74]. He says that every so often there is a generation that comes that shifts something. "They had gold sown into their cloaks for those who did not have gold." And it is like, there was once a time that homeopathy was quite big and maybe it won't crumble or maybe it will. I don't know.

ROWENA: What ingredients do you think make a good, successful homeopath – one that practises, earns money and can actually sustain him or herself?

GORDON: You have to love other people, whoever they are; otherwise you get bored of it. It is that simple.

ROWENA: What about business skills; do you teach those?

GORDON: Yes, we do. To be successful you do need to be quite pushy. You need to believe in yourself and that can come from natural enthusiasm and love for the subject. So you need love for people and love for the subject. Being aware of boundaries is also important and you have to have the ability to sit with others and let your own ego go. You have to focus on another, like a mother with a newborn baby. Your time is focused twenty four hours on that baby and your ego is removed. If you sit eight hours a day with patients you have to surrender your ego and be with the other.

This can be an area of difficulty for some and so they give up. When you surrender the ego, what comes up? Your shadow and it says things like, "Let's try something else", "Let's go to India", "Let's go travelling", "Let's go and do a seminar" or "Let's go and take up golf". Your shadow is where all the desires that you have never fulfilled in your life, come up and grab you. And then you say, "Hi shadow, what's your game?" and you play with it. That is what happens with homeopaths. You practise and sit with others; your shadow comes up and then most of the work is negotiating the shadow.

You sit and analyse a case and decide for example that it is dragonfly but the thing you don't analyse is, why you got this case to begin with. We should question what each case is telling us about ourselves. When you honour that, it is easier to sit with compassion.

ROWENA: What kind of books do you think are really must reads for homeopaths when they study? The *Organon*[4]?

GORDON: I wrote it out, word for word. I just sat down and wrote every aphorism. I have still got it somewhere around but I haven't picked it up since. I needed to make sense of what Hahnemann was talking about.

ROWENA: Wonderful. Would you recommend your students do that?

GORDON: They might all leave the course if I asked them to! You have got to make it easy for them. When I was studying I had a lot of time on my hands and I was very committed. I fell in love with it; it was like my first romance. I think Kent's *Lectures* [61] are great. He really had amazing insight into homeopathy and was an incredible homeopath. He totally changed the game, as did Rajan Sankaran. But bring Rajan Sankaran over to London now and he wouldn't know what to do. He would come up with some good ideas but following a case through for six months or a year, would be difficult because of all the allopathic intervention and pollution. I think he says himself he wouldn't want to practise here. I like Martin Miles' book *Homoeopathy and Human Evolution*[75], especially the beginning. It is a great book and he is a lovely man.

ROWENA: We are very lucky to be homeopaths, aren't we Gordon? It gives us that opportunity endlessly to.....

GORDON: Critique!

ROWENA: Yes! That is why I like my subject area of practitioner development because process will come up the whole time.

GORDON: It will do. It always comes up and it is almost denied in homeopathy and yet it is such a big part. There are two ways to work, you can see twenty people a day or you can work more on process and spend longer with each person.

ROWENA: Do you work more on process then?

GORDON: Generally, yes. I like to see eight people a day.

ROWENA: That is still a lot.

GORDON: I know it is a lot.

ROWENA: And it is exhausting.

GORDON: Oh God, I have been doing it for years. Sometimes I don't know how I do it.

ROWENA: Sometimes I see five cancer patients one after another because I work in a complementary cancer care centre.

GORDON: Oh God, that is exhausting. Working with cancer patients is big.

ROWENA: They have such huge stories.

GORDON: It is great that you are working in a cancer care centre. Are you doing it because it is a great job, it makes you a bit of money or you are helping people? What is your spiritual intention? Is it to do with your own growth and development?

ROWENA: This is what I am meant to be doing. I was led in this direction. You know how it is! Gordon, thank you, it has been great chatting with you today.

CHAPTER 15: SHEILAGH CREASY

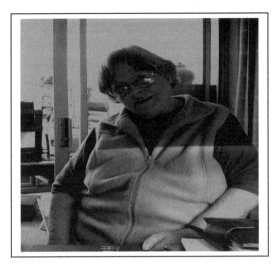

Tuesday 26 April 2005 took me to the home of Sheilagh Creasy. She was what the London College of Classical Homeopathy (LCCH) was all about for me. Inspiring, passionate, strong, experienced and endlessly knowledgeable; I learned so much from her. I have also attended several of her postgraduate seminars in Euston since graduating and admire her dedication and perseverance unconditionally. For me there is also something about her energy, perhaps she reminds me of my grandmother when I was a child, but she brings up memories in me of feeling protected and listened to. She is a lady whom I truly admire and have a lot to be grateful for.

"To cut a long story short, my grandmother taught me from about the age of eight, nine or ten what this thing called homeopathy was about so I was imbued with the idea from then."
Sheilagh Creasy, April 2005

"The starting point of my teaching is always, of course, the Organon[4]. You have to study the different editions and know where he was coming from. The same as you have to study his Chronic Diseases [76] and the Pura[77] and know in which era it was written. He was an innovator and as an innovator he experimented in producing something different because he found it was an improvement on what he had said previously."   *Sheilagh Creasy, April 2005*

"When classicists are accused of being rigid and inflexible, I feel like this is throwing bricks in total ignorance."
Sheilagh Creasy, April 2005

"The idea is not to teach too much, too soon as students don't know where they are. They need to learn the straight and narrow and then gradually that broadens."
Sheilagh Creasy, April 2005

CHAPTER 15   SHEILAGH CREASY

ROWENA: Tell me how you got into homeopathy, Sheilagh.

SHEILAGH: My grandfather was a doctor and my grandmother married him knowing homeopathy. And so she pretty well told him, and that was in those days, that she was going to continue with her practice. Meanwhile, they couldn't make ends meet in Ireland – that is where they were, in Cork. Of course there was incessant famine; he used bacon, scones and eggs and whatever the farm produced to feed the family but thought, "This is not good enough for my three boys", so he applied for the Foreign Service. Through the Foreign Service they were posted to the Andaman Islands, a colony of India when the British colonials were out there. He was the doctor there on the island, employed by the state and my grandmother continued as ever, with her homeopathy. The three boys eventually were sent to Edinburgh for their university training and my grandmother continued. To cut a long story short, my grandmother taught me from about the age of eight, nine or ten what this thing called homeopathy was about so I was imbued with the idea from then. When it came to me needing homeopathy myself, I was still pretty young so then I immediately sought the books and that is how it started.

ROWENA: Please carry on; tell me more……

SHEILAGH: I thought that I must be a doctor in order to learn homeopathy but, of course, circumstances, including the war, got in the way and I went into British Intelligence. After the war ended my husband's firm requested that he return to Shanghai. He had legged it from Shanghai away from the Japanese and got on to a Yangtze boat and boarded a ship with five others, and they joined up the minute they got to India and Bangalore. So his firm requested that he return to China to help release those who had been caught and were imprisoned and had had a very bad time.

We returned on a troop ship and if you have never been on a troop ship you haven't experienced anything! I was surrounded by men, nothing but men, and they wanted to sing all night and go sentimental or something like that and it was six weeks to Shanghai! The first thing that hit me is that I had got used to the smell of India, but the new smell of China was something else that was really new. We had a company house all ready and waiting for us but a terrible tragedy happened there. The firm had a wool making factory and the Japanese who took over these beautiful houses decided the only way to deal with the heads of the wool firm was to behead the leaders of every department. So the managers of every department were beheaded in the field near by. So that is what we were told.

ROWENA: Keep going Sheilagh please; your story is fascinating. Were you practising homeopathy at this time?

SHEILAGH: Not officially. I was practising just as an ordinary person but not officially.

ROWENA: So what inspired you in those days?

SHEILAGH: Right from the beginning I was fortunate, putting my hands on the right books precipitated by the *Organon*[4]. The *Organon*[4], Clarke's *Materia Medica*[28], Boericke[39], Kent's *Lectures*[61] and later on the other physicians. I thought, "Well, when I know more than Kent I will beg to differ." So I was always struggling to know how this man knew as much as he did. And I went on and on struggling and whatever he said and did, I followed it up. I kept on following up any lead including the Swedenborg reference. By then we had returned to England.

ROWENA: So what did you think of Swedenborg?

SHEILAGH: I have got all his books there behind you. Fascinating. He is called a mystic, but I soon realised that this man was a scientist. He was sent by the King of Sweden to further his research over here in England. In Swedenborg House in London, you can pick up the threads of a fellow called Frederick Quin who was the first to bring homeopathy over here. Skinner was another early one too. I soon realised that Swedenborg had got an awful lot of information but I wondered where he got it from. So I got digging and I found that its roots were from ancient Judaism. So I then started a new quest and started reading the ancient Jewish books and the Kabbalah[78]. Eventually I discovered and studied The Tanya[79] and that was the only one that really resonated; it was just like homeopathy. The principles of homeopathy are all in there.

ROWENA: Do you think Hahnemann read those books?

SHEILAGH: In my opinion Hahnemann was Jewish and I will tell you why. For sixteen or seventeen years I gave seminars in Europe and the USA. At a seminar in Germany two women with a sort of cross and a neat uniform asked me if I would come to their monastery to help treat their patients whenever I returned. I said yes, provided they pick me up at the airport and drop me back. They agreed and that is what took place. When I came to Hamburg, they used to attend the seminar and then we would drive towards Belarus and the monastery was there. They were all medical doctors and we would be talking all the way in the car. The monastery was in a very old agricultural area and I noticed there were stones sitting in the middle of a field. I enquired about them and was told that they were for the various spirits to bless the crops. The monastery consisted of three, enormous, beautiful Tudor barns. And the farmers, as soon as they knew this group of doctors wanted to administer to the poor and look after them, donated a barn which they converted and then they gave another barn and so on and so on. The whole thing built up from these barns including a little chapel.

We used to have meetings and then in the evening there would be the homeopathic sessions treating people who had come. They would ring the bell at the gate and the gate would be opened and they would say, "Come", and a group of us would be sitting about taking the case. It would be German translated and later on it became Russian, German and English, and we would be taking the most interesting cases all by candlelight. I went to the chapel and attended the services and they asked me to talk at their little meetings. There would be a group of us and endless cups of tea but you know in Germany, in the cold weather, they had their little cups of tea on the burners, so it was perpetually hot.

ROWENA: Fabulous.

SHEILAGH: I loved it. So when I was talking, the leader of this monastery, the one who escorted me everywhere, suddenly went "Ah" and she said in German, as she couldn't speak any English, "Ask her where she gets it from." I thought that I had been caught this time because it was not Hahnemann but Swedenborg through Hahnemann. So I had to say, "It was Swedenborg", and immediately I heard back, "Yes, but Swedenborg got it from where?" and I replied, "Well, it is from the ancient Jewish sources." That is when she told me she was Jewish and she had started this Judea-Christian community of doctors and that got her telling this other tale. She had started it because she had been exiled from France because she was Jewish and had literally legged it. She was allowed to practise because she was a doctor, but they were after her because of her Jewish ancestry. So we went full tilt and discussed that I thought Hahnemann was Jewish. I said, "Because he uses certain phrases; there are, to my knowledge, four references in the *Organon*[4] in terms of spheres but they are hidden away."

ROWENA: What do you mean by spheres?

SHEILAGH: They are the shells of the Jewish words and they are beautiful. The unravelling is one word, the shell itself is another word and the potencies are all there too.

ROWENA: I know that he influenced potencies.

SHEILAGH: So the potencies are there, the degrees are there, the spheres are there and the Law of Similars is there too.

ROWENA: All in the *Tanya*[79]?

SHEILAGH: All in the *Tanya*[79]. This has been a study of mine for thirty five years but I have had to shut up; I haven't been able to speak about this.

ROWENA: Why?

203

SHEILAGH: You cannot speak about this kind of thing in homeopathy colleges. For example, there are volumes of Swedenborg's *Concordance*[80]. If you say to me a word, like 'suffering' I could look it up in the *Concordance*[80] and it would give me my references in the Old Testament. That is Swedenborg; how he had time to write it all, God only knows. All the principles, the laws and the potencies are all there.

ROWENA: So this was a big area for you. Did that get you more into homeopathy?

SHEILAGH: For thirty five years I just was buried in it. Kent led me to Swedenborg. I always thought homeopathy was very spiritual in many ways but I did not understand why I felt dissatisfaction? But I discovered in time that the dissatisfaction was the fact that I did not understand where he got all his information. And I went on and on trailing it.

ROWENA: So why do you think it took so long for homeopathy to come about?

SHEILAGH: Because that is homeopathy. Knowledge is one thing but these are the degrees I am talking about. Knowledge is an outer degree; understanding is the inner degree.

ROWENA: So we weren't ready?

SHEILAGH: Yes, we weren't ready. So the outer degrees were all there, but I had to get to this inner degree, which was the understanding. So when the understanding opened, the new search started.

ROWENA: Why Hahnemann?

SHEILAGH: Throughout the ages from time immemorial, there has always been in the forefront the Jewish leader in whatever field; from literature and music to science and medicine. I come from no Jewish background at all so I am not biased but this is what I firmly believe. I have tried to trail the story of Judaism and how they had to trek, trek, trek because they were always being hounded. So I read this historically, and I thought, "Here they pop up again, why?" And that started this trail of thinking and I believe that they have always been chosen to lead in whatever the field.

ROWENA: I do remember you touching on this at LCCH fleetingly. How on earth do you avoid it when you are teaching?

SHEILAGH: God, I have a hard time.

ROWENA: I imagine so. I guess it is like missing out on sharing a huge part of your soul.

SHEILAGH: I would have been hauled over the coals if I were to bring religion into it.

ROWENA: That is true. Ok, so going back to your journey, how long ago were you working in the monastery?

SHEILAGH: It was comparatively recently. It was after the Chernobyl disaster and I was brought in on the cases of those who were affected by it. And that reminds me of another story. From the monastery they would go and collect thirty to forty people and bring them down from Belarus on the buses. They had to bribe their way past the guards and bring them to the monastery where they recovered. They were given food and lodging, and only one request was asked of them; a little work to help the monastery. Some helped out in the agricultural area. Anybody from the farms among the Russians, the first thing they wanted was to be with the cows and the goats outside. We had refectory tables, as it was communal eating, and we would first pray and then eat; beautiful food straight off the farm. Nothing was ever wasted.

ROWENA: And they were being treated with homeopathy?

SHEILAGH: The only treatment they received was homeopathy. We would be discussing it in the mornings and meet again in the evenings after supper at four o'clock. The nights were our own to do with what we wished. The others loved the nights but I am not a late night one as I am an early riser so that was the hard part where I was concerned. Otherwise the Chernobyl cases were fascinating. These people were very ill and there were one or two deaths there. A Hodgkinson's one was a direct result of the Chernobyl disaster; yes we were really nurturing them for months on end.

ROWENA: Did you feel homeopathy made a big difference?

SHEILAGH: Homeopathy did a lot for them; that is all they were getting. They were getting nothing else. Strange things happened there also. I would ask the leader of the house, "Where do you get your money from? I mean this place needs money to survive." At one of our meetings this radiant, typical German housefrau with red cheeks came in beaming from ear to ear. She had letters with her and the leader of the community opened them and she would hold up a cheque and another cheque and the cheques would keep coming. And the architects who did the renovation to the barns would take no money for their services.

ROWENA: Does this place still exist?

SHEILAGH: Yes it does. What else do you want me to tell you?

ROWENA: So tell me Sheilagh, who have you studied with?

SHEILAGH: Noel Puddephatt. I wanted to have somebody here in England to study with. At the time my husband's firm had sent us out to South Africa to open up the market there. It must have been in the 1950s. There I really did a lot of homeopathy. Our contract was that we lived there for three and half years and then we would get leave back to England for six months and then the cycle would be repeated. While in South Africa I decided I needed a contact in England and Noel came my way and I thought, "Oh, this is interesting. He knows Kent well." Then I wrote to *Health Science Press*[81] and through them, communicated with Phyllis Speight. Phyllis Speight and Noel had been in clinic working together.

Health Science Press[81] used to put out a magazine, which Noel Puddephatt used to write in. When I came to England I contacted Noel and I found him quite knowledgeable on homeopathy, more than I was.

ROWENA: So he was a lay homeopath as well? Where did he learn homeopathy from?

SHEILAGH: He had learnt from John Clarke. So I was now really pleased with this connection because years later, Ted, my husband who wasn't in the homeopathic thinking field, when I brandished my Clarke's *Materia Medica*[28] he said, "That's funny, I remember John Clarke coming to my grandparents home, he was a homeopath, yes I remember now, a homeopathic doctor'. It is Clarke's *Materia Medica*[28] that I find interesting. His *Repertory*[82] is too awful for words but his *Materia Medica*[28] is good. Why there should be this discrepancy between them, I don't know. Perhaps he wrote one years before the other.

So Noel Puddephatt and I would discuss problematic cases. I would write to Noel and Noel then said to me, "I have another student by the name of George Vithoulkas, an electrical engineer, and he has accepted a post in South Africa and I have given him your name and address. He will be contacting you because he is very eager and very keen on homeopathy. Soon enough, every Saturday, George and I would meet at my flat around the dining room to talk homeopathy.

ROWENA: Where?

SHEILAGH: In Johannesburg, South Africa. I have got marks on the table where we were laying down the law one to the other, quoting this and quoting that. We were absolutely meticulous like two bulldogs!

ROWENA: Were you in agreement with each other?

SHEILAGH: Yes, he was very keen and he knew his stuff. We were heading in the same direction and Noel Puddephatt was guiding us but we were naturally there. One day Noel said that he had had enough of the cold weather in England; he and his wife were suffering a bit of ill health. At that time his wife got a telegram from a solicitor in the USA, from a solicitor asking her to please come to the USA immediately. Her flight, accommodation and everything would be seen to and it would be to her advantage. So both of them set off to New York I think and while there she received the good news that she had inherited the whole of the Singer sewing machine empire. She was sixteenth in line of next of kin; not the first, second or third but sixteenth. They couldn't trail those closer; perhaps they had all died. So they got back to England and Noel, who was working for the Shell Company at the time, had to pack up and leave because of super bracket tax. And that is when he really concentrated on homeopathy. He then put the idea into her head that they needed the warmth and they came out to South Africa, at the drop of a hat.

ROWENA: So there was Noel Puddephatt, you and George.

SHEILAGH: First of all it was George Vithoulkas and I for two years, then Noel Puddephatt said, "Now get ready, when I come there had best be a group of people." So I had already organised a group of people. At that time radionics had loomed fast here and was used among the GPs in the UK.

ROWENA: Could you explain a little bit about what that is?

SHEILAGH: It was a De La Warr machine. First of all it was the Abrams machine, then it became the Rae machine and then it became the De La Warr. It is rife now. I thought the best way to find out about it at the time was on plants, not human beings. I knew that certain plants had growths and fungus and I would experiment but in the end I just threw it all in the dustbin because I though it better and more reliable to use my intellect and understanding rather than using strange psychic phenomena. I had at least tried it so I was open-minded. Then I kept my own records and I did so for twenty years.

ROWENA: Records of what?

SHEILAGH: Everyone who used the De La Warr or radionics developed growths and tumours.

ROWENA: The practitioners?

SHEILAGH: Yes. I kept records in South Africa and when I came here I thought that I better start again since I was back into the homeopathic swing. The same thing was soon revealed; they developed growths and tumours, usually in or on the head.

ROWENA: Not the patients but the homeopaths and the doctors that were using the radionics machines; like the machines that are used nowadays?

SHEILAGH: That is right.

ROWENA: So what do you think that is about?

SHEILAGH: I don't know and I don't understand it. Anyway, back to Noel Puddephatt in South Africa; I formed the group with George Vithoulkas for Noel and we would be doing this and we would be doing that and then George announced he couldn't learn anymore and was going off to India to meet his guru, Jiddu Krishnamurti. So off to India he went and then the tales from India came back which they always do and they were picked up by those who were coming here to the UK to teach.

ROWENA: So what kind of tales?

SHEILAGH: Platinum tales. You know *Platina* so you know what I mean by Platinum Tales.

ROWENA: I though that is what you meant.

SHEILAGH: I think a couple of years went by and the next thing was a letter from George Vithoulkas from the USA or Greece I cannot remember now. He had now teamed up with the American GPs.

ROWENA: Roger Morrison?

SHEILAGH: Yes and others too who were very eager to start a homeopathic forum. I was giving seminars in Germany at the time so I was picking up what was happening and heard that they were collecting money, in the USA, to build George Vithoulkas' clinic and his school in Alonissos. And so that is the tale that was told, which lasted over a period of a few years. And then Noel Puddephatt said to me one day that the weather was stinking hot and he was wearing this English tweeds waistcoat and coat and I thought he must be really cold. I realised that something was the matter and it was his liver. He was now in a bad way and within forty hours he was hospitalised as he was haemorrhaging and he died of cirrhosis of the liver. That was that. Meanwhile George Vithoulkas was installed in Greece. The clinic hadn't started then, he was just giving seminars and teaching and he was writing his two books with the help of Vassilis Ghegas. They are a very good introduction to homeopathy.

ROWENA: The *Science of Homeopathy*[31]?

SHEILAGH: Yes, yes.

ROWENA: And the *Essence of Materia Medica*[30], what do you think of those?

SHEILAGH: I don't. They are all stereotypes and in practice you don't find your essences like that. Those whose practise is only essences are not in practice.

ROWENA: Is that when you started feeling differently towards George Vithoulkas or was that earlier?

SHEILAGH: I never felt anything, I just thought that he had gone that way and I had gone this way. But information kept on coming back and then finally there was the New Zealand historian who wrote his book, *The Faces of Homeopathy*[43].

ROWENA: Ok, Julian Winston.

SHEILAGH: Yes. It transpired that George Vithoulkas had said that he had taught me. And so I got a message back to Julian Winston asking him if he had done his research to which he replied that he had. I then asked him, if he was going to use my name, why did not interview me. So that is how that came to a head. None of this is true and what is more is that there are at least four homeopaths alive who knew about George and me meeting regularly to study.

ROWENA: I suppose it makes him the leader. There is no one who came before him that is still around.

SHEILAGH: But the tragedy is that the practitioner here in England has a great deal of responsibility when they take on cases; they need to work directly with the patients and make many responsible decisions. In Greece it really is paper cases; you can only legally work through a doctor. So you get the GP coming to the seminar with the case and George Vithoulkas deals through the doctor. That is three-way; it is not a direct responsibility. I think it is a different sort of homeopathy here in comparison with there, with another kind of learning.

ROWENA: So what do you think about the state of homeopathy in our country now?

SHEILAGH: The latest *CORH booklet*[83] was not a shock; it was heading that way.

ROWENA: Which bit?

SHEILAGH: The questionnaire; to reply to all those questions, which took about three or four days, I knew very well I was doing it with my tongue in my cheek because it was just like an audit. And what is an audit? The lowest common denominator in the end; that is what this is and this is what it is going to be. The lowest common denominator which means that trash can join and trash can be homeopathy.

ROWENA: So my next question is how do you think we can stop homeopathy becoming dormant again?

SHEILAGH: I think every homeopath should read Harris Coulter's *Divided Legacy*[56] from start to finish and they will see that the USA went right through this; the world went right through all this already. The allopathic doctors took over because they had the means, the money, the schools, the colleges and so students studied naturopathy, medical sciences and the naturopathic way of doing homeopathy and that is not homeopathy.

ROWENA: So what do you think homeopathy education should be? If you were to design a course what would it be?

SHEILAGH: Well I have designed it; I designed the original course.

ROWENA: Ok, talk me through that. Was this when you came back from South Africa?

SHEILAGH: Oh yes, it has to be with the *Organon*[4] as your basis.

ROWENA: Let us just go back, because I have missed a huge piece of your history here. When did you come back from South Africa?

SHEILAGH: After my husband's retirement. Initially we semi-retired; we went to our holiday home, which was a sort of little chalet overlooking the lake and the sea in the Cape. Originally we were in Johannesburg.

ROWENA: How long did you live in South Africa?

SHEILAGH: About sixteen years. We lived at this chalet where I practised a lot of homeopathy in as much as I was dealing with totally different cases to the Johannesburg scene.

ROWENA: Was it all private practise in South Africa?

SHEILAGH: Yes.

ROWENA: Different in what way?

SHEILAGH: Now I was dealing with farms; not cattle but the labourers. The truck would drive up and it would be full of the patients that you would see during the day. The cases were just unreal; I would treat worms that came from the nose and yaws on the legs; syphilis in children.

ROWENA: Was this the time of Apartheid?

SHEILAGH: Yes it was the time of Apartheid; the ANC were loud and clear up north.

ROWENA: Did you treat black people as well?

SHEILAGH: Yes, always and there I was able to really understand the miasms because I saw them coming up.

ROWENA: And the Afrikaaners?

SHEILAGH: Yes. There were quite a few Germans who owned the farm.

ROWENA: So that was some huge learning for you.

SHEILAGH: That was a big learning for me, yes.

ROWENA: So is your husband interested in homeopathy?

SHEILAGH: He is very interested but he never takes part because it is just not his scene.

ROWENA: Is he open-minded?

SHEILAGH: Very, oh Lord yes, the whole family have been brought up this way; he is very open-minded.

ROWENA: And you have a daughter?

SHEILAGH: Two.

ROWENA: Two daughters - are they this way inclined?

SHEILAGH: One is still in South Africa. She was at Guy's hospital and specialises in resuscitation or whatever name they gave it. So she went back to South Africa but then went on to Zimbabwe because in South Africa, there was a requirement to speak and write Afrikaans. In Zimbabwe she joined a hospital; the war started and she was dealing directly with the war injured, the mines and blasting. She fled soon after because the war had got too intense, joined the Kensington General Hospital in Johannesburg and was doing resuscitation. She used to come back with tales galore. Once they pulled the plug out of the electricity but had to revive this fellow. They had used everything including jolts but he had flat lined. Then the next thing, the so-called dead person's eyes opened and he said, "Could I not have a pillow?"

ROWENA: So not with homeopathy?

SHEILAGH: Not with homeopathy. Then she realised that other than her field, which was really resuscitation, she wasn't interested in ordinary nursing. She would do it, but her fascination was in resuscitation. She started going through my books and demanding I teach her. She now practices homeopathy in South Africa. And now comes the South African tale; legislation came just like in the USA.

ROWENA: So you cannot practise unless you are.....?

SHEILAGH: No legislation came when I was there, so if you practised, you practised illegally. So I continued to do so for years. Then they brought back legislation after fifteen years they had a system; 'A' register, 'B' register or 'C' register. 'A' register is if you had any medical background and homeopathy, so she is in on the 'A' register with the entitlement of doctor. 'B' register is without the medical background but if you have done homeopathy and gone through a college. 'C' register is if you want to practise and have done some studying here and there; it is called mongrel homeopathy. And that is how you come in. They had to do this because of the witch doctors that by entitlement would be treating thousands, passed on by word of mouth from grandmother to grandmother.

ROWENA: Did the witch doctors practise homeopathy?

SHEILAGH: No, but they had their entitlement on an 'A' register or 'B' register or 'C' register. This worked for disciplines such as herbalism, which is more like what they practised. It proved to be a good system. I then took a degree in philosophy and that is when I did my medical sciences at a university in South Africa as a sort of manoeuvring. I had to take sixteen subjects; I took art and I used it to teach art to disabled and mentally disturbed people. So that was another area of fascination for me because I was using homeopathy as well as the art to bring out their issues.

ROWENA: So the art gave you a useful tool to see what was going on?

SHEILAGH: Yes. When I was in the Cape, I ran quite a lot of workshops on art for homeopathy and I held exhibitions of the work. It was a fascinating area, seeing it all the way through, teaching them and then giving them an incentive for exhibitions for sale.

ROWENA: Do you know Brian Kaplan?

SHEILAGH: Yes, I have heard of him.

ROWENA: His wife is a South African art therapist. I recently went to a seminar and she was explaining that some of his patients he refers to her and she sends the art back to him.

SHEILAGH: It is a field that could easily be used here but abused as well if we are not careful. It is a very interesting field. I always give pieces of paper to little children for their drawings and see how they develop.

ROWENA: So when did you come back here?

SHEILAGH: I cannot remember when it was but we have been in this house for twenty years. When I came back I joined and was a director of the Society of Homeopaths. At that time both leaders in our field over here had died: Thomas Maughan and John Damonte.

ROWENA: That was in the early 70s, I think.

SHEILAGH: There were a few floating ones like Jeremy Sherr and Misha Norland.

ROWENA: And Robert Davidson.

SHEILAGH: When I say floating, it is because there had been these two leaders and now there was a sort of a hole. Robert Davidson and Martin Miles set up the first college, the College of Homeopathy, at Imperial College and that is when I came in on the scene. Wendy Singer spoke to Robert Davidson about me and said that I had been practising for many years and I got an invitation to come and teach at the College of Homeopathy. And if only you saw the hundreds...

ROWENA: Of students every year?

SHEILAGH: Imperial College is big enough, but when you came up those stairs the whole foyer was full of students; every classroom was packed.

ROWENA: So you taught there.

SHEILAGH: Yes. Robert Davidson always kept aloof but he was very polite and always kind to me, as was Barbara Harwood. Before Barbara came Anne Saunders. She was Anne Bickley then, Anthony Bickley's wife. Jeremy Sherr seemed to be holding well, knowing exactly where he was going. He was also very nice. Misha Norland, likewise. Murray Feldman was around too. I taught at the Tiverton College of Classical Homeopathy for some time and by then I had already started the seminars in the USA and Europe. I did that for sixteen years.

ROWENA: So are you still teaching internationally then?

SHEILAGH: No, I stopped all international teaching at the same time. Too much was going on here and I was away about four to five days a month. When I went to the USA it was for longer as I started a school there called The Northern California Institute of Classical Homeopathy. And I was involved with Anne Larkin's London College of Classical Homeopathy (LCCH).

ROWENA: Where I studied and met you.

SHEILAGH: Yes. Then Lesley Gregerson, who I taught in her third year at Robert Davidson's, started her school, the London School of Classical Homoeopathy (LSCH)) and Ernest Roberts started the North West College of Homoeopathy (NWCH).

ROWENA: I really enjoyed your strong opinions when I was at LCCH, because it was kind of a wake up call. Your passion and love for homeopathy shone through your teaching.

SHEILAGH: Thank you. The starting point of my teaching is always, of course, the *Organon*[4]. You have to study the different editions and know where he was coming from. The same as you have to study his *Chronic Diseases*[76] and the *Pura*[77] and know which era he wrote that. He was an innovator and as an innovator he experimented in producing something different because he found it was an improvement on what he had said previously. Originally, everything came under psora until he learnt that there were other miasms. So we have got to know the chronological order of when he wrote about his findings. It doesn't mean to say we have got to be rigid because in *Aphorism*[4] straight away he said, "You must stick to the principles and the principles which can be clearly adapted...." When he speaks of the succussions and potencies; the pharmaceutical procedure, he says, "My exact procedure". So they are exact, whereas the methodology, so to speak, is adaptable.

ROWENA: That is interesting.

SHEILAGH: When you have advanced enough, I use the word 'advanced' because years 1, 2 and 3 are hardly advanced...

ROWENA: I am in complete agreement with you. At college even though we were told that it is just the beginning, you feel that when you get to the end, you know a fair amount. After a while in practice, I realised that I had only just started my journey.

SHEILAGH: Yes, it is left in your lap. That is why I am a firm believer that some issues should be left to postgraduate years; hence my workshops. Now the postgraduate years are based on a practitioner's experience in clinic, in other words inductive not deductive.

214

Homeopaths soon realise there are different cases, everyone being an individual, and the idea is to follow Hahnemann's principles but learn to adapt according to that patient's vital force.

ROWENA: So at undergraduate level, you teach in a basic and thorough way so that the students learn the fundamentals. Then when they are out in practice you teach practitioners how to individualise and adapt.

SHEILAGH: That is right. Then you can sort it out, because now you are working with a mixed bag of clinic cases, which usually have had masses of suppression, not only allopathically but today homeopathically as well. You are just thrown in at the deep end and you have got to begin to sort this out. So you have got to learn to adapt your cases and ask yourself how you are going to tackle the totality from start to finish.

ROWENA: So if a case comes to you, do you see it in layers?

SHEILAGH: No, there is no such thing as layers.

ROWENA: One totality?

SHEILAGH: It is a totality, but it is like a hologram - spatial and constant fluctuation according to life, circumstances and environment. So this constant fluctuation, like a hologram, will present an uppermost now, and the patient is screaming their pains and aches at you, but there is a lot going on here, which you cannot sort out because it has been suppressed. Now how do you deal with it? And then as things go on, so it moves and that is what you meet with; this hologram.

ROWENA: So, the hologram, would you say that is a relationship of certain remedies that are connected?

SHEILAGH: I work with the relationship of remedies, but it is more than that. I work in the miasmatic unfolding, and it is not like the next one comes along and then the next one; it is nothing like that. It is a hologram, and that is *Aphorism 103*[4] where Hahnemann says that portions appear and disappear. The degrees and spheres must be taken into cognition in every single case, so where to start is the big problem now that you are dealing with a particular case. This is where you learn to adapt and you now start practising from experience. You know when someone comes along and they say that they have got nothing physically wrong with them but they have panic attacks. You know very well that it is more than just a panic attack and that you can end up with a pack of lies, because that is the nature of a mentally disturbed case.

ROWENA: So what do you do with someone who is telling you lies?

SHEILAGH: You get started. Because of the different characteristics, it unravels it. You see them again and they don't remember anything about those packs of lies. It wasn't lies where they were concerned, it was real; but you put that to one side and now you are getting the real story coming up.

ROWENA: When people call to book in with you, do you tell them that it is a process they are going to go through?

SHEILAGH: Yes. I warn them that they cannot expect a miracle and if that is what they want they better go somewhere else. There are no miracles.

ROWENA: I remember you teaching us that if somebody was on the Pill that you wouldn't see them. Is that still the case?

SHEILAGH: They can start their treatment as long as they have an idea that they are going to come off it, because you cannot go bashing your head against the wall. Remedies will only do so much and no more because of the Pill.

ROWENA: Remedies like *Folliculinum;* do you use those?

SHEILAGH: No, I don't because it was not adequately proven.

ROWENA: So you are clear that the remedies you use have to be well proved?

SHEILAGH: Yes. In terms of potencies though, I use homeopathic tinctures all the way through to 50MM.

ROWENA: Would you work up to a 50MM, or would you prescribe them because somebody was that vital that they could cope with such a high potency?

SHEILAGH: I would work up to if the case demanded it. I can only go with what the vital force tells me and that is another lesson. Don't think you are so superior that you can tell that person's vital force how to go about it and what to do. It is the vital force that tells you what to do.

ROWENA: From your postgraduate group I learned how to use LMs without aggravating the case, so I have you to thank for that. For LMs, which I have to say I use a great deal, I have a protocol of prescribing one dose and asking them to call me two day's after with an update on how they are feeling on all levels. In that way we proceed empowered to monitor how the patient's vital force dances with the remedy assessing how frequently they will need a dose to stimulate a healing response gently and without aggravation.

SHEILAGH: You cannot bash away at a vital force without feeling your way as to how that vital force is going to react.

ROWENA: So tell me Sheilagh, what are your views on tautopathy - giving back the allopathic drug in potency to clear the case?

SHEILAGH: Allopathic drugs obviously confuse the case and are a menace.

ROWENA: So if someone comes to you having had breast cancer and is now on Tamoxifen because they have been told that the drug is their best bet in not having a relapse in the future and they have been instilled with fear; what would you say to them?

SHEILAGH: I say after taking the case that I cannot predict a prognosis for their homeopathy treatment until after the remedy. There is no such thing as prognosis before. I only know in my mind's eye, that the case might have gone a bit far if there has been surgery or drugs such as chemotherapy. Now I do wonder what hope there is if the case has metastasised which is often caused by surgery and drug intervention.

ROWENA: So if someone comes to you and they have their lumps removed, and have had radio and chemotherapies and now they are on Tamoxifen; how would you deal with a case like that?

SHEILAGH: Well, in cases like that, I cannot take them off any drug unless they come to that decision themselves, in which case they have to sign a consent form with me. If they want to stay on their drugs I will do my best to keep up their vital force but I will then draw illustrations for them of how homeopathy works to show them what could possibly happen when stimulating the vital force to cure itself.

ROWENA: You draw that so they can understand it?

SHEILAGH: That is why I have those pieces of paper here on the table. I just keep on drawing the circle showing how it started off with a certain symptom and that was treated. Then another symptom arose and that was treated and so on. So I give them at least fifteen minutes of education on homeopathy philosophy and then we go from there. I have got too many like that and they all want the disease treated, not the patient who had it in the first place.

ROWENA: So when you give them remedies, how does it work? Are you looking at a part of the hologram that is uppermost?

SHEILAGH: I have got three approaches: 1) Palliation, 2) Recovery and 3) Cure. Now, common sense tells me what the realistic chance of cure is when there is a lot of suppression in the case. Palliation is mainly where there is a lot of pain; pain or urgency, for example haemorrhage. A person cannot go on and on in pain; they will go down, so in order to keep that vital energy coming up I have got to deal with pain. So here is my totality in that particular instance.

When classicists are accused of being rigid and inflexible, I feel like this is throwing bricks in total ignorance. It is the total ignorance of homeopathy philosophy. Hahnemann's homeopathy has stood two hundred years of the test of time and it was even around before him. The rows that have taken place in the homeopathic world have been about methodology, nothing else - without any knowledge of the inheritances and this palliation, recovery and cure. A cure literally means a return of old symptoms. Now in a cancer case, for treatment to be curative, the patient will have to get a return of old symptoms.

ROWENA: So if someone has had a mastectomy, how would that work?

SHEILAGH: Well, I have treated mastectomy and it has returned to where it originally started with a fury second to none with all the lumps reappearing, and on the back; buboes appearing and that kind of thing.

ROWENA: And then what?

SHEILAGH: Well, you try to deal with all that comes up. There might be pus and haemorrhage, and the patient will need the support of a nurse to change the dressings etc.

ROWENA: That sounds challenging.

SHEILAGH: Yes, it can be.

ROWENA: It puts things into perspective, doesn't it? I work in a cancer care centre established by a general hospital and I had two cases last Friday that came back for their follow ups and I had given them constitutional treatment, one *Lycopodium* and the other *Natrum muriaticum*, and it is amazing to see the process that they are going through and the connections that they are making as to why they got cancer in the first place.

SHEILAGH: But, you have got to now be ready for the relationship of remedies if there is pain, haemorrhage or if there are any other problems.

ROWENA: Which we don't get taught so much at college, but you teach that at your group, don't you?

SHEILAGH: Oh yes. On the road to cure you see all the physical processes of the lump appearing and the discoloration. Eventually you will see the areola enlarging and then the indurations and ulceration.

ROWENA: So has that really got to happen after the remedy for the treatment to be curative?

SHEILAGH: If the body wants it to come out, it won't just choose the exact spot; it can choose the back or another localisation. It has to localise if there is a cure. But if you want to stop this, you can by not treating the whole totality. You can keep to recovery and palliation. Sometimes you cannot take the risk, as the patient will go down with too much coming up. In terms of potency, you definitely do not prescribe LMs or one off doses. You avoid the over stimulus of the vital force and if you can see that they are sensitive then you lay off the deeper remedies. This is when you need to understand the relationship of remedies.

ROWENA: So where do we find more information about the relationship of remedies?

SHEILAGH: It is in our books, one just needs to take the time and effort to study it and to use it. It is important too, though, for it to be used and not abused, because this could easily happen.

ROWENA: So I need to go and look back in Kent and I also need to attend your postgraduate seminars!

SHEILAGH: Also read Farrington[84] and Boenninghausen[85]. These books need study; they each have a merit of their own. It is still homeopathy; just adapting what Hahnemann meant. It is not the methodology that matters; it's the case that matters.

ROWENA: And justifying your actions?

SHEILAGH: Absolutely.

ROWENA: So why do you think you have a reputation of not adapting, moving with the times and being flexible?

SHEILAGH: It is stated in ignorance. If they don't know miasms, if they don't know relationship of remedies, if they don't know about adapting according to each individual case, where do you start talking? You have got no grounds to talk on. Therefore those statements that are made are pure ignorance because they are using methodology as the be all and end all of homeopathy instead of the philosophy. The Society of Homeopaths has got rid of all the principles one by one.

ROWENA: Is that why you moved away from them and left their register?

SHEILAGH: Oh yes. The signs were on the wall a long while ago. All they wanted to do was find new methodologies. Everything is new; it is like the fashion industry. The philosophy is one where you should move with it and not get stuck. Move where and in what direction? How? Principles should not be plucked out of the air. It is fine to innovate, by all means, but see if it works in other cases before making statements.

ROWENA: So, if you were to design a course now, what would it include?

SHEILAGH: First of all read *Divided Legacy*[56], all four volumes. This is going to take them many, many years. I would like them to learn the background of Swedenborg; what he meant and why Kent quotes him. Also why Hahnemann was torn to shreds in Kent's time and the criticism Hahnemann received.

ROWENA: I need to follow that through as well. I have got so much to study!

SHEILAGH: The idea is not to teach too much, too soon as students don't know where they are. They need to learn the straight and narrow and then gradually that broadens. Then when we are into clinic cases, their knowledge and experience broadens more and more because decisions have to be made. For example, which way are we going to get at the totality and then what potencies? Then we are being so broad, that we are really adapting.

ROWENA: Classicists have the reputation that we give one remedy and then wait forever. I know, I know, I hear this all the time. People say, "You're still practising in a classical way? What, you just give one dose of a remedy and wait six months?" And I am thinking, "I never do that, actually."

SHEILAGH: It is such ignorance; this is the tragedy.

ROWENA: Yes, it is. It is very frustrating. So do you think it is unlikely that homeopathy is going to become dormant again? What do you think?

SHEILAGH: It may go through exactly the same sequence of events as the USA, and there will be a few lone voices that will carry it on, and these lone voices, through the history of time, will keep the flame burning.

ROWENA: Like we had with you in the last century.

SHEILAGH: Just the lone voices will carry it on until the lone voices increase again and then another load of rubbish will come in again.

ROWENA: So what do you think are the ingredients that make a successful homeopath now? You know it is pretty much a struggle for people coming out of college.

SHEILAGH: You cannot stand at your clinic door and say, "You are an eczema case and therefore I don't want you." You cannot choose your patients, you have got to take what comes. But just don't try and go beyond your capacity without seeking help, particularly the cases of today, because you can land yourself in it. You have got to be very careful.

ROWENA: And financially successful?

SHEILAGH: You have got to have two jobs. You have got to be either a teacher or have another job outside of homeopathy. I have always said that homeopathy will not earn enough and the Institute of Complementary Medicine, to which I belong to and have done for twenty years, has shown horror at this remark.

ROWENA: Of having two jobs?

SHEILAGH: Yes. A homeopath cannot exist just as a homeopath. They cannot.

ROWENA: Because?

SHEILAGH: The length of time of consultations. There is a limit to how much you can charge. The average person is not going to Harley Street. The reason why those homeopaths there charge so much is that they have got to have a secretary, a nurse and pay that rent. So you have got a poorer circumstance to exist in and you try and keep it as cheap as you can, meeting your VAT, etc. So you realise when sitting down with an accountant as to how much your limitation is in charging patients, and there is a limit.

Then there are certain cases where you offer a concession when you understand their predicament. I work on there being a limit. One could say that if they went to the pharmacist and bought this and bought that, they would soon reach that limit but that is not really an argument against there being a limit. Here is this person struggling and in need and they are ill. They can barely make ends meet so there is a limit. Together with an accountant one needs to work out how much is your legitimate charging for an hour's work in keeping with others. Then you have got a seventeen and a half percent VAT on it and your rental if you are renting a room. This is why you really have to have two jobs and supplement your income in some way or other. I know somebody who charges one hundred and twenty pounds. I do not have many people on my patient list that could pay one hundred and twenty pounds.

I have been busy writing a book *The Integrity of Homeopathy*[86] and it is just about completed.

ROWENA: Great. What is it about?

SHEILAGH: All that I have been talking to you about.

ROWENA: Fabulous Sheilagh, I cannot wait to read it. Thank you so much for sharing all your wonderful stories with me; it has been such a pleasure.

CHAPTER 16:   KATE CHATFIELD

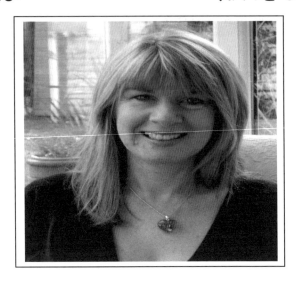

I interviewed Kate Chatfield on Thursday 28 April 2005 on the telephone. We had previously met at the teachers' seminar in Malvern and shared many a meal together, so it was easy to reconnect with her. She spoke to me about her personal experiences as well as on behalf of the course at the University of Central Lancashire where she co-directs the degree with Ian Townsend and Jean Duckworth.

"I am inspired by anybody who can commit their lives to the study and the expansion of the use of homeopathy."   *Kate Chatfield, April 2005*

"I couldn't really say that we produce a particular kind of graduate. What I hope for is that we produce a free thinking graduate who also knows how to reflect on what they are doing."   *Kate Chatfield, April 2005*

"There are all kinds of things that make a successful homeopath. It has got to be something to do with having their basic education, but also being able to adapt and be flexible, so that when they get difficult patients, they know how to find new information, a different style, or a different approach. They need not to be scared or fearful of anything that is coming in. Hopefully our students, our graduates, would not worry about what kind of level of pathology the patients have got, be it on a physical, emotional or mental level."   *Kate Chatfield, April 2005*

CHAPTER 16: KATE CHATFIELD

ROWENA: So my first question to you is, how did you get into homeopathy in the beginning?

KATE: I was eighteen years old and thinking about becoming a medical doctor. While I was doing my science A Level, I won an honour in school to spend some time working in a pharmaceutical company. I went and worked there in the laboratory as a work placement and was really appalled by how they produced drugs and marketed them; you get to know the whole story when you work there.

At the age of eighteen, when I was young and idealistic, I had just thought that all drugs grew on trees. But working in the chemistry laboratory we were playing around with the molecular structures of various medicines, synthesising different products and sending them down to try out on the animals in the biology laboratories to see what they did. It was hit and miss. Then they would adjust them and repeat the process and that went on until they got an interesting result on the animals and then they tried it on humans. It was all about marketing and money and how you had to offer doctors incentives to take on your product and that kind of thing.

ROWENA: So pretty much what is rumoured actually is true from your experience.

KATE: Well it was at that time. So it was a bit shocking for me. And also at the same time, my mother developed breast cancer. Well, she had had it for two years but the doctor had kept turning her away, saying there was nothing wrong with her and that it was in her mind. Then eventually, when he did feel the lump in her breast, he sent her for tests and she had invasive breast cancer. So those two things combined had a big impact on me. Also, at the same time, someone gave me an article on homeopathy to read. So the three things all happened in the same year.

ROWENA: So what year is this?

KATE: 1980. I decided at that point that I wanted to study homeopathy, but I was only eighteen, I didn't have any money, and there were only private colleges around that you had to pay for. I realised I was just going to have to do it later in life after I had my children. So I went and studied philosophy and did some wild things first and then I came back to it.

ROWENA: Where and when did you study?

KATE: I studied at Ernest Roberts" North West College of Homoeopathy (NWCH) in Manchester and started in 1990; I was twenty eight then. I spent ten years waiting to do it but I was reading books around the subject beforehand.

ROWENA: So you have done a lot in the last fifteen years then.

KATE: Yes.

ROWENA: What was your experience like at Manchester?

KATE: Great fun. It was like coming home, being surrounded by a load of other nutcases. When you are out on your own thinking these things, you feel like a real fringe person. It is not that I don't enjoy that, but it is occasionally very nice to go to a place where you can be surrounded by people who are like you. It sort of puts you into a comfort zone.

ROWENA: It is a strange path we have chosen in some ways. It is interesting, isn't it? Who studied with you at that time? Are there any other homeopaths that you know who are still practising from your year?

KATE: My best friend at college was Clare Relton.

ROWENA: Who were your teachers, who inspired you the most?

KATE: I had lots of good teachers, in and out. Dave Mundy was a key teacher at the NWCH. Also Tony Hurley, Anne Saunders and Murray Feldman.

ROWENA: Oh really, he was still teaching then.

KATE: Yes. He was there in my early years. Ian Watson did a bit of teaching for us. I cannot remember anyone else.

ROWENA: Do you remember who had the biggest influence on you, if anyone?

KATE: No. I just took little bits from everybody.

ROWENA: And what about the books that you read; was there something back then that you read and thought, "Yes, this really makes sense to me"?

KATE: Well that would have been before I even studied, when I read George Vithoulkas' *The Science of Homeopathy*[31]. I do remember walking around the house reading bits out to people saying, "You have got to listen to this!" It was driving everybody crazy. So for me, suddenly it clicked. When I read that I thought, yes, that makes sense to me. I cannot remember what year that was.

ROWENA: So who inspires you now, within your practice and your teaching?

KATE: I wouldn't say I have one particular field of inspiration. I am inspired by anybody who can commit their lives to the study and the expansion of the use of homeopathy. I find them all inspiring, but I am not the kind of person that would hook herself into one particular guru. I do love to listen to Rajan Sankaran's teachings, and I think George Vithoulkas has done a lot. I think all of these people are fabulous, but I wouldn't say that I particularly put one above another.

ROWENA: Ok. And how do you practise? It is a really difficult question, isn't it?

KATE: It is eclectic, they way I practise. I know people expect it to be quite classical, but it is not really. I think I am very lucky, in that I had a very solid classical foundation in my education, but I have explored just about every other way. Well of course not every other way, but lots of other ways of practising. Because when you have got a patient that one method is not working for, it makes you look at other ways, and so I have just gone on and on and on. And I would say I have always tried to update what I am doing; my skills. I am a person who loves to go to conferences and seminars; to listen to new things and read new books. So the way I practise is constantly changing.

ROWENA: Are you appreciative of your classical foundations?

KATE: I think it is good to have a way to practise that you can always go back to; that is good. But what I don't like is when people teach that one way is the only way. I think it is great to have a foundation, but it allows you the freedom to go off and explore other areas.

ROWENA: So if you were to have your time again studying, where would you choose? I guess you will say the University of Central Lancashire!

KATE: Yes, you are not kidding! I think the students that come out of our course are so much better educated than I was. It is just much more rounded. With a university approach to education, it is just totally different. You learn so much from working there. It is about freeing up people's minds, rather than stuffing them full of facts.

ROWENA: How did they do that?

KATE: Well, we start off in the first year with encouraging the students to gather facts and learn how to understand the basic principles. When students come in the first year they want black and white, right and wrong. They want to know how the teachers practise and what they would prescribe. They think there is one way, they only want one way. In the first year that is just about all they can cope with. I mean a little bit of challenge, but not too much, otherwise they would all run away scared. But by the time they get into the second year, you want it to be more in some kind of holistic perspective. There is this way, but you have all these other things to think about as well. It is not just about right and wrong. Every case is individual; every person is in their own world and there is a bigger world out there. So you have to put it into the wider perspective.

By the time they get to the third year they need the ability to critically evaluate and reflect on everything that they do. That I think is the key difference in this kind of course. So students write an essay, and they make a sweeping generalisation, they will get a big line through it and me asking them to justify what they have said. Who said this? How do you know that? Where is your evidence? It is about continuously looking at where the information comes from, and constantly thinking about it. Is that right? How do we know that? So, it is just a slightly different emphasis I suppose; teaching them how to be critical and reflective thinkers.

ROWENA: So, how do you feel about colleges that throw their students into the deep end? Classical colleges have the reputation, as I am sure you are aware, of making their students fearful. How do you feel about that?

KATE: I think it is appalling. I really do. Those colleges that teach one way as if it is the way are stuck at first base. It is about giving the students information, and not really expecting them to question it too much. It is a kind of fundamentalist teaching.

ROWENA: And do you think that is still out there?

KATE: I don't know. I wouldn't like to say that because I don't go along to other colleges. It was rumoured to be that way when I was at college. This was the way it was done, no-one questioned it.

ROWENA: At colleges that teach in a 'practical' way; right from the start the students are prescribing remedies. What do you feel about that?

KATE: I am not overly happy with that either. I think students need a little bit of security before they start getting out there. All I can talk about is my own experience, and from my experience the practitioners we produce from our course are really much more confident than graduates that I have seen, say, from other courses. I don't want to mention any names.

ROWENA: Good, nor do I. I am just trying to get your views. I don't want the book to be everybody criticising each other and it hasn't been actually. Otherwise it just gets unpleasant and that is not what it is about at all. It is for raising awareness because there is a lot of confusion out there. I hear it all the time because I have got a classical background and people ask me if I give one remedy and wait six months. It is like, er.....no! I actually give LMs mostly, thanks to Ian Townsend's influence. So tell me about the team that work at the University of Central Lancashire.

KATE: Well we have a core teaching team of three – Ian Townsend, Jean Duckworth and I. The three of us complement each other really well. Now this kind of core team teaching, I suppose, is very different from the private colleges because the three of us will do the bulk of the homeopathy teaching. Of course the students have lots of other teachers, because they have other teachers for the other modules; for their biology, pathology, philosophy, nutrition, and all of those other subjects. The three of us do most of the homeopathy teaching and I was a little bit worried about that at first, because I wondered if they were just going to get our three points of view. But actually it makes it easier to be congruent in the areas that we are covering and the way we are delivering. The students find it hard enough to accept our three different views, let alone twenty perspectives.

ROWENA: It is really confusing when that happens.

KATE: Yes, yes, we have all got our own way, but what we do is communicate a lot, because we share an office all the time. So we see each other on so many days a week that there is an ongoing conversation about how classes are working, what we have just taught, what the next lesson is, and it helps it to flow. We always know if there is something going on in the class. That way we are quick to respond to the students' needs and it does keep us in touch with what the other tutors are teaching. We do complement each other's skills, I think. Ian Townsend is really good on all the reflective stuff.

ROWENA: Yes I know. I had him for a whole year. I think I was very lucky in that respect.

KATE: He does loads of work on the therapeutic relationship. I do most of the philosophy, because my background was in general philosophy, although it is nothing like general philosophy obviously. I also like to do some of the third year stuff; looking at different methods and challenging the students to make them look at things in a different way.

ROWENA: What kind of methods?

KATE: I like to look at all kinds of things, so within one of my modules we look in detail at Burnett and organ support, and how that fits in with homeopathy. I get students to write an essay about whether they think it is homeopathy or not, which always brings up some very interesting discussions. We look at the use of the chakra diagnosis and meditative provings. If they want to they can explore and write about their findings. I think it teaches them how to critically evaluate different methods; how to compare it to what Hahnemann said, and whether they think it is right for them in their practice - and not to just accept things blindly.

ROWENA: Do you think most come out practising in a classical way?

KATE: I think they come out practising in all different ways. There are some who will come out and practise very classically, particularly those who have been strongly influenced by Ian Townsend. There are those who will come out having embraced the organ support system and go that way. Some come out far more esoteric and use their intuitive skills. So I couldn't really say that we produce a particular kind of graduate. What I hope for is that we produce a free thinking graduate who also knows how to reflect on what they are doing.

ROWENA: Dead Poets Society[87] - that film had such a big impact on me. Have you seen it?

KATE: Yes, yes.

ROWENA: So if anyone says 'free thinking' I am there. And Jean Duckworth, what does she teach?

KATE: Jean Duckworth teaches all kinds of stuff. She is the filling in a sandwich. She does mostly second year and is really good on the practice management side of things because her background is in law, so she does all the legal issues. She also does all the miasm work and then a bit of everything.

ROWENA: So how did you three come together?

KATE: Ian Townsend was brought in from the London College of Classical Homeopathy (LCCH). I was working in Preston anyway. There weren't many homeopaths locally and Jean Duckworth lives quite close to Preston. So when LCCH merged, they wanted to bring Ian in and they wanted two other local homeopaths to teach on the course. So they looked around and Jean and I were the two that they chose. And that was because, I think, we both had a first degree, we were both qualified as teachers and homeopaths, and just loved the subject. It was clear to them, I suppose, that we felt passionately about it.

ROWENA: So they approached you, or did you hear about it?

KATE: Well, they contacted all the homeopaths in the area, and we all got together for a meeting. That is how it happened. It wasn't a closed shop thing; it is not that they just picked on us. At the big meeting, we all went along to hear what was going on. And I had been involved with the university for the previous two years, trying to design a course anyway. So I was already trying to get a homeopathy degree here.

ROWENA: Ah right, ok. So there was a branch of LCCH in Preston? I don't really know the history, could you tell me?

KATE: Well, what happened was there was a woman at the University of Central Lancashire in Preston, who worked in the nursing department, who had this vision of a homeopathy degree here and she contacted me, and a couple of other homeopaths who lived locally to write the course and we did start designing a course. And then she met with LCCH in London, who said to her, "Why not become partners with us and you can have our course?" The University of Central Lancashire set up a memorandum of co-operation with LCCH and at first we adopted their course. And we did teach that for, I think it was three years. Then LCCH were having financial problems in London under Mary Hood. She was quite ill as well through that time. Also there was a problem in as much as we were teaching a curriculum that wasn't really right for us, or at least Jean Duckworth and I thought so. Ian Townsend was teaching for LCCH anyway and he is fairly classical, so he was more comfortable with it, but Jean and I didn't feel comfortable.

It was also difficult working with people who weren't actually physically present. They were in London and paying our wages, but we didn't really have anything else to do with them. So there we were in Preston, teaching a course that we didn't really like and being paid by people from London who didn't really have much to do with us. And then when they started having problems – Mary Hood became ill and Barbara Harwood took over LCCH - it was just all very complicated. What happened in the end was that they wanted more money from the university, but the university was already making a loss on the course. So that is when we rewrote the course ourselves and had it revalidated. We wrote a different course that was less classical, which was what I wanted.

ROWENA: So how long ago was that?

KATE: 2002.

ROWENA: How is it going now?

KATE: Great. This is the time of year when we give students their module evaluation forms. So, for each module they have been taught they have to fill in these very long evaluation forms that ask them about their experience, the quality of the teaching, things they have enjoyed, and what we could make better. They have to rate it and give comments. So we get a lot of feedback from the students and in response to that feedback, each year obviously, we have tweaked the course. Not to give the students what they want so much, because we cannot just give them exactly what they want, but just responding to their feedback. So if there is something that they really like, we might give them a bit more of it. And we have put in place different teaching methods that work.

ROWENA: What kind of things do you find they are requesting?

KATE: They do like different teaching methods. They don't like us standing in front of the class lecturing them and saying this is the way. We use lots of different teaching methods.

ROWENA: Like what?

KATE: Like small groups, interactive work and asking them to put on presentations. We give our students games and quizzes; all kinds of different ways of learning the material to stimulate them. We work in three hour blocks so we need to keep them awake!

ROWENA: Yes, I remember I struggled.

KATE: Yes, I cannot concentrate for more than ten minutes! And so I cannot expect them to. So there is a lot of interactive teaching. It looks, I suppose when you are in there, like the tutor is not doing an awful lot, because they are not talking for three hours. But all the preparation comes beforehand.

ROWENA: Yes, I know.

KATE: So, you have to be really well prepared beforehand, to know exactly what you want to do.

ROWENA: I have a teaching background myself and the emphasis in my training was student-centred. So I know it is a huge amount of work in advance. And it is a lot of work at the time, but it is not the same as lecturing but certainly more enjoyable for students. And for me as a student, I have always learnt by experience. If someone just lectures to me, it doesn't work for me.

KATE: Well, you might as well just go and read a book.

ROWENA: Yes.

KATE: That is what I think about lecturing, it is a boring alternative to reading. I hate it. Occasionally you get really good lecturers who are entertainers, and that is different. If you have got an entertainer, you can sit and listen to them. But we cannot all perform all the time. So you have to have other ways.

ROWENA: So how many students do you have, approximately, in each year?

KATE: About twenty in each year.

ROWENA: I thought you probably would say that. Which is a nice number to teach isn't it?

KATE: We are limited by the clinical training that we offer, because it can only hold so many. Because all the clinical training is done in the room with the clinician, we don't do any video link.

ROWENA: And again, is that the three of you that do that?

KATE: No. We have got two different clinicians, who are also teachers as well as clinicians. So they are absolutely fabulous. It really is a teaching clinic. And the students sit in small groups with the clinicians.

ROWENA: And because you are attached to the University of Central Lancashire, do you find it easier to get patients?

KATE: Yes. We don't have any problems getting patients. The students always evaluate their clinical experience very well. As they do with their module evaluations. The feedback we got recently was fantastic. So we never have anybody saying they are dissatisfied, apart from about things like the accommodation, that they didn't like the room. I have a lot of fun with them; we laugh a lot and I think that is really important.

ROWENA: Yes, definitely. We all need more of that.

KATE: Laughing is good.

ROWENA: Homeopathy is obviously in a boom phase, not that we necessarily feel it in our practices because most people still find that quite a challenge. What do you think makes a successful homeopath, and a successful homeopath financially?

KATE: That is an interesting question. There are all kinds of things that make a successful homeopath. It has got to be something to do with having their basic education, but also being able to adapt and be flexible, so that when they get difficult patients, they know how to find new information, a different style, or a different approach. They need not to be scared or fearful of anything that is coming in. Hopefully our students, our graduates, would not worry about what kind of level of pathology the patients have got, be it at a physical, emotional or mental level.

ROWENA: Because they are equipped.

KATE: Yes, I hope so. When I interviewed my students as they finished the course some years ago, I asked them about their experience of studying the science in the course, because we have more science in the course than you would in a private college. I was worried about that when we first started but the students felt that it made them more confident. That word 'confident', came up in just about every interview I did.

ROWENA: Oh, that is very interesting.

KATE: They had confidence because they understood disease process and because they could communicate with other health care practitioners. And so if a patient came to them and they said they had this particular physical pathology, they knew what they were talking about. And if they said they were taking a particular drug, they knew what that was, too, and they knew what kind of side effects it might cause.

ROWENA: So do you think this is the way forward? To have courses validated by universities and to have these other modules, other than the homeopathy ones?

KATE: I think that helps. I don't think it necessarily needs to be done through a university. I have a private college in Galway, Ireland and we are going through the process of applying for degree status out there. We can apply directly to a government body to get degree validation. You don't have to be affiliated to a university.

ROWENA: Very interesting. So that is a first?

KATE: It will be.

ROWENA: Well done.

KATE: Don't say well done yet, I haven't achieved it yet. But that is the next thing.

ROWENA: Well it is out there.

KATE: It is one of my projects at the moment. I am writing the documentation for that process. It is a lengthy procedure but the students in Ireland seem to want the degree status, so that is what we are trying to provide.

ROWENA: So how did you get involved with the Society of Homeopaths?

KATE: Just through the college I went to. I automatically assumed that the Society of Homeopaths was the register to join.

ROWENA: Me too.

KATE: So I did, and that was it. I just knew that they were the best; the most professional. That is how I got involved with them.

ROWENA: And when did you become a director?

KATE: Three years ago from this year.

ROWENA: What was your role as a director?

KATE: When I first joined the board the directors all had individual roles. My area of interest is research and so I got involved in that area because I very much wanted to get things going there. So while I was on the board we established the new research committee and got the nationwide project established. Now we have a very active research committee with clear terms of reference. I ended up being involved in all kinds of stuff including chairing the membership committee and being Vice-Chair. I need five lives for all that I want to do.

ROWENA: What do you think makes for a financially successful homeopath?

KATE: It is difficult to say from my own perspective because I have never been a poor homeopath. I didn't have any problems building my practice and I do lots of other work as well. So that is my own experience and I don't understand why others are poor. In a very simplistic way, I went out and gave lots of talks and ran little courses when I first started building my practice and I soon had loads of patients. But I think fearful homeopaths, homeopaths that never really make a commitment, who don't put themselves out, they won't ever be successful. I think you have to work doubly as hard as a homeopath because it is alternative as well. People don't want to pay for healthcare.

ROWENA: Yes, so we are fighting against so many different obstacles.

KATE: We are and we need so many different skills. Hopefully we can start to address those in our courses. But they have got to expect to earn a living. I don't like the idea that we need to be poor and I don't think we do.

ROWENA: No. I agree with you. But do you think there is a ceiling on how much we can charge?

KATE: No. Is there?

ROWENA: I don't think so.

KATE: I don't think so either. If you charge too much people won't pay it I guess.

ROWENA: Well many of the central London homeopaths, I think, are doing very well and I am sure they charge above the average.

KATE: If they charge an absolutely astronomical amount I might start thinking it is unethical.

ROWENA: What do you think is astronomical?

KATE: I have been told there is someone in the USA who charges over one thousand US dollars for a consultation. I don't like that. I mean, that is really setting yourself up on a pedestal isn't it?

ROWENA: I know what you mean. Do you think homeopathy will become dormant again? Can you see that happening?

KATE: I wouldn't like to say because things come and go, don't they? They go in a cycle. I don't think it would disappear, I think it would be transformed into something different. I don't see that homeopathy, the influence of homeopathy and homeopaths now, could completely disappear. If it does diminish in its present state it will live in some other form. Homeopathy, to me, is still in its infancy. We have got a long way to go, before we start dying.

ROWENA: Good, good.

KATE: And we have a lot to learn. It is still a baby at the moment.

ROWENA: Yes, absolutely. I was speaking to Sheilagh Creasy the other day and she believes that homeopathy has been around since day one of our creation. It came through Hahnemann because we were more ready then to accept and appreciate it. She traces it all back through *the Bible*[27] - even the Law of Similars.

KATE: It is fascinating and it is never going to disappear completely, is it?

ROWENA: I don't think so, because it is of the universe, so how can it?

KATE: We just might call it a different thing and look at it in a different way.

ROWENA: I think we are very lucky, don't you?

KATE: Absolutely. I think I am the luckiest person in the world, I do. I love my life and I wouldn't exchange it with anyone.

ROWENA: That is so nice to hear. How many people would say that? Not many.

KATE: No.

ROWENA: I have to say, I am in agreement with you and I have said exactly those same words, but I do think it is unusual. It has been so nice talking with you. I am sure our paths will cross again.

KATE: Undoubtedly.

CHAPTER 17: ROGER SAVAGE

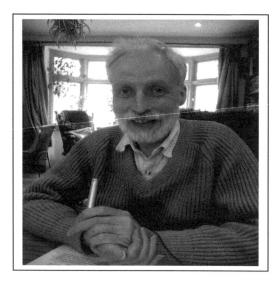

I met Roger Savage, a Fellow of the Society of Homeopaths, at the Alliance of Registered Homeopaths' (ARH) Spring Conference. We just got chatting, as you do; I told him about my book and because he has been in and around the profession for a number of years as a teacher and practitioner, I him if we would like to be included. A few weeks later, on Wednesday 4 May 2005, he came up to my house for lunch and a chat.

"Patients may present to us in 'layers', but we don't need to use these labels, because just as we are urged not to treat disease labels, so maybe if we did a little less labelling of philosophical concepts in our work there would be slightly fewer arguments."

Roger Savage, May 2005

"Really honest senior practitioners, of whom you must have already interviewed a few, have said we probably very rarely hit the simillimum. Most of the time we are doing, we hope, pretty good work, but not going through the centre of the core of the apple on the boy's head. William Tell may not always be that good a shot! When I first heard Jeremy Sherr say that he thought he hit the simillimum twenty per cent I was startled, thinking, 'What a low average!' How little I understood in those early days of what he was saying – that percentage of simillimum prescribing is really good!"
Roger Savage, May 2005

"To think we are barefoot doctors who should apologise for charging five or ten pounds is a big mistake, and is doing us all a disservice. If we have worked hard with a case we deserve a bigger thank you!"
Roger Savage, May 2005

CHAPTER 17: ROGER SAVAGE

ROGER: Well Rowena, I read through the synopsis to your book again this morning and noted that all this began with an interview with George Vithoulkas. I think what is amusing is that he says that in Belgium and Germany there are some who are following what he is teaching to the letter. As you know, George is vociferously and vehemently against so much of the new research being done, which I regard as basic core work now. I do feel that homeopaths arguing and fighting with each other on a big scale is not helpful. It is tiresome and just causes confusion, because I agree with those who say that all that members of the public want is to be made better. They are not interested in, I say this, and, you say that, and the in-house fights that go on within our profession.

ROWENA: Actually it is more than them not being interested; it is off-putting.

ROGER: It is very off-putting. I think we fight because all of us are keen to get a really good understanding of homeopathy. There is a tendency in our eagerness to be really good homeopaths for us to feel that there is one right approach or answer and anybody thinking differently is wrong. I feel that we can learn so much from other homeopaths who are trying to change that way of thinking, and to name one I would pick out Jan Scholten. As well as creating some revolutionary thoughts, he is inclusive and co-operative, which is encouraging, and gives us less of a sense of feeling guilty if there is anything we are doing that isn't already in one of the old books.

It is good to have principles and basics, but I suppose we need to face the fact that in these days even those are not completely agreed. Maybe all of them need discussion but so long as we have a clear idea of what we consider to be wrong with a patient, who is to say whether there is only one totally correct answer for them? Jeremy Sherr, in my opinion, rightly says that we should prescribe on the greatest totality that we can see. That definition, by somebody who would be thought by most to be a pretty straight classical homeopath, is non-judgemental, because it immediately takes the guilt and the fear out the prescribing process.

We will aim to perceive as broadly and as deeply as we can, and if we have assessed a case without our own preconceptions diverting us, then our prescription will turn out to be a deeply long-term curative remedy or else from that dose another remedy picture will emerge. That is attested to frequently in Kent's *Lectures on Homeopathic Materia Medica*[88], which I have just been re-editing. He does not talk endlessly about there being one remedy for a person and only one forever – not at all. We have to be very practical people dealing with the situations that we face. Patients may present to us in 'layers', but we don't need to use these labels, because just as we are urged not to treat disease labels, so maybe if we did a little less labelling of philosophical concepts in our work there would be slightly fewer arguments. Now that was quite a long monologue as a start to our conversation!

ROWENA: Yes it was, and interesting too. There are homeopaths who say that if you see the totality, sometimes you shouldn't go there at that point because it could be too deep if there is a lot of pathology, and could create chaos. How do you feel about that?

ROGER: This ties in with something I was going to say. Where Rajan Sankaran talks about the idea of going back to a very early symptom picture of a patient, he says that although he can sympathise with that, he can only regard it as not logical, because what we need to treat is what is in front of us now. And probably that will answer the theory about going too deep. Suppose at the moment I am suffering from great chilliness, extreme sensitivity to draughts, jumping every time there is the slightest noise, detesting chocolate and wanting slices of raw lime; if ten years ago I was the exact opposite of all that, do I treat the ten years ago picture or what is current now? Sheilagh Creasy valuably pointed out to us in her classes that one of the best guides to what is going on with a patient and what treatment they need is, can we see a point at which their story and their state changed? If so, that is what we should treat initially – and as she often used to quote, "The acute often points the way to the chronic".

If we don't talk of theories but just look at the person, we can then see more clearly. Now, if the person has obvious symptoms and the vitality, as opposed to the energy, is good because the symptoms are clear, we are safe treating them with a major remedy and possibly a high potency. But if we already have found a few remedies have caused upset in the person and the picture isn't clear anyway, we may be suspecting that their vitality is compromised. That is when we are going to have to be careful what we do, and maybe we will have to begin by some partial treatment or even palliation. Kent says that in these difficult or threatening cases we are correct to palliate; I read it again yesterday. So, Kent was also very practical.

ROWENA: So how does one palliate; how do you know that is what you are doing?

ROGER: I think one of my first criteria of palliation is that the symptoms simply abate and the person just feels a relief from the intensity of what they were suffering.

ROWENA: So would that be because the homeopath knows in advance that they are going to be palliating?

ROGER: I hope we may know it if we are really, really astute, but in many cases it happens by accident. Really honest senior practitioners, of whom you must have already interviewed a few, have said we probably very rarely hit the simillimum. Most of the time we are doing, we hope, pretty good work, but too often we are not going through the centre of the core of the apple on the boy's head. William Tell may not always be that good a shot! When I first heard Jeremy Sherr say that he thought he hit the simillimum twenty per cent of the time I was startled, thinking, "What a low percentage!" How little I understood in those early days of what he was saying - that percentage of simillimum prescribing is really good!

This brings me on to the concept of cure. Are our goals realistic? Are we expecting every single sign of aging to reverse and go back to a state of vigorous youth? If we are, we may be asking the frankly unrealistic and if we look back at what Sheilagh Creasy calls 'the classic writers', they weren't talking of this, either. They were talking of clearing pathology that was in front of them in a patient without something worse following on. Maybe we could call it 'serial clearing', and maybe 'serial palliation'; it depends exactly what the outcome is. And by that process we may move in steps to a deeper state being cleared. I have had it happen with some patients, but if we imagine that with one dose of the perfect remedy we are going to shatter every aspect of the malady and the person is going to emerge with unfurled wings one week later, which I think is often what we do put upon ourselves to achieve, this is frankly unrealistic.

I had an eighty year old patient to whom I gave *Nux vomica*, having honestly wondered if it was *Stramonium* and seriously considered *Anacardium orientale*. But on reviewing everything, *Nux vomica* seemed to win. But I was a little concerned because that very day he started to feel better and one week later was still feeling magnificent. Now I may have shot through the core of the apple, and if he stayed fine like this for a month, for two months, three months and so on, then I did. But if other things had crept up insidiously and he went downhill and a repeat didn't bring anything like the same effect, then I would know after the event that I had merely palliated and something else was required. He went after some time for an injection for his prostate cancer, and no, I am not expecting to make all his pathology vanish, and it just doesn't quite happen like that. But even that treatment didn't pull him down and his spirits remained good and his energy, up. All around him were calling this miraculous. Miracles worry me because they can be the hallmark of a palliation. But maybe we have shot through the apple and done better than we dared hope!

On another subject, I even come across homeopaths going along with the idea that above 12C potency there is nothing traceable in the remedy, and I am wishing to say, in a very loud voice, this must be untrue, because if there were nothing there, nothing would happen. I think we should look back in science two hundred years to William Crookes who lived in the late eighteenth century, around about the time Hahnemann was beginning his research. As I recall, he said we have solids, liquids, gases and the radiant state (I believe scientists nowadays regard his ideas as disproved!). I decided to do my own experiment and I got a lady with very sharp clairvoyant vision to look at bottles of LM1, LM2 and LM3 and I asked her to tell me what the differences were, if any, that she could observe. I didn't tell her which was LM1, 2 or 3. She fed back to me that number 2 had a slightly finer resolution than number 1, and number 3 slightly finer than number 2. By 'fine', I mean in the sense of comparing the coarse image of an old style newspaper photograph with a modern high resolution picture that has millions of pixels.

For the moment I think the safe thing to say is that our present-day laboratory equipment is too crude to see what is contained in a potency higher than 12C. In potentising *Lycopodium*, the club moss, what is seen under the electron microscope is that the spores break up and open out like flower buds to reveal the petals within, which is why the inert substance becomes full of energy. So, when we go past the point of statistical probability of molecules, we perhaps are finding ourselves in that 'radiant' state. In the future some finer kind of electron microscope will have been created which will show what is there and people will laugh and say, "You realise that up until the year two thousand and whatever they couldn't see this and some of them even said there is nothing there!"

So, we homeopaths should be very careful what we say and shoot down this idea every time it comes up, because we are not treating with nothing and we know that, because homeopathy works on babies who are not known to be susceptible to bedside manner, and it works on animals, too. And if we give the wrong remedy, usually nothing happens. Homeopathy works on people who are definitely not susceptible to the power of positive thinking. Hahnemann posited the presence of germs but couldn't see them. We also know that electricity happens, but it is invisible. Radiation is not generally visible; we need special equipment to see it. So we homeopaths need to fight that scientific corner much better.

ROWENA: How did you come into homeopathy, Roger?

ROGER: In childhood, whenever my tonsillitis or earache didn't resolve with penicillin, my parents took me to a Faculty homeopath, Charles Oliver Kennedy, who I think has died since. This was fifty years ago now and I don't know what he gave me, because of course in those days they all followed Hahnemann's remarkable dictum, "The name of your remedy, Madam, is no more your concern than the name of your disease is mine!" These days we would regard his comments as jolly arrogant and they would be contrary to the revised *Code of Ethics*[47], but one can see why the early prescribers took that view. So I don't know what he gave me, but each time the tonsillitis and the earache were resolved and I never did have any organs cut out. My parents were unusual in not agreeing to this very fashionable operation of the 1950s, so I am very fortunate.

Then at university, several years later, I met a young student who had just been to an ashram in India where his interest in homeopathy was awakened. By then, having had some unhappy things happen to me, I wasn't very well and he carefully went through Boericke[39] and selected for me *Silica terra* as the remedy in a 200C potency and it definitely had an effect. In those days I had been sleeping until ten o'clock on those dark winter mornings. After the remedy I was suddenly awake at six, full of vitality, and went in to college breakfast for the first time in months despite the dark morning! A few months later, when I had a dreadful eruption on the knuckles, I noticed in *Boericke*[39] the symptom, 'cannot eat onion' listed in *Thuja occidentalis*, and took it with dramatic effect. So, these experiences made an impression.

I studied Classics - Latin and Greek - and then switched to English for the third year, so I am an arts graduate who is now doing something totally different. I was bad at mathematics, detested physics and never seriously did chemistry, so these are the changes life brings in our maturity. I am grateful for a classical background, because it means the names and our old-world terminology hold no terrors. I read Plato recently and found the following: "Just as one wouldn't stop at treating individual citizens but then would look to treating the whole state, so we wouldn't seek to treat just part of a person but would look to treat the whole person". That is actually the first statement I have found of holism.

After university I, again, had some unpleasant skin problem and went to see a homeopath who, amusingly, was a struck off doctor in northeast London. He gave me *Hepar sulphuris calcareum* 6C and told me to take it every two hours but with no time limit. This was certainly not classical thinking; it eventually produced severe aggravation and I had a flash of intuition and thought, "This is making me really ill: apart from anything else I am now morbidly sensitive to sugar and the skin isn't resolving." So I went back to him but he said to carry on taking it, and I was sure this was wrong. So I ordered from Nelsons Homeopathic Pharmacy *Hepar sulphuris calcareum* 1M and took a dose and it rapidly antidoted the ill effects of the endless 6Cs. But as a result I was on the underground train and suddenly had an enormous pressing need for emptying the lowest chakra. I raced back urgently to the necessary facilities only just in time, but the upset was cured.

I went back to the homeopath and he said, "Don't worry about it, I am going to retire and would you like to buy my practice? I can give you easy terms." As I gulped he said, "You needn't do the acupuncture, or you could do if you liked." But I just knew at the age of twenty two that this was far too soon and the wrong way to go into practice, so I said to him, with one of those amazing moments of wisdom that are very rare in my life, "I am too young and I need to learn something of life first."

So I went off and taught English to foreign students for eight years, until I became frustrated at just teaching them language when they were sitting in front of me telling me their illnesses and problems. So then when some more disasters happened in my life, I switched from teaching, but I switched to homeopathy via a route that many of the strictly classical only homeopaths would disapprove of greatly. I wanted to try to find the answer to some mysterious and unpleasant symptoms in a loved one, had an intuitive conviction about where to turn, so I went off and studied radionics with someone whose main treatment modality was homeopathy, but according to specific indications and often in combination formulae, which brought up struggles within me over methodology even though I saw successes with his way of working!

ROWENA: Sheilagh Creasy started to talk about radionics last week. Could you explain it to me?

ROGER: Did she speak favourably about it? Sheilagh Creasy always seemed implacably against radionics and intuitive ways of working and at the time, so was Robert Davidson (though he has changed a lot of his views very radically since then!) Throughout the 1970s I was slowly building up a store of remedies and prescribing for myself and family members. I was encouraged by a friend who is a very pragmatic user of homeopathy and has, to this day, a remarkable method of keeping up vitality even in her mid-nineties, treating constantly what we would call partial symptom pictures. I am saying that we can argue out the supremacy of 'unicism', as the French call our classical homeopathy, but somebody else who eats remedies like 'Smarties' is doing so well on this regime that they can say they are getting better and better! So, there are many ways to reach the goal, even though we may not feel comfortable with all of them.

On finishing language teaching I went to Tenerife at the end of 1980 to study radionics intensively with a man who was a very strange person but a brilliant practitioner. His method of practice was to use plenty of specific 'homeopathic' remedies for named conditions. This may very well work, but the debate would be, is this homeopathy? Remedies are effective against named diseases, there are correlations, but probably this is palliation. It could be curative by accident and it may be suppression, but we may choose in certain situations to do both of these, and these approaches can in some situations be jolly useful.

This could be called a homeotherapeutic way of working, and actually it is really useful to know about therapeutics, because if there is an acute crisis we haven't time to discuss the person's tendency to be a sun worshipper, for example, in order to fill in the deeper yet more remote picture. They want the violent pain or the profuse bleeding dealt with dramatically fast. So to know, for example, that *Hypericum* is the emergency remedy of choice for injuries to fingertips or *Bellis perennis* for deep bruising to the back is valuable knowledge, and we are not going to worry about the mental match; we will sort that out later.

So therapeutics indeed has its place, and in a sense this person has lived on lifelong therapeutics, and maintained good mental health and managed to make a complete recovery from serious illness. It is humbling, because every time I am asked to provide a batch of remedies I gulp, and I have tried offering single remedy treatment but the effects aren't sufficient. I have observed that those who live on remedies have to continue living on them; once you start that course you have limited their action and you have to go on that way, and such patients often cannot give us the 'complete symptoms' we are looking for. Which is why many of us ask patients not to add in a few remedies of their own when we are treating them. It shouldn't be because of personal power issues, it should be so that as far as possible there is a clear field in which to work.

ROWENA: Who introduced you to radionics?

ROGER: I knew that a naturopath in north London had such a device. A radionic session revealed where the deficiencies and problems lay hidden in a very difficult case and he was able to select treatments and remedies by 'resonance'.

The disadvantage of radionics, and why I gave it up, is that I found I became somehow 'hooked into' the malady of the patient. So if I was treating cancer patients, I would feel sick and if I was treating MS patients, I would feel dizzy, and I knew one day I must stop doing this as I felt I was draining my heart chakra. There are, as I now know, ways one could insulate oneself from the disease vibrations passing through the radionic instrument. Anyway, one day I found myself opening my pad at a blank page and asking the patient to tell me their story. That was my first unaided case taking and it just happened, and I knew this would be the better way, and it is.

As Robert Davidson put it, homeopathy is at the highest level because it is what he calls 'informational' medicine whilst radionics and bioresonance are the next level down being 'energetic medicine'. Energetic methods can be very helpful and supportive, but we can get a far broader picture of a patient by using more outward and interpersonal methods. Nowadays the computerised successor to radionics is bioresonance. With bioresonance, the testing is done by sending the patient very brief bursts of micro energies and finding out where and to what degree their reactions occur. So, radionics and bioresonance work by a resonating principle and homeopaths work by the totality and/or similarity of as much of the picture of the person as we can establish.

I would regard radionics and bioresonance as back up methods when we just cannot get the information or just cannot sort it out. It is there as a reserve, and I am grateful for bioresonance because, with its help, I found the remedy that got me out of severe multiple food allergies when no-one found the right remedy by normal outward homeopathic methods didn't. The remedy was *Candida albicans 9C* and one dose held for fourteen months.

I once had a boy who was cured on one dose of *Hepar sulphuris calcareum 3C*, so this says something about potency. It dealt with both his dream of nasty ghosts and the eruption on his hands, and he never needed anything else. So it just depends where the level of disturbance is within the person. We cannot say that all low potencies are short acting and brief. Kent says that the Milk remedies need to be in high potencies, which makes sense, as in their low potencies they are a food and therefore less active. It is probably a matter of the degree of remedy similarity and the vitality of the patient. Candida, a fungus, is in its crude form an invader and will credibly have a strong action even in low potency. So in my case I felt really quite awful for an hour or two after it, as though I would faint, and then I had a vast range of my old symptoms come up, one by one, like a series of echoes.

The worst interpretation of my experience is that it was positive palliation, but I think it was a good partial cure or a good layer clearance. I was so sensitive that one grain of wheat would produce a near death experience with unbelievably appalling headache for twenty four hours. Nowadays, to my astonishment, I can eat course stoneground wholemeal bread, and although I don't vastly like it, there is no ill effect at all. I am still sensitive to sugar, and to alkaloids as in tea, coffee and chocolate, so it will be interesting to see by what method the remedy for that state will be found! At the time, *Candida albicans* was not a well-known remedy. I am grateful that I was pointed towards that remedy, even though it was not by another method.

Mostly for people with allergies, a quick dose or two of *Candida albicans* 30C acts as a stepping stone on to something else, but my experience was profound, and when we have that experience we know it. I have had this with one or two other remedies, with dramatic effects on the emotional level but also the release of two decades of hay fever. The research of radionics and bioresonance as well as orthodox medicine tells us that there is quite a link between mercury poisoning and fungus. Mercury toxicity affects the system and can make us more susceptible to a fungus state.

ROWENA: Interesting. So what encouraged you to study homeopathy?

ROGER: I just knew I must do and I had put off doing it for two to three years until dramatic events in my life forced me to make the change from teaching. It was as if I was following the guidance, 'If you are thinking of something, resist it until you can resist no longer'.

ROWENA: Where did you study, and when?

ROGER: With Misha Norland. At the time he was living in London and I was going to set up a course in Cambridge for him to teach. Suddenly he moved to Devon, so a year or so later, although it was a jolly long way from Cambridge, I travelled to Devon twice a month, for teaching weekends and clinics, for three whole years. Once that journeying was over I didn't travel any long distance for a whole year!

Misha Norland was the main teacher and Janet Snowdon was the Dean of Studies. They were a good team. Janet has for some years been closely following Rajan Sankaran's school, and she has wide experience and a great grasp of the principles.

Sheilagh Creasy came and taught us sometimes. She aimed to shake us by the roots, for after forty years of homeopathy experience she clearly knew what she was talking about. I wanted more, so I also started going to her group in London, where she showed us in detail how to follow the homeopathic principles in daily practice. So these were my teachers.

ROWENA: Which other teachers have inspired you?

ROGER: Misha Norland, Jeremy Sherr and then, just before I qualified, Rajan Sankaran came over from India and he was indeed a huge influence and a great inspiration. When I took over running training events for the Society of Homeopaths' Continuous Professional Development programme, I was very keen to maximise our involvement with him and other people who knew him or who had trained or worked with him. Whatever one's particular homeopathic angle, these practitioners had vast experience and were faithfully incorporating the best of the teachings they had been given. They were also applying it to their experience of life and they had patient numbers that could only have our jaws dropping. Like you, I would call twelve or so patients a day a very busy day. He would have, in those days, one hundred and twenty follow ups in one day!

Jan Scholten has also been an inspiration – he has opened up the mineral table for us in his very special way and, controversial as his approach is to many, his predictive pictures of many of the previously unknown remedy minerals have been vindicated. Now he is taking us into the plant kingdom. Jeremy Sherr is another to inspire us – just studying homeopathy was a big undertaking for most of us, but he at the same time qualified in acupuncture too! He is continued to be a major figure in homeopathy, restoring the art of proving as a major part of our work – many of us have had cause to be so grateful for remedies he has introduced, for instance *Scorpion (Androctonos amurreuxi hebraeus)* and *Chocolate*. There were other teachers too, of course, but this begins to answer your question!

ROWENA: So what do you think are the important qualities of a successful homeopath, Roger?

ROGER: Oh golly, all the things I fail to do and be! Being empathic is a major feature of being a homeopath, just like a counsellor. Your patients must want to talk to you. We try to be the 'unprejudiced' case-taker in every case, but they say that for each of us there is a proportion of the population we cannot make headway with.

You said to me when we met a few weeks ago, surely everybody likes me; well, not everybody does! One patient, I remember, in London, and I had an observer sitting in at the time, came to see me and we had a really difficult session. She came back and we had another horrid session, and I said to her, "I need to ask you honestly, am I right that you have come here today because you told yourself you must manage it and you will somehow make it work, but despite your best efforts you just cannot stand me and you are coming up against a block?" She said, "Honestly, that is the truth." I said, "All right, we must acknowledge this. You and I, by accident, are like two north poles of a magnet with each other and I am trying to make it nice to receive your story, but unfortunately my very being is jarring to you." "Yes", she said. It can happen, so we just had to close the session! It was just obvious we were going nowhere. Sometimes it can be like trying to run an engine with sugar and sand in the petrol.

I have to watch out not to get too excited when taking a case and then throwing out some question which may be intuitive but also may be felt as invasive. I need to remember what Rajan Sankaran says, "We should just 'ah ha' and 'oh ho', and risk atrophy of the vocal chords!" That can sometimes be hard. He says that we should just nod and look encouraging. As Rajan Sankaran says, "They want to feel we are their friend - not too much of their friend, but non-judgemental." And that means that we should be, in our homeopathic point of view, sociologically, culturally and politically neutral. We may find we are dealing not only with suffering but with cases of abuse. So we really have to be pretty flexible and adaptable, and it can be quite tricky, pushing us sometimes to our very limits.

ROWENA: Agreed. And of course cases like that raise issues about what cases we have to report to the social services, but we have the *Code of Ethics*[47] to guide us there. Do you think it is possible to make a fruitful income from practising homeopathy?

ROGER: Ah Rowena, yes, this is a big question. Would you like a reasonably full answer? The majority of our practitioners are women, and for many their practice may be a way of earning their own money or extra money rather than the main income for the household. Perhaps this is what leads to the idea that somehow one cannot charge 'too much'. One international homeopath said, "It is my husband's business that brings home the real money". The consequence is one thinks it is all right to charge thirty pounds for a new session and fifteen or twenty for a follow up, and through doing three or four of these appointments a day to feel one has worked hard and perhaps earned quite well.

I was fortunate that in my early days of practise, a friend called me to London and said, "My clinic is overflowing; I need you to come and help." There I was trained into seeing six, eight, ten, twelve or more people in a day. Working at this intensity develops one's 'mental muscle', but I think most people don't see that number in a day. We should probably consider trying to charge more than we do, especially because homeopaths generally see people at a longer interval than acupuncturists, osteopaths and the like; so we should see whether we can charge more than they do per session because the patient's income can stand it at our longer intervals. Perhaps we should try to find out what other people are charging in our area and charge no less than them or 'the going rate', and if we have experience in practice, to charge more.

ROWENA: So what do you think an experienced homeopath should charge?

ROGER: This depends on geography. In central London, a new appointment can be a hundred pounds or more, and follow ups might be sixty, seventy five or more pounds. But somebody practising out in rural Wales, for example, unless they have forty or fifty years experience and a great reputation so patients will make a pilgrimage to them countrywide, will find that level of charge is a non-starter. So we have to be practical but also have courage. We also have to have successes and be known to be good.

The highest charging American homeopath commands a fee of over one thousand US dollars for a new patient and about two hundred for follow ups. Now you are grinning, which is what many people do. This person is criticised strongly for this by many in the USA as well as here, but actually charging at the level of a senior consultant means they are putting themselves on the line by making that charge, because it is a statement that they are accepting a tremendous degree of responsibility. It would worry me a lot; it might worry you even more, if I was charging anything like that without having a resounding success in every case. But ironically, when the new fee was put up from fifteen hundred to two thousand US dollars per person the clinic got busier; people travelled across the USA to see her.

Charges on that scale would just not work here – we have to be somewhat in line with the perceived going rate, but also to feel we are worth what we want to charge. It is also ironic that the most rewarding patients are often those with little money. Wealth can somehow bring in its train a more closed attitude! Each of us, like the international teachers, have to find a way of earning enough, whether by clinical work alone or also by teaching or lecturing or writing. Each of us has to set the level at which we feel we have the potential to earn well, but won't be too mortified if we have a failure. To think we are barefoot doctors who should apologise for charging even five or ten pounds is a big mistake, and is doing us all a disservice. If we have worked hard with a case we deserve a bigger thank you!

ROWENA: I am in agreement, but I think there is more to it than that. Sheilagh Creasy, for example, was saying you cannot be a homeopath without taking on another job alongside it.

ROGER: Oh dear! And that is from the voice of experience! Well, fortunately that isn't true for everyone, but I am still trying to ascertain what makes some practitioners really busy, even soon after graduating, whilst others in the same district, even after years of experience, may always struggle financially. There is no shortage of potential patients, but we somehow have to attract them and keep them.

ROWENA: Other homeopaths will say you have to teach and write as well.

ROGER: That may be the case; we have to find a way of 'making up our portfolio'. It may also depend on how big our debts and our outgoings are and how much we need to earn. A person who is seeing patients three or four days a week and teaching once or twice a month, if they are not living an otherwise riotous lifestyle, should be doing fine; assuming their clinic isn't full at just ten pounds a patient. In other words, it should be possible to earn at least two hundred a day, and for some practitioners even more. Feelings of unworthiness have to be resolved and then you 'go for it'! Many practitioners are also finding that co-operation with other homeopaths in their area actually helps their business rather than the opposite.

ROWENA: Roger, how do you think we, as a profession, can avoid slipping into a dormant state again?

ROGER: Well, I don't think we are doing so and I don't think we will. There may be discouragement among some practitioners, but that may be connected with low income and quite a lot of public attacks on homeopathy. Homeopathy is doing quite well in this country; unlike some other countries where many practitioners work in near total isolation, we here have the benefit of quite an active and sizeable homeopathic community. We have made efforts to become visible to the public and I think we are now quite widely known about, and as this has resulted in an increased level of media interest and attack from many quarters, we are now on our mettle, so dormant is not the word that comes to mind.

ROWENA: Roger, thank you for your time and sharing your story with me today.

CHAPTER 18: SUBRATA KUMAR BANERJEA

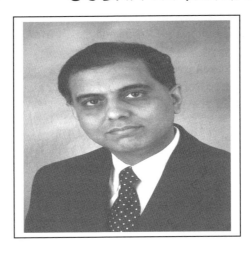

Thursday 12 May 2005 took me to see Subrata Banerjea. I first met him while still at London College of Classical Homeopathy (LCCH). He came to give us a lecture on miasms and made a big impression on me. A few years later I made his acquaintance again when I worked alongside him as his education adviser for the Society of Homeopaths. I travelled to Chelmsford to the Allen College of Homoeopathy, watched him teach in the morning and then he spared some time for me to have a fascinating conversation with him in the afternoon.

"If you throw a stone in a crowd in India, it will hit a homeopath!"

Subrata Banerjea, May 2005

"Homeopathy has survived in India for two hundred years, because it has been dealt with like a science." Subrata Banerjea, May 2005

"There are cases where we have waited six months or even twelve months, and the patient is still improving; so why should we give another remedy? Anybody who challenges this, I welcome to sit in at our teaching clinic in Essex. I sometimes hear homeopaths say that people from the East are more patient and tolerant and in the West they want much more of a quick fix. To be honest, as I have practices in both parts of the world, from my experience I would say that patients are the same; they all want relief as soon as possible. It is a question of prescribing the right remedy with confidence, which we openly demonstrate in our teaching clinic. Our message to the students is, "If the patient is improving, don't interfere with the process." And that is classical training and prescribing."

Subrata Banerjea, May 2005

CHAPTER 18:   SUBRATA KUMAR BANERJEA

ROWENA: How did you get into homeopathy initially, Subrata?

SUBRATA: Homeopathy has been in my family for four generations. My great grandfather was a homeopath. He practised for about forty four years and passed his wisdom to his son, my grandfather, who had the privilege to go to the USA and study with John Henry Allen.

ROWENA: So when was this?

SUBRATA: I presume between 1910 and 1920; sometime about then.

ROWENA: Was homeopathy always popular in India?

SUBRATA: Homeopathy came to India during the era of Hahnemann himself, and you know in those days India was a land of kings and maharajahs, so training in homeopathy became available if any of the kings or maharajahs became interested in it. I remember a person called John Martin Honigberger who came to India around 1830. He was a Hahnemannian disciple and he treated Maharajah of Patiala who was cured and homeopathy, as a result, spread. In the western world, during 1940 and 1965, homeopathy really declined to a low ebb. All the USA colleges shut down, and there were problems in Central Europe. But in India, homeopathy never got to that low ebb, which is an interesting comparison.

ROWENA: And is homeopathy the main medicine in India?

SUBRATA: I would say homeopathy is not the main medicine. Because all the multinationals are pumping in money, conventional medicine is the main system of treatment. But if you throw a stone in a crowd in India, it will hit a homeopath!

ROWENA: Is there a national health service?

SUBRATA: Yes there is and homeopathy is offered within it. On every corner there is a homeopathic clinic; in a square kilometre in an inner city, you will find at least twenty or more, especially in cities like Calcutta and Mumbai.

ROWENA: What makes somebody choose orthodox medicine over homeopathy?

SUBRATA: To a certain extent, I would say, there are three issues. One, orthodox medicine is free on the Indian national health service or in government hospitals in India, as it is here in this country, and is more readily (widespread) available, because multinational drug companies pump money into the government, and they set up these conventional medical facilities everywhere. Two, it is a quick fix; if you have poor people pulling a rickshaw or bullock cart, they cannot afford to take two days off sick. And, three, there is widespread advertising for orthodox medicine everywhere you look.

ROWENA: And for chronic disease as well; do people go for radiotherapy and chemotherapy for cancer?

SUBRATA: I would like to make the Indian approach a little clearer. In terms of conventional medicine, it is very developed if you are prepared to pay but the government hospital facilities are very poor. In the private facilities you even have people from the UK going over there for hip replacements, and it costs them a quarter of how much it would in Central Europe. There are plenty of private hospitals and private nursing homes where you get very up to date modern techniques. The Indian doctors come over here and go back again with their fellowships. Just for your information, an MRI scan in India would cost one hundred and twenty pounds, and a CT scan, a maximum of sixty to seventy pounds.

ROWENA: Ok. Well I don't know what it would cost here, but I know it is much more expensive!

SUBRATA: It is much cheaper in India, and, in answer to your question, there is a trend for people to choose chemotherapy or other conventional treatments but I have to say that it is quite divided. I would guess almost thirty to thirty five percent come for homeopathy as their first option. In India, homeopathy is being taught as a regular university degree. It is an intensive four and a half year full-time programme, eight hours a day, five days a week; in my day it was five years. In the first and second year we will have done dissection of a cadaver; that is how extensive our anatomy and physiology is. They achieve a Bachelor in Homeopathy, Medicine and Surgery, which means they have a licence to even write a death certificate.

If a person comes for homeopathic treatment and is not going for chemotherapy, he can have it, and if any problem arises, the homeopath is guarded by his licence. So you understand, there is quite a bit of difference and by nature of the way the system is set up, the homeopath gets much more confidence to practise. Also patients have the clear choice and right to decide and there is no threat to a homeopath from GPs or consultants, as the homeopaths are guarded by their license as well.

ROWENA: So if you had the choice here, would you teach at the Allen College in the same way that they do in India?

SUBRATA: Obviously but with certain limitations and taking into consideration the law here in the UK. I clearly explain to my patients in the UK about the effects of conventional drugs. I refer them to books and websites, and leave it in their hands as to what to do, in terms of weaning themselves off conventional drugs. You understand the Council of Organisations Registering Homeopaths (CORH) is trying to adopt all the organisations under one umbrella, and it will be a great thing, if we can all be unified. But I am really against degrading the standards of homeopaths, as a result. Anybody can be in CORH, and that shouldn't be the case. Homeopathy should have the proper status and standards so that homeopaths can stand on a par with other professionals.

ROWENA: And do you think we should be aiming for even a higher standard of education than we have now?

SUBRATA: Exactly. We should know what our limitations are. In India, we were being taught extensively but not for us to then go and perform surgery. It was so that we could understand our limitations and in that way we can be very clear and homeopathy will become much more popular. If I say, "Well, look, I can do up to this, and after that you have to go to the GP or your consultant", I think the patients will have much more confidence in us, rather than if we give false hope and try to treat them up to the end.

ROWENA: I agree.

SUBRATA: So, I will come back to your original question. My great grandfather studied in India in Calcutta and passed on his interest to his son who studied with John Henry Allen in the USA. Actually, this is also very interesting because there were two friends, my grandfather and another person, N M Choudhuri. He wrote A *Study on Materia Medica with Repertory*[89], which is quite popular in the UK and many people have read it. So my grandfather and Choudhuri went to the USA together, and Choudhuri studied with Kent and my grandfather with John Henry Allen. So it was almost like, "You get what you can from Kent and I will get what I can from Allen, and we will share."

And they went back to India and set up a school together, which goes by the name of the Bengal Allen Homeopathic College. 'Allen' is to pay tribute to the guru that was John Henry Allen. Perhaps my grandfather learned the miasmatic technique from Allen, because he was known for discovering the fourth miasm; the tubercular miasm. So he brought back that wisdom and then passed it on to his son, my uncle; so he was the third generation. My dad narrowly escaped - he is a microbiologist - but later on he became a very strong supporter of homeopathy; he even lectured in the homeopathy college. And I am the fourth generation.

ROWENA: Were you always interested?

SUBRATA: To be honest, it was very difficult to escape because in those days we had a joint family; all the cousins and uncles were in one kitchen and I was brought up hearing stories of the homeopathic cures from my uncle at the age of two, and I knew perhaps the name of *Arnica* at about the same time. So it was difficult to escape really. My dad wanted me to study medicine, and do homeopathy as a postgraduate, but my uncle wanted me to do homeopathy straight away. When I finished my A levels in 1974, by strange coincidence, the University of Calcutta took up homeopathy as a graduation course, so it was good timing! And I can draw on the knowledge of the thousands of homeopathic books in our own library for my studies.

ROWENA: Homeopathy has its own pull, doesn't it?

SUBRATA: Yes, it does.

ROWENA: And in your teaching now, your emphasis is on miasms, isn't it?

SUBRATA: Yes, more on miasms; that I have got from the family heritage, really. My approach is called 'MTEK.' M is for the miasmatic diagnosis, which I do first of all, and the TEK is the Totality Essence Keynote; so I combine this information. So many times these days, when the patient is drug dependent, there is a scarcity of symptoms but, of course, Hahnemann did mention this in his *Organon*[4] in *Aphorism 173*.

ROWENA: So how do you treat those cases?

SUBRATA: I use a tool called MTEK, which I would appreciate if you could include as an appendix in your book.

ROWENA: I would be happy too and I will include it at this point in the interview so that it is easy to refer to.

SUBRATA: Thanks that is great. Here it is.

APPROACH- A

UNSUPPRESSED CASES: CASES WITH CLARITY OF SYMPTOMS:

MTEK is a useful memory aid for arriving at a correct prescription.

M = Miasmatic Totality
T = Totality of symptoms
E = Essence (should include gestures, postures, behaviours etc)
K = Keynotes (which should encompass PQRS symptoms(SRP symptoms (strange, rare and peculiar symptoms)), refer to *Aphorisms 153 and 209* of Hahnemann's *Organon*[4])

When the above criteria are considered and the steps below followed, a correct prescription can be made.

Step-I: Make the miasmatic diagnosis of the case i.e. ascertain the surface miasm.

Step-II: Assess the Totality of symptoms + Essence + Keynotes and PQRS (if any) of the case and formulate the indicated remedy.

Step-III: Ensure that the indicated remedy covers the surface miasm, as diagnosed in Step I.

Step-IV: Administer the remedy, which encompasses the miasm as well as the Totality of symptoms.

Step-I:

Make the miasmatic diagnosis of the case i.e. ascertain the surface miasm, this can be done by:

(a)   Head to foot assessment of symptoms (please refer to *Miasmatic Prescribing, Its Philosophy, Diagnostic Classification, Clinical Tips, Miasmatic Repertory and Miasmatic Weightage of Medicines*[90] by Subrata K Banerjea).

(b)   Through clinical manifestation of disease, e.g. hypo/scanty/less are psora (e.g. hypotension, atrophy, anaemia etc); hypers are sycotic (e.g. hypertension, hypertrophy, hyperplasia etc.); dyses are syphilitic (e.g. dystrophy, dysplasia etc.) and allergies and haemorrhages are tubercular (e.g. hay fever, menorrhagia etc).

(c)   Through psychic essence, nature and character of the individual case (e.g. suspicious, jealous and exploiting in nature represents sycosis; destructive and cruel to animals represents syphilis; stubborn, changeable and impatient natures are tubercular etc.)

(d)   We can diagnose the miasm from other, different aspects, e.g. reference to hair falling: alopecia with dry lustreless hair and bran-like dandruff is psora; circular or spotty baldness is sycotic; diffused hair falling is syphilitic, and thick yellow crusts in the hair are tubercular; in reference to taste: burnt is psoric; fishy is sycotic; metallic is syphilitic and taste of pus is tubercular; in reference to pulse: bradycardia is psoric; tachycardia is sycotic and irregular pulse is syphilitic; in reference to bowels: constipation is psoric; diarrhoea is sycotic; dysentery is syphilitic and malaena is tubercular; in reference to pains: neuralgic pains are psoric; joint pains are sycotic; bone pains are syphilitic and pains with exhaustion are tubercular.

(e)   Diathesis (tendencies/predisposition) can also hint the miasm: eruptive diathesis is psoric; rheumatic-gouty, lithic-uric acid or proliferative diathesis is sycotic; suppurative-ulcerative is syphilitic and haemorrhagic diathesis is tubercular.

(f)   Psoric secretions are watery and mucussy; serous sycotics are purulent, yellowish; sticky, acrid, putrid and offensive whilst syphilitic and haemorrhagic secretions/discharges are tubercular.

(g)   If you ask your patient what his hobbies are: 'hunting' reflects syphilitic taint; 'travelling' is tubercular, whereas 'gambling' is sycotic!

(h)   Ask your patient: "If you could take a week off and money would be no object, what would you do?" Mr. Psora is lazy and will do nothing; Mr Tubercular will go on a round the world trip! Thereby you understand the innate dyscrasia and miasmatic nature of your patient.

(i)   Miasmatic diagnosis can be made from nail appearance; e.g. dry harsh nails are psoric; thick, wavy, ribbed, corrugated, convex nails are sycotic; thin, spoon shaped concave nails are syphilitic and glossy and spotted nails are tubercular.

(j)   Miasmatic observation of children: nervous, anxious, constipated children are psoric; restless, hyperactive (ADHD), colicky, diarrhoeic children are sycotic; withdrawn, dull, extremely forgetful, convulsive, dysenteric children are syphilitic and allergic, haemorrhagic, stubborn, impatient children are tubercular.

By such a prescription, which covers the miasmatic dyscrasia of the person, the chances of recurrence are eradicated and the axiom of 'rapid, gentle and permanent recovery' (Hahnemann's *Organon*[4] Aphorism 3) is encompassed. In cases of one-sided disease with a scarcity of symptoms, the action of the antimiasmatic remedy is centrifugal, and by bringing the suppressed symptoms to the surface, allows a proper totality to be framed.

The miasmatic consideration is therefore of great importance as demonstrated in the following example:-

A person is suffering from features of gastric ulcer, which has been confirmed by radiography. As ulceration is syphilitic, the surface miasm is therefore syphilitic also. Let us say that the totality of symptoms (physical, emotional and essence) of the person reflects towards *Kali bichromicum*, an antisyphilitic remedy. The choice of remedy is therefore simple, as *Kali bichromicum* covers both the totality of symptoms and the surface miasm of this gastric ulcer case. *Kali bichromicum* will peel away the outer layer and reveal a second layer underneath. This second layer may perhaps manifest through the appearance of warts or moles on the face, an indication of suppressed sycosis and the next assessment of the case should include this new surface totality. Following Kentian ideology we now know that there needs to be a change in the plan of treatment, that is, the previous syphilitic plan needs to change to a current sycotic plan, and a new antisycotic medicine needs to be selected based on the presenting totality.

Step II:

Assess the Totality of symptoms + Essence + Keynotes and PQRS (if any) of the case and formulate the indicated remedy.

Totality of symptoms:

(1) Each of the symptoms must be complete with regard to its location, sensation, modality and concomitant (My addition: Cause and onset, duration of the suffering and treatments he/she had in the past.)

(2)   The symptoms should have a chronological order of development and progression.

(3)   Environmental, occupational and other exogenous influences on the case must be evaluated.

(4)   Then the background of the case from (a) the past history (with special reference to various forms of suppressions) and (b) the family history (inherited miasmatic influences), must be in the purview.

(5)   The qualitative totality of all the symptoms (outwardly reflected picture of the internal essence of the disease) is the sole indication for the choice of the remedy.

Essence:

i)   Acquaintance with the psychic essences and personification of 'Drug Pictures' [e.g. Mr Lycopodiums are teachers, doctors, successful dictators, and politicians; and their personality characteristics reflect they are careful, cautious, conscientious, conservative, courteous, contained, avoid risk and commitments - Mr Safe; Mr Nux vomicas are CEO, share brokers, salesman, and their personality characteristics reflect they are ambitious, impatient, arrogant, charismatic, aggressive, independent, confident, courteous, workaholics and perfectionists; Mrs Pulsatillas are nursery nurses, teachers and carers and their personality characteristics reflect they are emotional, tearful, moody, changeable, pleasing, perceptive, affectionate, caring, forsaken, worriers; and Miss Phosphorus can be artists, actors, receptionists, maitre d'hotel and politicians and their personality characteristics reflect they are expressive, emotional, social, artistic, impressionable, gregarious, sympathetic and sensitive] with modern interpretations of old proving symptoms;

ii)   To ascertain a clearer picture for the constitutional medicine e.g. ask about the innate nature of the person, for example, "Give ten words to describe yourself" and when the patient says, "I am COMPASSIONATE"; - e.g. *Argentum nitricum, Belladonna, Calcarea carbonica, Calcarea phosphorica, Carcinosin, Causticum, Cocculus indicus, Graphites, Ignatia amara, Lachesis muta, Natrum carbonicum, Natrum muriaticum, Nitricum acidum, Nux vomica, Phosphorus, Pulsatilla nigricans, Sulphur;* "DUTIFUL":- *Calcarea carbonica, Calcarea iodata, Carcinosin, Cocculus indicus, Ignatia, Kali arsenicosum, Kali carbonicum, Kali iodatum, Lycopodium, Natrum muriaticum, Pulsatilla nigricans;* "EASY GOING":- *Arsenicum album, Calcarea carbonica, Carcinosin, Lilium tigrinum, Lycopodium, Magnesia muriatica, Natrum muriaticum, Nux vomica, Phosphoricum acidum, Phosphorus, Pulsatilla nigricans, Rhus toxicodendron, Sepia succus, Silica terra, Sulphur, Thuja occidentalis,* "FAMILY ORIENTED":- *Aceticum acidum, Anacardium orientale, Arsenicum album, Baryta carbonica, Calcarea carbonica, Calcarea iodata, Calcarea silicata, Carcinosin, Graphites, Hepar sulphuris calcareumuris calcareum, Ignatia, Iodium, Kali bromatum, Kali nitricum, Kali phosphoricum, Lycopodium, Magnesia carbonica, Natrum carbonicum, Natrum muriaticum, Petroleum, Phosphorus, Phosphoricum acidum, Pulsatilla nigricans, Psorinum, Rhus toxicodendron, Sulphur* etc. These are modern extensions/ interpretations of old proving symptoms and not found in the repertory books and I have developed an extensive repertory of personality characters.

APPROACH- B

CONTAMINATED DRUG DEPENDENT CASES - CASES WITHOUT CLARITY OF SYMPTOMS:

i)   In drug dependent cases placing emphasis on Lesser Known Medicines (e.g. *Franciscaea uniflora, Ginseng, Pimpinella saxifraga, Stellaria media, Viola* etc. to open the steroid dependent arthritic cases with few uncontaminated symptoms and absence of clear modalities, can prove beneficial; such lesser known organopathic medicines have the capability to alleviate symptoms to a certain extent, thereby giving the patient the chance to wean off their conventional medication, and experience shows that after forty to fifty percent weaning off; uncontaminated symptoms of the natural disease surface and give scope for constitutional prescribing) can succeed when well selected remedies fail;

ii)   For example, in drug dependent asthma cases, when the patient is on an inhaler and/or steroids; in such cases it is very difficult to get a clear picture of the case. The artificial chronic disease is superimposed on the original natural disease, therefore symptoms are contaminated or suppressed and the patient cannot give a clear picture e.g., modalities, etc. In such cases, homeopathic bronchodilators e.g., *Aralia racemosa, Blatta orientalis, Aspidosperma, Cassia sophera, Eriodictyon, Pothos foetidus* etc, can be prescribed on the basis of few available symptoms (according to *Aphorisms 173 to 178[4]*) and gradually the conventional allopathic bronchodilator is withdrawn. I ask the patient to sip the homeopathic medicine prescribed on the basis of symptomatic similarity, when the patient is out of breath and in need of conventional bronchodilator. The patient takes the homeopathic medicine and tries to defer the conventional medicine as much as s/he can. In this way, a steroid dependent patient who used to take a steroid/inhaler eight hourly; can, with the help of homeopathic medicine now defer the steroids to twelve hourly. This is the way conventional medication is gradually weaned off.

In the same way, for painkiller dependent migraine cases, the artificial chronic disease is superimposed on the original natural disease, therefore symptoms are contaminated or suppressed and the patient cannot give a clear picture for a constitutional medicine as well as the modalities of the pain are masked. Therefore, the following medicines can be selected on the basis of few available symptoms, e.g., *Acetanilidum, Anagyris, Bromium, Chionanthus virginica, Epiphegus, Ferrum phosphoricum, Indium metallicum, Iris versicolor, Kalmia latifolia, Lac defloratum, Melilotus officinalis, Menispernum canadense, Menynanthes trifoliate, Oleum animale aethereum dippeli, Onosmodium virginianum, Saponinum, Usnea barbata, Yucca filamentosa*. Accordingly the conventional allopathic painkiller is gradually withdrawn and after approximately fifty percent weaning off of the conventional medicine, suppressed symptoms surface and now the patient can give much clearer modalities. This will lead to making a change in the plan of treatment and on the basis of `MTEK' a constitutional prescription can now be made.

A similar example of difficult cases are the drug dependent hypertensive ones where the following medicines (*Allium sativa, Crataegus oxyacantha, Eel serum (Serum anguillae ichthyotoxinum), Ergotinum, Lycopus virginicus, Rauwolfia serpentina, Spartium scoparium, Strophanthus hispidus*) are capable of gradually weaning them off the conventional medication.

iii)   Generally experience shows after approximately fifty percent weaning off of the conventional medicine, suppressed symptoms surface and now the patient can give much clearer modalities. This will lead to making a change in the plan of treatment and on the basis of `MTEK' a constitutional prescription can now be made. Through this approach, not only does the patient gain immediate confidence that homeopathy works, but can also wean off the conventional medication to certain extent.

ROWENA: Thanks Subrata; I am going to find what you have said very useful to refer to. Do you believe that miasms move from being dormant to active with the consequence, therefore, that we are not always resonating in the same miasm?

SUBRATA: Physical, emotional and environmental influences change a person, so accordingly there is a change of miasm as we go through the different phases. I always compare that to the lotus, which throws petals to the surface. Different layers come to the surface and we have to act accordingly. But we don't have to change the prescription all the time, because many medicines are multimiasmatic, so that can take care of the miasm. In fact, I don't change my prescription very often, really.

ROWENA: Do you think people change state?

SUBRATA: Yes, they change according to their external environmental influences, and we have to change our approach accordingly. Say, for instance, our patient as a young boy was extremely restless and screaming, like a *Chamomilla* child. Then his parents split up and that was a real shock; I would take that shock or grief as an exciting factor. Then, let us say, the boy becomes introverted and depressed. Obviously here, that shock has triggered a suppressed syphilitic miasm to come to the surface, and accordingly we treat the miasm and the corresponding symptoms.

ROWENA: I was thinking of *Natrum muriaticum* when you said that but it isn't a syphilitic remedy, is it?

SUBRATA: No; but it is a multimiasmatic; so that is the reason that the remedy can take care of that. In other words, if you think of an unhappy person with a traumatic childhood, *Carcinosin* might come up. Obviously, I do believe the miasm changes. I will tell you a story; when I first graduated in 1982-83, I told my uncle, "I have already sat in with you for a couple of years, so could you send me to one of your friends around Calcutta with whom I can sit for one year or so and start my practice?" As a result, he sent me to a person who was about fifty miles away from the city of Calcutta and he said I should learn from him. In those days, travelling fifty miles in India took hours! So I had to get up at about five in the morning to reach him to start at half eight.

The first day I arrived I walked into a tiny consulting room, and this person, who was late middle aged, was sitting at a small table with a stool for his patients. I was offered a tiny stool and I thought, "Oh, my God, I am going to be sitting on this stool from eight thity in the morning until six in the afternoon" I was quiet, polite and dedicated, if you like, and I sat there and took it all in. He had a brass bell on his table, like they might have in a B&B on the counter, and you tap on it and it makes the sound, "Tung". He also had a helper who stood in the doorway where there was just a curtain. His appointment system was to put a piece of paper outside the consulting room the night before, at say ten, and the first one hundred he would see the following day. People would queue from three or four o'clock in the morning, and if you were one hundred and one, you had to come back the day after. There were no appointments or anything like that. Perhaps it was a test of patience before you could try homeopathy!

Outside there was a big field where there were people selling Indian Chai, samosas and onion bhajis; initially I wondered if it was some sort of fair. Later on I discovered this was actually his waiting area because the official room was tiny and could accommodate a maximum of five or six patients. All these people were waiting outside, and as we are about fifty miles out of the city, they couldn't go back and forth, so they wrote their names on the list and were stuck there for the whole day until they were seen.

Anyway, to make a long story short, the patient would come in, start telling one or two symptoms and the homeopath would grab their hand, look at the nails, ask one or two questions and write out a prescription. "Tung. Next". So I am sitting there, and I am thinking, "What the hell am I doing here? This man doesn't ask questions, he is not caring for the totality or anything. He gives five minutes, maximum, for a new patient, looks at the nails, and comes up with *Bryonia* or *Natrum muriaticum*. How can he do that?" But in those days it was more like a guru and disciple relationship in India, and I was not going to be rude or ask any questions; I just sat and observed.

So at the weekend I met my uncle and I said, "I thought you loved me". He asked, "What happened?" and I replied, "You sent me to this man, and I spent a whole week observing him but learned nothing. He basically looks at the fingernails, and sometimes the toenails, and writes a prescription. One hundred people a day are queuing for that." My uncle advised, "You go back there and you will learn from him." He and this homeopath were good friends, so he sent me back there, and basically he told him, "My nephew couldn't understand you, so could you please explain how you practise to him?"

So the next Monday I arrived, and he looked at me and said, "You don't understand what I do", and I said, "No, sir, I am sorry", and he replied, "I look at the nails and I diagnose the miasm." Basically, he taught me that dry nails indicate psora, and when you find peaked or ribbed nails, which are a proliferation, they are sycotic. He taught me wavy nails are sycotic and, when you get potholes, pockmarks, ridges or inward indentations and grooves in the nails, this is destructive and therefore syphilitic. I have discussed in detail about this miasmatic diagnostic technique in my book *Miasmatic Prescribing, Its Philosophy, Diagnostic Classification, Clinical Tips, Miasmatic Repertory and Miasmatic Weightage of Medicines*[90].

ROWENA: What about white marks on the nails?

SUBRATA: He taught me white marks or any marks on the nails are tubercular, as are glossy nails. If you raise a little bit of the nail and leave it and it starts flushing up, the tubercular miasm is responsible for this flush.

So, just to finish this story, a patient would come and say, "My GP has diagnosed I have a gastric ulcer", and he would ask, "Where is your pain?" Perhaps he is showing his pain with the tip of his finger on his tummy in the epigastric area. He will look at the nails, and if it is a syphilitic nail, within two minutes he will write out a prescription for *Kali bichromicum* 200C. He is coming from the knowledge of the following symptoms, pain can be covered by the tip of the finger and ulceration. *Kali bichromicum* is a syphilitic medicine, so with his observations he is discovering the symptoms covered by the medicine. He is doing the MTEK!

Believe me, I stayed with him for about a year, and later on I took steps to record how many of his patients were improving and he had an eighty percent plus success rate. Later on, when he gained confidence in me, I used to take the case as well, and he used to do his two minute diagnosis and come up with the same prescription. So he had masses of experience combining the miasm with the materia medica; it was just amazing. He was so confident and if, within three prescriptions, the patient hadn't got better, he would say, "I am not treating you anymore; I have done my best. Go somewhere else!"

ROWENA: I think we miss out here in the UK in not having an apprentice scheme.

SUBRATA: Yes, definitely. My uncle used to say that there is a gap between the cup and the lip when you study. In the Allen College we have a compulsory teaching clinic right from the first day, with experienced clinicians guiding and supervising. Going through cases is the best way of learning.

ROWENA: So what made you come over here to the UK?

SUBRATA: I first came to England in 1985. I had started lecturing on miasms in Calcutta and I wanted to understand what was going on over here. I met Linda Shannon and she said, "Would you like to address one of the groups here?" Sheilagh Creasy was in that group, and she was one of their mentors; it was just a small group, and I talked about homeopathy and miasms. At that time I was running a free clinic in India and they asked me if they could visit the clinic and see more cases. As you say, the apprenticeship scheme is missing over here so they were keen to come, and in 1986 the first intake arrived in Calcutta.

They were a group of twelve homeopaths; including Linda Shannon, Francis Treuherz, Carol Boyce, Carol Wise, Hilery Dorrian and some others. The clinic was a very busy one; we would see about thirty people in an hour with very fast prescribing. And I also organised a few lectures with my colleagues, and since then we have been running this Calcutta clinical course for three weeks, every winter in January and it is non-stop. Just this winter we had twenty two people, so it is growing. I don't live in India anymore but Janet and I visit and run the clinic and we have our assistants, too. Janet came to do this Calcutta programme in 1992, and we got together in 1995 and set up the Allen College in Chelmsford here in the UK.

ROWENA: And you got married this year! So when did you set up the Allen College?

SUBRATA: We started the Allen College in 1997-1998, and once again, we were debating the name. I thought perhaps as we have a long history with John Henry Allen it would be good to pay tribute to him.

ROWENA: So what is it about the Allen College that draws students, do you think?

SUBRATA: What we teach at the Allen College, we demonstrate practically through homeopathically cured cases, so that is our primary strength; it is not a theoretical training. We have about a hundred cases on our website and they are accessible to everybody all over the world. I believe that homeopathy should be presented on a par with medical science. If a conventional doctor challenges us, there are medical records, such as CT scans, before and after treatment. Our basic point is, we demonstrate what we teach. The second point is, we believe in homeopathy as a science and we don't believe you can dream up a medicine and prescribe that; it is a science and it should be dealt with like a science. That is the way it survived in India for two hundred years, because it has been dealt with like a science. George Vithoulkas is one of the great modern teachers of homeopathy, because he sticks to the principles.

ROWENA: Did he teach you?

SUBRATA: I have attended one of his seminars.

ROWENA: So he didn't come to India when you were studying?

SUBRATA: No. My major teachers were B K Bose, who was a direct student of Kent, and my uncle who had a Master of Science background, so he was always very careful in promoting homeopathy as a science, and he was very scientifically minded. He won't believe anything that is not proven by X-ray and things like that; it would have to be very authentic and proven.

ROWENA: Are there many colleges in India now?

SUBRATA: Things have changed a bit now. In our day, Calcutta was known as a centre for homeopathy because all the big homeopaths of the country were taught there. The approach to homeopathy in Calcutta is still totally different from that of the Mumbai and Delhi because you will find that they use the repertory, like in the West, and that is how they find the medicine. But in Calcutta, the emphasis is mainly on materia medica; you have to know your medicines, and the repertory is just your final aid. And we do the same in the Allen College. We introduce repertory late in the second year.

ROWENA: So it is about having the remedies inside your head?

SUBRATA: We try not to put too much of a burden on our students. In the fourth year, they have to sit an exam covering all the materia medica they have learned throughout their training. It covers about two hundred remedies and they have complained that it is too much. I say to them that they are well trained and that I feel confident that they can do it. We teach them *Organon*[4] thoroughly and I personally spend lot of time on comparative materia medica so that they have solid foundations and no confusion, at all! But I also give them a list of thirty to forty, and say that if they learn those, they will do well in homeopathy as their career, but only if they are learned as a mother knows her baby. I also present medicines with keywords, for example, 'discontented and unfulfilled' for Tuberculinum, which expresses its need for stimulating experiences like travelling and drugs and how it is superstitious, changeable and ritualistic by nature.

ROWENA: I think that is great because I know that in my second year, when we had materia medica exams, I learnt how to learn them, and I learnt remedies. I missed not having them in my third year. If someone said to me now, "Sit down and learn your materia medica; devote some time to it every day", I know it would benefit my practice. Perhaps this is a project I could move on to after I finish this book!

SUBRATA: I think I can safely say this to you, Rowena, some colleges don't believe in exams. Having now lived in this country for the past twelve years and being married to a British woman, I understand the difference in the philosophy in terms of understanding and learning. But, in my opinion, materia medica is a subject that you have to sit and learn. My uncle used to say that the repertory is a quantitative totality but homeopathy is a qualitative totality. I think that is very important. You feel like giving *Natrum muriaticum* to the *Natrum muriaticum* qualities of the patient. Kent was a master prescriber not because of his repertory but for his grasp over the nuances of materia medica.

ROWENA: It just becomes obvious, doesn't it? It is a remedy that I am very familiar with, and I do get a lot of *Natrum muriaticum* patients; not because I am projecting that they need it, because they do really well on it. You just know it, and it is because I have learnt that from experience, but also I learnt the remedy very well at college.

SUBRATA: Exactly. And that experience that you spoke about is very important. You know, I always present *Natrum muriaticum* with the word 'retention', and the retention is physical, emotional and in every aspect. Emotional retention is characterised by keeping everything in; even the hands are crossed and put away, and they are leaning back from you. These are observations, and with them you should come up with the prescription.

ROWENA: So which teachers have inspired and influenced you, Subrata?

SUBRATA: I like George Vithoulkas' philosophy; but these days what I am trying to do is combine the old knowledge of the classic masters of the West - Kent, John Henry Allen and Eugene Beauharnais Nash - with the more modern writings of *George Vithoulkas*, Roger Morrison and *Frans Vermeulen*. Some of these modern materia medicas are great in terms of their interpretation and presenting symptoms. In my opinion, students should learn the old literature first, and on top of that the modern literature so that they know what the Hahnemannian proving was. Many of the modern materia medicas are made up of third grade clinical symptoms but we must also know what the first grade proving symptoms are.

ROWENA: So what books do you recommend to your students when they are studying with you?

SUBRATA: Initially, we strongly recommend Nash as a starting book[91,92] in the first year because it is easy to read. We then move onto Margaret Tyler's wonderful book *Drug Pictures*[93]. In the second year we strongly recommend *Kent*, because in the first year Kent can be boring as he spends twenty five pages just on *Sulphur*! From the third year we recommend Frans Vermeulen, Roger Morrison and Jan Scholten.

ROWENA: And Rajan Sankaran?

SUBRATA: Rajan Sankaran is there, but not in our recommended curriculum. But we encourage reading his books in our library.

ROWENA: What is your opinion on whether homeopathy will become dormant again? Obviously it hasn't done so in India. Do you think we are on the up in the UK and it is going to ebb again?

SUBRATA: I have mentioned a little bit about how in India homeopathy never became dormant. Here in the West, and especially in the UK, after the second Great War there was a stage where homeopathy was not that popular. Then it came up again in Margaret Tyler's time, from the 1960s onwards. However, when I first came to this country in 1985, when I would say, "I am a homeopath", people would ask, "What is that?" but there is much more awareness about it these days. Basically I think that one of the ways of saving homeopathy is adhering to the principles and this is reflected in our history. The French schools of homeopathy taught mixing all the tinctures together and doing drainage, and the German schools taught combinations and mixtures and homeopathy went down possibly as a result.

ROWENA: So do you think there is a place for prescribing like that in the way you practise, or do you think it is not necessary?

SUBRATA: I cannot support polypharmacy. In my opinion, it cannot hold the case. When you mix all the medicines together, you don't know the result and effect of it. The very basis of homeopathy is the similar simplex, and the similar simplex has been diluted.

ROWENA: Do you treat patients with cancer?

SUBRATA: I do treat many advanced and terminally ill cases in this country.

ROWENA: And do you find homeopathy successful?

SUBRATA: It depends. If it is a very early stage breast malignancy, and the patient is opting to try homeopathy for a couple of months, delaying the radiotherapy, chemotherapy or mastectomy, I will obviously take the symptoms, and if there is less suppression I will go for the totality, include the miasm and prescribe on that. But say for a terminally ill patient, where the cure is not possible, we have to palliate and give comfort. In those cases I will treat with a low dose and sometimes even with tinctures to support the organs but still with the indicated medicine according to the symptoms.

I may use *Phosphorus* 6C for stimulating the liver and tinctures such as *Chelidonium*, *Myrica cerifera* or *Hydrastis* in terminal cases. The patient can take other medication as well because it will act on a different level. So that is the way I will progress.

ROWENA: And in India, is there a divide between practical and classical homeopathy, or is it all taught classically?

SUBRATA: In every college it is taught classically; that is number one. In Bengal there are about twelve colleges. Bengal is like a county, but a county the size of England, and Calcutta is the capital of Bengal. In Calcutta alone there are four colleges, and I can say that in every college it is taught classically in the Kentian approach. But there are homeopaths that do practise polypharmacy and give two or three medicines at a time; but they are not the majority and classical homeopathy is widely respected.

Polypharmacy is getting more popular here, but I would say that it is not the right way to keep the flag of homeopathy flying in the twentieth century. I strongly believe if we stick to the principles, homeopathy will survive. Newtonian gravitation cannot change and nor can the homeopathic law. We can adapt with modern provings, but we should adhere to the principles.

ROWENA: So you do prescribe newer remedies?

SUBRATA: Not very often, but I do. I just always make sure that the medicine has been proved authentically, according to the Hahnemannian technique. I don't use remedies proved by meditative proving. I think there is great scope for homeopathy here in this country, if the students are less confused. I run several postgraduate programmes in different parts of the UK, which attract students from other colleges and sometimes they come to me very confused. This should not happen after four years of study, if they have been taught the solid foundations of homeopathy. In the Allen College we teach the *Organon*[4] in a very practical way, and we really teach every section. Many of the modern readers of the *Organon*[4] say that even today, when they restudy *Aphorism 1*[4], they feel there is something new to learn.

We use the words practical and classical quite often in the UK but I think homeopathy that cures is practical, so the practical aspect is not a separate effect.

ROWENA: I agree completely. I was aware of that when I asked the question earlier and I wondered how else to phrase it to you.

SUBRATA: At the Allen College we receive enquiries, like, "Do you teach practical homeopathy?" Our curriculum is very well structured; when you enter the first year, you know what will be taught in the last session of the fourth year, because we have a set curriculum broken up each week listing what we are going to teach. We never say *Arnica* can do it unless we can demonstrate it. I think practical versus classical is an interesting and debatable topic. I want it to be known that the practical way is the way you are curing, and you are doing that in the classical way. Classical is practical.

In our teaching clinic, which is open to students because we believe that they should interact with the patients, if there is improvement, we wait and we wait. There are cases where we have waited six months or even twelve months, and the patient is still improving; so why should we give another remedy? Anybody who challenges this, I welcome to sit in at our teaching clinic in Essex. I sometimes hear homeopaths say that people from the East are more patient and tolerant and in the West they want much more of a quick fix. To be honest, as I have practices in both parts of the world, from my experience I would say that patients are the same; they all want relief as soon as possible. It is a question of prescribing the right remedy with confidence, which we openly demonstrate in our teaching clinic. Our message to the students is, "If the patient is improving, don't interfere with the process." And that is classical training and prescribing.

I have covered quite a lot of ground in this interview, haven't I?

ROWENA: You have and it has been great! I have learnt a lot, and I have really enjoyed it, too. Thank you so much for your time, Subrata.

CHAPTER 19:   YUBRAJ SHARMA

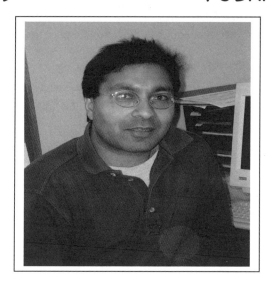

Saturday 14 May 2005 took me through the back streets of Wembley to the School of Shamanic Homoeopathy to meet its principal Yubraj Sharma. In the streets nearby, a market was in full swing accompanied by the colours, sounds and smells of India. I was now totally in the mood to interview this mysterious man who has Masters from the past such as Jesus Christ, Buddha and Hahnemann himself to critique his book, *Spiritual Bioenergetics of Homoeopathic Materia Medica*[94].

I found him in a converted lot in an industrial estate. He had a class of ten students sitting in a circle of chairs fully participating in his lecture on genetics. I sat in for the morning class with a library of books stacked behind me, including several copies of his rather large and eye-catching materia medica. You can see there is something of the driven workaholic about him. He kindly spent his brief lunch break with me in his clinic room next to his pharmacy downstairs, answering my numerous questions on what he is all about.

"I am bringing in the spiritual concepts from the beginning, and bringing in the medical diseases and the models from an allopathic and esoteric perspective, and then getting people to grasp the spiritual anatomy."   *Yubraj Sharma, May 2005*

"So what I am doing is to show people that although Hahnemann explained vital energy and said you cannot see it, I am saying that you can see it, you can feel it and you can perceive it - whether that is with machines, dowsing, pendulums or direct energy work. It is intuitive. If you feel one patient with cancer, you can feel it as a sticky, stagnant, damp energy that feels out of sync with the rest of the energy field. Then after a while it is in your library; your vibrational library of memories."   *Yubraj Sharma, May 2005*

CHAPTER 19:   YUBRAJ SHARMA

ROWENA: How did you get into homeopathy, how do you practise and how do you teach?

YUBRAJ: Firstly I don't see that in a biographical way. So I wouldn't see the answer to your question as I did this, then I did that, then that person said this etc. To me it is more channelled; it is more a spiritual awakening. At any moment something new can come flooding down without any prior training or precedence.

ROWENA: Ok, I understand what you mean. So when did that start?

YUBRAJ: I went to work at the Royal London Homeopathic Hospital to convert from western allopathic medicine. I trained with the Faculty and got my qualification in 1996 and stayed there.

ROWENA: What encouraged you to get into homeopathy?

YUBRAJ: Well, like any doctor who goes into homeopathy, they start getting disenchanted by allopathy and by the consequences of suppression. They may not understand all the details, but they have a knowingness already then of the suppression of disease, and so they want to find something that is more meaningful and curative. So homeopathy is a very good choice, because it is quite scientific anyway, if someone thinks like that, but also there is a training route through the Royal London Homeopathic Hospital without needing to take a break in career. That is quite useful for medical doctors.

During the training I already knew there were other influences without seeing exact sources in the material. It is more the spiritual. I was already channelling anthroposophical medicine and then reading all about it.

ROWENA: What do you mean by anthroposophical medicine?

YUBRAJ: Well, the works based on Rudolph Steiner and the philosophy of a spiritual science - understanding the human being in terms of cosmosgenesis, world forces and cycles of spiritual beings; understanding the subtle bodies, the astral body, the ego, the identity in relation to the etheric and the physical. As a consequence all the concepts of anthroposophical medicine had started to dawn on me. There is a rich scientific and spiritual kind of way of looking at homeopathy and anthroposophical medicine. And then I started to understand Chinese Medicine, and it seemed quite simple. I gained this understanding through an appreciation of spiritual and esoteric philosophy which is mostly theosophical and the works of Alice Bailey, Douglas Baker and the *Secret Doctrine of Madam Blavatsky*[95]. This was followed by any other spiritual book, new age textbook that grabbed me, then integrating it all into a spiritual knowledge. So again, it is not something for which there is one source, it is not something I am doing differently to anyone else. I am just stitching together bits of information from many paradigms. And then it dawned on me after a few years of private practice after leaving the Royal London Homeopathic Hospital that I should teach this.

ROWENA: Where do you practise?

YUBRAJ: Here, privately. I have done work before, subcontracted in Greenwich and Dartford, but now I am only in private practice, which is fine because you cannot run too many sites as well as be a principal. I have been running a course since 1998 and generally speaking, I don't advertise much, the budget isn't there as I keep the charges low. So far I have charged seven hundred and fifty pounds a year, which is about a third of the price of most courses (but due to rise to eight hundred and fifty pounds).

ROWENA: How many weekends a year do you teach?

YUBRAJ: Ten weekends a year over four years. In between, people can come to the clinics and I organise lots of retreats and trips out to places like Kew Gardens.

ROWENA: Have you applied for recognition with the Society of Homeopaths and the ARH?

YUBRAJ: I gave up on the Society of Homeopaths. Well we mutually gave up on each other, back in 1999 because I teach single handed and because there is far too much of a spiritual content outside of the field of homeopathy. So they were a bit concerned. I am not going to water down or change the course, so there is no point going down the Society of Homeopaths' route. And eventually, as you know, the Alliance of Registered Homeopaths (ARH)) came into existence. They are promoting a diversity of training, and as long as someone has the homeopathic training, then if they are also a spiritual worker or healer or interested in esoteric medicine, then they can still be on their register.

ROWENA: So you are on their list of colleges?

YUBRAJ: Yes. Most of my graduates either go to the ARH or join the Association of Natural Medicine, but the Homeopathic Medical Association (HMA) also recognises me. The new accrediting body when it is in force, as a new registering body, will have to reaccredit all colleges as you probably know. Their mission statement is to have openness and diversity of training and not to have a closed system anymore, so there isn't going to be the same Society model. I partly know that because I am involved in the Registration and Continuous Professional Development working groups, through the Council for Homeopathic Colleges (CHC).

It was an interesting time, when I was in the Accreditation Working Group for a few sessions, to fill in for some missing CHC members, because we were put into small teams and asked to get together some of the principles of the new accreditation process. The one I was asked to do was write up the teaching and learning methodology, so the accreditation system could look at how a college taught and how students learnt to see if that was the way they should teach and learn for this accreditation model. So of course what I could have done, which would have been presumably the Society of Homeopaths route or something like that, would have been to document every single way of learning, every single way a student could learn both intellectually and intuitively, imaginatively, every single way. Document every single way a college and tutors could teach, whether that is through verbal, lecture or seminar and role play and case studies and video cases. And just put it all into a big hefty kind of listing, and if a college fulfils a certain number of them and so on.

But of course I didn't. I just wrote just half a page, a very simple two part test. If a college met the learning and teaching requirements of the future accrediting body, all they had to show were two things - one was that whatever method of teaching they taught and whatever method of learning students adopted, they were free to do whatever they wanted as long as they fulfilled the two part test which was a) they achieved basic National Occupational Standards (NOS)[96] at the end, and b) they promoted the self-development of the student. And then that was it, the college decides, the student decides and it is open.

ROWENA: So how was that received?

YUBRAJ: Very well. Because people were really tired of going through, slogging out every single possibility and then realising there is still some other possibilities that could exist. Jerome Whitney, Christopher Hammond of the Homeopathy College (which used to be known as the College of Practical Homeopathy in the Midlands (CPH Midlands)), and Anne Waters of the Lakeland College of Homeopathy are all part of this group.

Although I have a programme that I follow, every time I tend to update it, bring in some new perspective and add some more material based on what is going on in the world. We have new remedies and new provings, so the first year is very much about basic, preclinical sciences - anatomy, physiology, like any other foundation course would have. But instead, I am bringing in the spiritual concepts from the beginning, and bringing in the medical diseases and the models from an allopathic and esoteric perspective, and then getting people to grasp the spiritual anatomy.

Then the second year tends to be about integrating. I then bring in the more esoteric models of herbalism, crystals, flower essences, iridology, cranial work, all the rest of it, so from the beginning there is homeopathy embedded into each class, but bringing in all these different paradigms from the second year. Then the third year is continuing, but with a bit more focus on looking at how to treat mother and child with all these different ways; how to treat a vaccinated person, hospital patient and so on. Then in the fourth year it is integrating it further; ethics and practitioner development. So hopefully by the end of it they are both a healer - they understand spirituality, they have done a lot of self-development - and they have got the basic NOS[96]. I am not training people up to be a herbalist, an iridologist or a flower essence practitioner. They kind of only touch on these areas, but it is more than usual and it is quite easy to integrate with homeopathy because herbalism really blends well with the use of mother tinctures.

ROWENA: So I am going to try and get a feel of how you practise. Someone comes to you with cancer, for example, how do you treat them?

YUBRAJ: Taking the case history will take no more than half an hour. If it goes beyond that, then I just cut it short and carry on with any case taking the next time. And usually it takes less than that, twenty minutes, for example, because after a while you kind of cut corners, and you know like passing a driving test, you don't ask all the modalities. And then I spend about half an hour doing hands on healing and I tend not to explain anything about the homeopathic or the alternative perspectives until after I have done the healing work, because only then do I get a real feeling for the energy. So what I am doing is to show people that although Hahnemann explained vital energy and said you cannot see it, I am saying that you can see it, you can feel it and you can perceive it - whether that is with machines, dowsing, pendulums or direct energy work.

ROWENA: So through that healing you get a sense of what remedy they need or remedies they need?

YUBRAJ: Quite possibly. Through the healing I will get a sense of what miasm they are in, where the active layers are, what is the active energy now, and I may actually then perceive the layers in the case energetically and work out what their soul purpose was for that disease. I work on karmic issues; going through past life work with them or in myself without necessarily telling them all the details. It depends on time and how much they can understand. I will also know what drug is doing what.

ROWENA: And how do you do that?

YUBRAJ: Well after years of it you get a feel for what a chemical or radiation feels like in the energy. You can often feel mercury or fluoride in the body, for example.

ROWENA: How do you feel that?

YUBRAJ: It is intuitive. If you feel one patient with cancer, you can feel it as a sticky, stagnant, damp energy that feels out of sync with the rest of the energy field. Then after a while it is in your library; your vibrational library of memories. Then you can feel someone else with the same pattern and you realise what it is. And if there is a new energy that you have never felt before you can ask it questions, as energy talks.

ROWENA: So how do you ask it questions?

YUBRAJ: You fire a question at it with your thoughts and you get an answer back and you use your internal dialogue or imagery. Everyone has their own psychic facilities. As you are healing, if you can get a handle on your thinking, through meditation work, then your thoughts will be clear. Then you can observe whatever thoughts you are getting while you are healing someone. If you listen to your thoughts while the person is talking to you then you will be actually listening to some of the patient's own inner dialogue.

ROWENA: So has this been channelled to you? Did you learn it somewhere?

YUBRAJ: Both, self learning, doing courses here and there, shamanic training, joining channelling courses, meditation groups and through teaching.

ROWENA: So that is how your students do their consultations - in the same way as you do?

YUBRAJ: Well, how they would want to.

ROWENA: But you are a role model for them.

YUBRAJ: One of the students prefers to dowse, another is very much kinaesthetic and another is very visual. So it is a matter of getting them to read their own psychic and spiritual impressions and to build that inner library of experiences. By the end of the four years I have hopefully exposed them to a wide variety of diseases and got them to grasp intuitively that as well as to intellectually know it.

ROWENA: So do you take cases in front of them, or do they take the cases?

YUBRAJ: I bring a patient in or they present a case that they have got, so usually every weekend somebody either is presenting a case, or I am presenting one or doing a slide show with clinical signs of scanned images from textbooks, showing them a jaundiced patient or a patient with a stroke and then explaining the energetics of it so they get a visual image.

ROWENA: So what would a prescription be like? I know that is a really difficult question to answer, but it is obviously not just one remedy?

YUBRAJ: Well, the remedy itself may shout at me from the healing and of course during the case taking and then I will usually go and make all my remedies. I prescribe on site from my own pharmacy from medicating tinctures in ninety six percent alcohol. I medicate my own sac lac and I have got about two thousand remedies in my pharmacy here now and that is just the homeopathics.

And I have also got about one thousand flower essences, a few hundred crystals, herbal tinctures and dried herbs. So from that I will either make a mother tincture or herbal tinctures to drain an organ. For example, if they have obviously got kidney problems I might make up a herbal formula with fennel, horsetail, nettle tea and dandelion. For homeopathy I usually use a 30C, and if they have got a chronic disease then I will repeat the dose. Occasionally I just do the one dose but I find people are multilayered so therefore I tend to use repeated dosing. Mostly, Robin Murphy influenced me, at least in the earlier days anyway.

ROWENA: Is this specifically for cancer or generally?

YUBRAJ: Generally. For a case of chronic rheumatoid arthritis for example, I might use 6C three times or twice a day and 30C once a day for a few weeks and then review.

ROWENA: The same remedy or different remedies?

YUBRAJ: The same remedy but at the same time, because I might not see that patient for two months, partly from clinic constraints and partly time availability. I often get a sense of the layers and the layer that is beneath the one that I am just treating and give them a remedy to start in three to four weeks so I am pre-empting the layers.

ROWENA: Which you have been able to sense...

YUBRAJ: Yes. And then the other thing I often do is use a high potency remedy and drain it with a low potency of the same or a different remedy. So I might give them *Nux vomica* to drain, while I am giving them *Diamond (Adamas)* or *Thymus gland* or a new remedy. And I use a lot of new remedies, because we make a lot of new remedies here anyway.

ROWENA: Do you prove and make them?

YUBRAJ: Both. We make them from the original samples, either we make the macerated solution or we triturate it down if it is insoluble. Generally speaking there are about one or two new remedies being made a week so we have got about three or four hundred new remedies.

ROWENA: So not remedies that have been made before?

YUBRAJ: No, they haven't been made anywhere. For example, we have made a few remedies from paintings. We have got *The Temptation* and *The Crucifixion*, from our visits to the National Gallery. We have got some sacred site remedies, for example, *The Sphinx* from Egypt when we went there.

ROWENA: So these were trips with students?

YUBRAJ: Yes.

ROWENA: Well I can see why the students come here then!

YUBRAJ: Yes. The whole overall experience is very different.

ROWENA: So if you don't advertise, where do people hear about you?

YUBRAJ: Word of mouth mostly. I used to advertise in *Caduceus*[97] and *Positive Health*[98], but because I haven't raised the fees I have to watch what I am spending on marketing. It works out because just by word of mouth there are enough students. At the moment there are about a hundred and twenty six students across the six years. It is a four year course, but people tend not to want to just go away and never come back again, so there are two post graduate years. About a quarter come back regularly to attend some of the postgraduate meetings. We have three or four a year, and the rest of them maintain contact either now and then by telephone or when they want a new remedy or advice.

ROWENA: So they are going off and being quite successful in their own practices?

YUBRAJ: I would say half the graduates work and build up a client base. The other half don't; you cannot make people. Primarily their intention is only self-development. They don't want to be homeopaths and because it is actually not just homeopathy, it is a lot of personal development, spiritual awareness and fun - people can come in late, they can miss classes, they can turn up to repeat sessions of classes they have missed - so it is very, very flexible for people.

ROWENA: So this afternoon with your genetics class, how does that work, what would you be covering and how does it enter the spiritual realm?

YUBRAJ: What I am doing today so far is starting with the scientific models, explaining genetics scientifically in quite lengthy details as you have seen, and then I will be explaining the *I Ching*[99] and how the Chinese saw the genetic code and I will explain the spiritual concepts that are well documented in various spiritual books including *The Book of Knowledge; Keys of Enoch*[100]. I am explaining the languages of light, colour and sound, and the frequencies and the mantras and how there are pyramid forces in the genetic code and so on and so forth. And then I will explain Atlantis and the history of the human race. I will start explaining twelve stranded DNA and go through New Age concepts of the genetic code, gene therapy and cloning and the relevance of these and how it is distorting the vital energy. By the end of it, they will have a grasp of both basic and spiritual genetics, the modern diseases that could come out of the way we approach genetics and how to look at diseases.

I will explain the remedies, including the miasms, and I will also be explaining other forces within the genetics and remedies. So I might look at *Obsidian, Jet* or *Berlin Wall*, or one that we have made, *Zubeneschamali*, for example, which is from the planet where the Grays come from and is involved in a lot of alien abduction. I go onto educational websites for scientific researchers and download genetic sequences for my students. Online Mendelian Inheritance in Man (OMIN) is affiliated to the National Institute of Health in America and on that site you can actually search on any disease to see if they have found the genetic sequence for it.

So I download the genetic sequence for a disease a patient might have, print it off on my printer, stick a bottle of alcohol on it, and make a remedy from it. Then I can give that remedy to people with that particular type of disease. I also downloaded one of the genes for hypertension and use it for some patients with high blood pressure. What we are going to do is download from the internet a few genes of certain diseases and get the students to do the provings, so we are building up a library of genetic remedies.

ROWENA: Fascinating.

YUBRAJ: Classically there is only DNA, which is in OA Julian's new remedies book *Materia Medica of New Homoeopathic Remedies*[101]. I think there is an *RNA remedy* too. What we have done is actually to make specific genes rather than some bog-standard generic DNA. So I have opened up the subject for people. We also do some gene healing techniques which I have developed to repair the genetic code, to clear ancestral mutations and to anchor extraterrestrial genes, to clear out latent karma, to repair ageing degenerative sequences, to unblock the DNA from human diseases and anchor a new blue print – the classic spiritual concept of the divine image of God in human or man. I am not Christian or religious, but feel if humans are made in God's image then clearly God's image is in a blueprint somewhere inherent in every human, so it is about bringing that inherent divine blueprint in. So I teach them some of these techniques.

ROWENA: Tell me about your book *Spiritual Bioenergetics of Homoeopathic Materia Medica*[94].

YUBRAJ: It explains one hundred and fifty one homeopathic remedies of which eight or nine are new ones including *Lac humanum, Ayahuasca, Moldavite* and the *Berlin Wall*. And the rest of them are classical *Aconitum napellus* to *Zincum*. I have made it a bit more reader friendly than perhaps some other materia medica. I draw on the Doctrine of Signatures, toxicology, the native botanies, zoology and geology of the substance, too. But rather than just saying it, I have also tried to explain the signatures. For example, in Sepia succus, if the male Sepia succus can lose its reproductive tentacle when it mates with the female, then I have related that to how the male can be feeling impotent, as if he has lost his drive, his tentacle, and his testes. Then there is a whole section on the spiritual aspects of the remedy, some of which is brand new and channelled, some of which is in existing material in anthroposophical textbooks or articles or journals here and there.

For each remedy I have explained an astrological profile, not just the idea that this remedy may be a Mars remedy but it also may be a Sun and Mars remedy where the Sun and Mars are in conjunction, or opposite each other, or in squares. So I am bringing in a more detailed astrological profile and also some of the new astrological data of asteroids and some esoteric planets. This is useful for the astrologer who may want to study homeopathy or if he is using it already. It is not necessarily for homeopaths who want to study astrology, as I have written it at the level an astrologer understands.

Then I wrote a little section on each remedy on the cranial sacral profile, again it is more for the cranial sacral practitioner who wants to know what the *Arnica* state would feel like in the cranial sacral system. Over time I am hoping that homeopaths will explore these other modalities and will then start wanting to use a materia medica that is a cross over as well. I explain the Chinese diagnosis that matches the remedy profile or the disease profiles. So again, some people actually have an affinity for oriental medicine whether or not they have studied it. They understand the concepts of damp and spleen, chi deficiency and all the rest of it very well. So clearly they have prior training or Oriental guides etc. And then there is a section on related remedies. Rather than just a list, I have actually given a more detailed profile of at least some of the related remedies and put in a few new remedies in there as well. And at the end of the book there is a glossary section, so people can read basic principles of astrology, cranial sacral and Chinese Medicine. I am working on Volume Two now.

ROWENA: How do you have time for everything?

YUBRAJ: It is a mystery! Volume two is a pictorial companion book with about eleven hundred pictures in it. I included caricature cartoons in Volume one for a bit of humour and because I think that some people actually find that the cartoons grasp the essence of the remedy.

ROWENA: You mentioned channelling earlier, do you channel through meditation then?

YUBRAJ: Yes, and also just by reading and listening to people.

ROWENA: So do you hear or do you see?

YUBRAJ: I perceive the thoughts.

ROWENA: How can you differentiate between your thoughts and the thoughts that are being channelled?

YUBRAJ: It takes years of discernment and just being clear.

ROWENA: So what was your background before all of this then - I know you were a doctor, but were you spiritual when you were growing up?

YUBRAJ: I was, but I also went out and played cricket.

ROWENA: Did you grow up here?

YUBRAJ: Yes, in England. It was just an ordinary background, nothing special. I got kind of symbolically hit on the head in the early twenties and woke up. I am now thirty seven. I chose the name the School of Shamanic Homoeopathy and people always ask me what does that mean, so I explain that I use the term Shamanic simply because I want graduates to feel empowered that they are a shaman and that they understand the laws of vibration and healing that are streaming from them and through them.

ROWENA: You have given me much food for thought here Yubraj. Thank you for allowing me to sit in on your class and giving me the little time you have for the interview. You have blown me away with your ideas! Thank you.

CHAPTER 20:   KAAREN WHITNEY

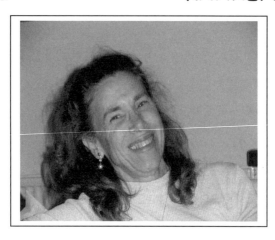

I had the pleasure of having a telephone conversation with Kaaren Whitney but our paths had crossed before when she spent a day teaching us in our final year at the London College of Classical Homeopathy (LCCH). She had spent the morning sharing her insights of *Carcinosin* and the afternoon practising dream analysis with us. The day was an interesting one and I did recall that Kaaren was one of those homeopaths that had been around since the start of it all back in the 1970s. Referred to by Jerome Whitney as 'my dear ex-wife' throughout my licentiate, it was wonderful to finally be on the receiving end of her teaching back in 2001 and the telephone with her four years later on Thursday 19 May 2005.

"Doing absolutely your best for each person who comes to you would be my criteria for success. That does not mean every patient is totally cured. That is quite unrealistic, as there are some things they need to work out in a long-term way, and I am just a step and I want to be the best step I can."   *Kaaren Whitney, May 2005*

"If your goal is to make a living, it is going to be a problem. If your goal is to do good homeopathy, then it is not going to be easy, but it will be wonderful. It depends on whether you want easy or wonderful."   *Kaaren Whitney, May 2005*

"By the end of the first consultation, I want to know about sleep, food and weather. And within the sleep area, I always ask about dreams; whether they have had any recurring dreams, if they have any dreams from childhood and if they have had any nightmares that have affected them in a particular way."   *Kaaren Whitney, May 2005*

"The study of people is more important than books. Books are needed, but the emphasis on people and how they work is a greater study than what can be obtained from books."   *Kaaren Whitney, May 2005*

CHAPTER 20: KAAREN WHITNEY

ROWENA: I would love to hear your story Kaaren. To go with the flow for however long we have and see where it takes us, but starting with how you got into homeopathy and what your journey has been like.

KAAREN: As did many people, I got into homeopathy because of not being well and was fortunate enough not to be well in the vicinity of Thomas Maughan!

ROWENA: Right. Had you met him before you were ill then?

KAAREN: It was very serendipitous. It was about time to 'do' Europe, and because you speak English here, I thought it would be easy. My cousin was here, and so we made this arrangement for a holiday. The day before we left we were at a mediation, and a woman that we knew had a friend with her who had just come back from England and she said, "If you are going to England you must try and meet this amazing old man. He might not answer his phone but if he does you might get invited to tea in his garden." So she wrote down the name and eventually when we got here, we rang up and luckily we were invited for tea in the garden.

ROWENA: Wonderful! He was meant to answer his phone that day and you were meant to meet him!

KAAREN: Yes, and it went from there. Since I only knew my cousin, and now Thomas, when I got ill, my first recourse was to go to homeopathy, although I knew nothing about it. So Thomas treated me until I recovered and our holiday instead of two weeks got extended to four or five.

ROWENA: What a holiday!

KAAREN: Yes, it was cold turkey, really. We also then got to go to Stonehenge and Jerome actually joined the Druid Order at that time, but I didn't because I didn't actually think I had anything to offer.

ROWENA: What were you doing in the USA before you came?

KAAREN: I was a children's librarian and I had a wonderful children's library with lots of staff and even more volunteers and had a really great time. When I came back from the UK I felt wonderful, but my skin was erupting all over the place and everyone said, "Are you all right, dear?" I was very good, but I might not at that point have looked the radiant self I felt. From then I very much wanted to learn more about homeopathy but it was 1970 and there were only five homeopaths in all of the USA!

ROWENA: Really!

KAAREN: At least on the register, anyway.

ROWENA: Did you know who they were at that time?

KAAREN: Well, one was Dr Davis who happened to be in my next town, which is again just miraculous. There was one in Washington and I don't remember where the others were, but they were hugely spread out in the country. But of course there is homeopathy and homeopathy, and Dr Davis was actually quite good but not Thomas Maughan. I went to him for some acutes subsequently but when it came to what I call 'real' treatment, I was back in England. We made several trips and eventually I also joined the Druid Order, appreciating that I had a lot to learn and well, things just went from there. I went to all the classes I could.

ROWENA: So how quickly did you move here?

KAAREN: It took about a year and a half. I had a very responsible job, so it took a while to tie everything up.

ROWENA: Did you move here because of Thomas Maughan?

KAAREN: I moved here because of homeopathy and the Druid Order.

ROWENA: Does the Druid Order exist in the USA?

KAAREN: No. There are groups that call themselves Druids, but like homeopathy, there are all kinds of variations.

ROWENA: OK. So when did the Druids first come about?

KAAREN: Egypt, Greece and Rome, but the Druid Order was reconstituted in 1717.

ROWENA: So, still a long time ago.

KAAREN: Yes.

ROWENA: And did it have a resurgence at the same time as homeopathy, in the 1970s?

KAAREN: I would say it probably did.

ROWENA: Do you think that that had something to do with homeopathy?

KAAREN: Only in the sense that the premise of the Druid Order is that life is good and people actually do try to be good, and their past, their habits and weaknesses hold them back from their basic aim.

ROWENA: Yes. Are there a lot of homeopaths involved in the Druid Order?

KAAREN: Quite a lot, yes.

ROWENA: But are there a lot of Druids who have nothing to do with homeopathy?

KAAREN: Yes. But because their main emphasis is on self-development, they will be interested in some aspect of healing; not necessarily as their life work, but they will probably choose acupuncture or something natural when any kind of trouble arises.

ROWENA: That makes sense. If they were putting loads of antibiotics into their system, they wouldn't necessarily feel they were following a good path, I would imagine.

KAAREN: Yes, but there is no rule that you have to do this but natural medicine ends up being the most logical choice for their health.

ROWENA: And they learn quite a lot within the Druid Order about nature and the spirit of plants and things like that?

KAAREN: Yes, if you are open to receive, yes. But there is nothing that you have to do or have to learn.

ROWENA: OK. So what was your involvement?

KAAREN: I was drawn to homeopathy and I was also drawn to the integrity of Thomas Maughan; not that he was a saint but he walked his talk, which is what integrity is all about. It wasn't a word that was bandied about in those days; it was just how I felt.

ROWENA: So where did you go from there?

KAAREN: Well, I suppose that the next phase was when Thomas died, and both Jerome and I, and a small group who had been studying intensely with him, took up the mantle, so to speak. It was a very strong, focused group; Peter Chappell, Robert Davidson, Mary Titchmarsh, Lynn Lovell who is not practising anymore, Jerome and I.

ROWENA: And Martin Miles?

KAAREN: Yes, very much so. We would go to all the classes we could and we would get together in between and work on taking cases of friends and relatives. We would get different views from each other and it was just a very intense time. This was before Thomas died. And then after, it was even more so. I think Robert Davidson took over the classes in the first instance and then Martin Miles did subsequently, and a few of us did it in between, as well.

ROWENA: And then he set up his school; the College of Homeopathy (COH).

KAAREN: Yes. And then we set up the Society of Homeopaths. Around the same time, just after Thomas died, there were a few people who wanted to know more about homeopathy, and so I started doing classes as well. So we are talking about 1976, now. The classes were small in the beginning and really exciting. Also at this time, a great lifelong wish was fulfilled and I became pregnant and had Alexandra. And that was done all with homeopathy, including being treated for septicaemia.

ROWENA: Oh my God! When did you get that?

KAAREN: After childbirth. Martin Miles was great! We had to create a hospital at home and the boiler went and the telephone went, and everything happened because that is how life is! It just gives you more challenges to work with.

ROWENA: I couldn't agree more.

KAAREN: And I continued practising and teaching in a relatively minor way, but the main thing was, however many or few patients I had, I gave my all. I think that is one of the mainstays of how homeopathy can continue and one can make a living out of it. Of course, that depends on what standard of living you aspire to. But doing absolutely your best for each person who comes to you would be my criteria for success. That does not mean every patient is totally cured. That is quite unrealistic, as there are some things they need to work out in a long-term way, and I am just a step and I want to be the best step I can.

ROWENA: That is beautifully put and I am in complete agreement, of course. So do you see patients at your home?

KAAREN: Yes. I have always worked from home.

ROWENA: OK, and where is that?

KAAREN: Now it is in Suffolk, but it used to be in London. Here I have a tree circle in a field that is separate from where my house is and I am walking there now as I am talking to you.

ROWENA: Is it like a labyrinth? Jack Temple used one as part of his work[102]. Are you influenced by him?

KAAREN: No. I actually don't know much about him, although I have heard much about him.

ROWENA: He is wonderful. In saying that, he is not in this realm anymore. He died, I think, last year.

KAAREN: Yes, and he had actually been to Suffolk and I wasn't able to go to the talk he did here. There are obviously insights that he learned from his patients that would have been great to hear about but the real thing is the inspiration that inspires us to practise. But inspiration isn't just received from a person. Inspiration occurred in the 1980s when we had classes in London in Ross Road. It was really a Golden Era, but it was not just me giving out; it was the exchange and it was the connection with the students. It was the give and take. I was inspired because they were inspired.

ROWENA: Yes, I know what you mean.

KAAREN: It was great working together. Thomas always talked about the Golden Age and he said, "You never think that you are in it. You think it is really hard work and you know nothing, which is quite true, but in retrospect you can look back and see what an amazing fruitful, shining time it was."

ROWENA: Do you think we are not in a Golden Age anymore, then?

KAAREN: I think it is possibly becoming 'gold oriented' rather than golden, and some of your questions you sent me ahead of the interview probably highlight that.

ROWENA: The one about it going dormant again, maybe?

KAAREN: And the one about how to make a living.

ROWENA: Do you think it was easier then?

KAAREN: No. If your goal is to make a living, it is going to be a problem. If your goal is to do good homeopathy, then it is not going to be easy, but it will be wonderful. It depends on whether you want easy or wonderful. And there is a lot of emphasis on going for less than golden.

ROWENA: It is really interesting having this conversation with you, because I can see it from a completely different point of view now. Back then there probably wasn't this whole emphasis that we have now about it being a career that you need to make a living from. I am getting a feeling that back then that probably wasn't even something that was talked about. Or was it?

KAAREN: No, it wasn't talked about, but it was lived. I mean, if you did make money, that was what you lived on. And if you didn't, as is the case with a tremendous amount of artists and musicians, you would do other things to support your passion.

ROWENA: Yes, so they don't have a sort of expectation necessarily of making money out of what they love.

KAAREN: No. It is not the prime goal. If it is the prime goal, then I have not really seen any successful homeopaths that have had it as such. I have seen homeopaths that have considerably more money than I do, but they may want or need more. I am very content with my level of income and I am living very well. There are actually a lot of homeopaths in this area but I don't find that at all a problem, because everyone is going to get the person they need at that time. And they might change, and people do change, and that is the whole point; to change.

ROWENA: Yes, exactly. Do you think we can outgrow our homeopaths, then?

KAAREN: Maybe not necessarily outgrow but as we change, a different kind of treatment is required.

ROWENA: And so in what sort of way do you prescribe? How would you describe the way that you practise?

KAAREN: Basically Hahnemannian, but I will do whatever is needed.

ROWENA: So what do you mean by whatever is needed?

KAAREN: If there is a desperate case and I feel that it might need three low potencies all at once, I will do that.

ROWENA: Why would you feel the case might need that?

KAAREN: Because the vital force might not be sufficient; or in the sense of allowing time for me to find the right remedy to use in a higher potency.

ROWENA: So those lower potencies will ideally up the vital force and get it to the point where either the one right remedy will show itself or.....

KAAREN: Or within those three might be the right remedy. Hopefully it is in those three. That is what I would do if I needed to, but that is not how I generally prescribe.

ROWENA: So generally it is one remedy, then?

KAAREN: Yes, one remedy, but quite often in a divided dose and mainly to take at bedtime. If it is a first appointment, I am generally looking at a very long-term kind of aspect. It depends on where they are, what their need is at the time and how I assess whether they will be able to use the remedy. If I think it will be too traumatic and they won't continue and they will just reject their rubbish that comes up, I might go quite slowly and prepare the way more, so it depends. My preference is to give one remedy and find the results, and in that line I don't generally tell patients the name of the remedy. Because like me, they are all interested and go and look it up and say, "That's not me" or "Oh, I didn't know that I had that".

ROWENA: Do you think that affects the case very much?

KAAREN: I think it does, and I know it is not a popular view, but it is still what I do.

ROWENA: Well, that works for you and that is what is important.

KAAREN: And there are some patients that it does not work for, and so I adapt and they can know it, but I generally ask for some time, and they generally find that OK.

ROWENA: And do you tell them at the right time?

KAAREN: Yes. I have no intention at all of keeping it from them. My only intention is that health will come about as soon as possible.

ROWENA: I understand. Do you use dream analysis in your practice?

KAAREN: A lot. Yes. Dreams can let me know how a remedy has worked much more quickly than physical symptoms. It takes time for the physical symptoms to change, but there is great information in the dreams. That is for my benefit in a sense, but as far as the patient goes, their dreams can also help lead to a remedy.

ROWENA: So in the first consultation, you ask about their dreams?

KAAREN: Oh, absolutely. And especially in the first consultation, because part of my procedure is letting them talk, but at the end of the day, I want three areas covered besides their history, which they give in varying forms. By the end of the first consultation, I want to know about sleep, food and weather. And within the sleep area, I always ask about dreams; whether they have had any recurring dreams, if they have any dreams from childhood and if they have had any nightmares that have affected them in a particular way.

ROWENA: And if they have had any bad dreams in childhood, which certainly I can remember that I did, do you see if people move out of that state? If I were to come to you and you were to ask me that question, I would probably mention a recurring dream I had as a child. Would you then think that is part of me now?

KAAREN: If you still remember that dream, yes.

ROWENA: OK, that is interesting.

KAAREN: It will be part of your present remedy because it is still within your consciousness.

ROWENA: And then how do you look that up in the repertory?

KAAREN: Well, that is the long-term skill and challenge. It is not necessarily direct, but there are three routes into the repertory with dreams. First of all there is the dream section and then there are fears and delusions. Also, depending on what the dream is about, it could just be an exemplar of a remedy. Like, to have dreamt of a huge stool, as in excrement, might indicate Mercury (*Mercurius solubilis*), which has that sort of aspect. That would probably be the sort of dream one might remember.

ROWENA: OK. Do you do some sort of dream analysis with patients like we did in class that day?

KAAREN: No. That would need a whole separate session, as it would take a minimum of forty five minute. There is definitely not time within the first appointment or subsequent appointments. Although if someone is coming up with significant dreams, I do ask them if they would like to work on it and even more so if I am stuck, but they have to be willing and really wanting to do that. Most people are fascinated, but they have the delusion that I will tell them what their dreams mean and they are always, always, always impressed that actually they know what their dreams mean themselves.

And people do not know that they know, and really it takes quite a lot to encourage their understanding to come out. I was doing a whole day, dream workshop and this woman brought a dream, and in just staying with the process and having her bring out what was within, the most amazing understanding came out of a stillbirth that was never acknowledged.

ROWENA: Oh, that is fantastic.

KAAREN: It was so powerful for all of us there. I wrote a ritual for her later and that had an aspect of completion for that phase of healing for her. So it was not only that dream work, but what happened subsequently.

ROWENA: Brilliant, brilliant. And so do you still teach?

KAAREN: In theory, yes. But I really don't enjoy the travel so much anymore. I love teaching in Ireland and I love teaching there because the pupils are so receptive. It is part of what Nuala Eising provided; she created that atmosphere. I really enjoyed teaching there because I really appreciated the exchange. I don't want to just lecture. It is give and take.

ROWENA: Is there anything else you want to share with me?

KAAREN: We have slightly covered it, but one of your questions was about books, and all I want to say about that is that the study of people is more important than books. Books are needed, but the emphasis on people and how they work is a greater study than what can be obtained from books.

ROWENA: So how do people do that? Obviously you get the experience of being with patients, but prior to that how does one get that?

KAAREN: Yes, that is an interesting question because that kind of study can come from every aspect of the person. The thing I try and encourage students to do most, is to study people on the tube to see, for example, how a certain kind of nose goes with a certain type of ears. Making observations is a skill homeopaths need and this is a good way to get used to it and connect it with people you know. Another way is looking at hands and another way is the study of astrology or the chakras. It is all in relation to understanding more about the person.

ROWENA: So do you do all that with your patients?

KAAREN: Not necessarily. These are just aspects of looking more deeply at people. And eventually it really just becomes second nature.

ROWENA: I have so enjoyed this conversation and personally I have got a lot out of it, and so I know that whoever ends up reading it will too. Thank you very much, keep well Kaaren and take care of yourself.

CHAPTER 21: ANNE WATERS

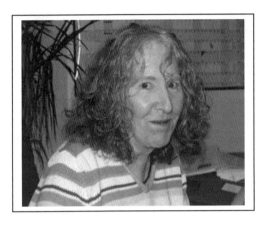

Saturday 21 May 2005 took me to the Lakeland College of Homeopathy at its Regent's College campus in London, home to the Centre for Homeopathic Education (CHE) as well. Its other campus is located in the Lake District, Cumbria (Lakes). After observing the comings and goings of many happy students in the reception area during their break, I joined Myriam Shivadikar's first year materia medica class where I gleaned some further insights into *Opium*, a remedy I haven't prescribed myself but felt like I needed a few years ago! I then met with Anne Waters, the principal and, with much laughter between us, she shared her experiences with me. Since completing the interview, Dave Evans is no longer a director at the Lakeland College, though he still teaches for them and he now owns and runs The North West College of Homoeopathy (NWCH) in Manchester. Anne's new co-director is Kay Hebbourn, one of the Lakeland College's first graduates.

"I am a peripatetic homeopath; I don't like clinics and much prefer home visiting. When I first started practising I wanted to work with children and see them in their natural environment where they were relaxed, comfortable and at ease. Where they didn't have to sit still, behave and play with a basket of toys that wasn't of their choice."
Anne Waters, May 2005

"We want our students to understand that if someone has a physical issue it often started as an energetic problem. So we teach people about the aura, and the chakras, and how the lungs in Chinese Medicine hold grief; the kidneys, fear and the liver, anger. We talk about how if someone is not speaking their truth, their throat chakra may be blocked, and how to open it up and get the energy flowing."
Anne Waters, May 2005

"I fundamentally believe that homeopathy is safe. I think you can have unsafe practitioners, but that is different."
Anne Waters, May 2005

CHAPTER 21:   ANNE WATERS

ROWENA: The first question to ask is how did you get into homeopathy originally?

ANNE: Well that is a really good story! I was the head of a residential special school for children with emotional and behavioural difficulties. It was an interesting and challenging job, and I thought I was doing it quite well. They were all seven to twelve year olds with blond hair and blue eyes, looking like angels. One day one of the mums came up to visit, and she went into the kitchen and through the kitchen cupboards. She was pulling things out of the drawers and asking me why I was giving them this and that. She was reading all the additives and E numbers, and demanding that I should know more about the Hyperactive Children Society. This was back in 1984 and I didn't know anything about such things. I was an educationalist and I wasn't into anything alternative and she made me feel very limited and inadequate.

And so, I started to research nutrition, and to take a great deal of interest in what I was feeding the youngsters. And that put my foot into the alternative world. I saw the effect the food changes had on making our life easier in school, and it also developed in me a grudging, respect for this mum who had really made me look at other things. And then she sent some *Sulphur 6C* for her son, for his dry skin and asked if I would please give him one three times a day. So I phoned the school doctor and said that I had got something called a homeopathic remedy, *Sulphur,* and he said that it was placebo and to throw it in a drawer. So then I phoned my dad, who was a pharmacist, and I told the same story to him, and he said it was a placebo as well! So I didn't give it to the child and then three weeks later, his mum started asking me how her son was getting on with his *Sulphur* and I absolutely couldn't justify myself and so for a second time this woman completely wrong-footed me.

So, I didn't know what homeopathy was, I had never heard the word. I went into the staff meeting, and I asked if anyone knew anything about homeopathy. My secretary replied that a friend of hers was studying homeopathy in London and was in her final year. So at my request my secretary brought Sally Holligan into school to see me, she was Sally Bennett at the time, and she was the girlfriend of Ian Watson. She told me a little bit about homeopathy, which just sounded totally ludicrous to me and I really wanted to prove that she was off the wall and bonkers. My son was three at the time, an asthmatic and on Ventolin. Sally talked about asthma and how she treated it so I asked her if she would take his case. She prescribed him *Tuberculinum bovinum 1M* and for the first time he stopped wheezing at night in bed; he could run, and do things without getting out of breath.

I invited her to come and look at the boys in school and tell me if she could do anything for them. When she came she brought Ian Watson with her and they watched the children. Sally Holligan decided that she would like to treat one of the children. She picked up a little boy who was talking to himself and to his shoulders. He was a much damaged child who had had a horrendous start in life, with failure to thrive with his natural mother, and lots of foster placements where he had been abused and burnt with cigarettes. He ended up in the psychiatric ward in hospital being drip-fed. When they released him from hospital, he was on very heavy medication.

He was one of the first ever children to be put on Ritalin, he was also on something called Methylphenidate and he had been on Haloperidol since he was only eight. I had to get the permission from his psychologist, psychiatrist, social workers, educational welfare officers and the school doctors for Sally Holligan to treat him. It took me about three months to get the permissions, and than Sally came in, and she spent just an hour with him. She didn't talk to him; she just stood and watched him and than she gave him a *Hyoscyamus 10M*. And I remember, at the time, thinking, "Only one tablet to suck before he goes to bed twenty minutes after he has brushed his teeth; this is ridiculous!"

And then the next morning, one of the care stuff rung me around seven in the morning, and said that he was running round in the yard in his pyjamas and asked what she should do. I said to leave him alone and if he comes in, just invite him to have a shower and I told her that I was on my way. I joined him running in the yard and we had our first conversation ever. I asked him why we were running and he said that he didn't know but he knew he had to run. And we negotiated our first agreement, and he said, "I just woke up and I just had to run" and I said "well, if you feel you need to run, just tell your teacher that you need to go out; you go and run and I will get your teacher to send someone for me and I will come and run with you."

And I got really fit because we had three weeks of running, and in that time he talked to me about all the things that had gone wrong in his life. I had given him a puppet to talk to because he was talking to himself and three weeks after that he gave me the puppet back, and said that he didn't need it anymore. He asked if I could give it to another little boy that needed help. He ended up back in mainstream school and I ended up in homeopathic training college.

ROWENA: Amazing.

ANNE: So it was a road to Damascus experience, well and truly. I had the good fortune that my secretary, who now runs the college office for me, was the best friend of Sally Holligan. Sally married Ian Watson a couple of years later but now they are divorced and both remarried. But that is where it started for me, with Ian standing in my school dining room looking out of the window. I went on to do a first aid for beginners course with him and one day he gave me this piece of paper and asked me to sign it. He said it was an application form to go and study homeopathy. I said that I couldn't go and study homeopathy and he replied that I was going to do it one day so I might as well do it now.

ROWENA: When I did a first aid course fifteen years ago, there were people going on from there to study full time, and I also thought, "No way; I am so not ready for that." But a few years later I was.

ANNE: Ian Watson was one of my teachers at the College of Practical Homeopathy in the Midlands (CPH Midlands) (now called the Homeopathy College) and for four years we travelled one weekend a month together to Birmingham. I would go there full of enthusiasm and come back not quite so positive. I couldn't understand why we were learning all this stuff that we would never use. For example, in-depth anatomy and physiology, taught by a fantastic guy who I love to bits, but, oh God it was so boring. I have files of information that I have never opened since. Poor Ian Watson, he had to listen to me whine all the way home.

Eventually Ian Watson just said to me, "Shall we design a course and start a college ourselves?" Ian, Sally Holligan, Anjie Jackson, Dave Evans, Beth Tyers, Deirdre Moon, who are all on our teaching team now but were our tutorial group at the time, just cooked the college up round Ian's kitchen table in evening tutorials and because of my background as a head teacher, I was just the obvious person to help to put it all together.

ROWENA: What year was this?

ANNE: We started the Lakeland College in September 1993 with sixteen students in the Lake District, one of which teaches for us now. We tend to nurture and grow our students and bring them in to teach when they graduate but we do have a lot of people who haven't trained with us teaching here too. We do refer to the college as the Lakeland family. On a regular basis, we still see people who graduated eight or nine years ago, or they run a clinic or a tutor group for us. We very much nurture that connection with our graduates and once they have got a couple of years' experience behind them they can become a mentor to our new students.

ROWENA: I heard that Ian Watson is not involved anymore. How did that come about?

ANNE: Ian Watson is an innovator, he starts things off; he is very tubercular! He puts a huge amount of energy into things and then moves on. We were very lucky to hold him with the Lakeland College for as long as we did, really.

ROWENA: For about ten years?

ANNE: Yes, but for the last four years he was slowly reducing his level of teaching and involvement in the administration and office, so that for the last few years he did mainly teaching. It felt like it became a bit of a one-man band really. Ian Watson has moved on a lot from homeopathy but is still one of the best homeopaths I know. He does a lot of other things, and the work that he wanted to do with the students, was taking us, as a college, away from what we were here for – which was the homeopathic training.

ROWENA: What kind of work is he doing?

ANNE: He is doing a lot of personal development and journey work. Ian Watson is a fantastic facilitator within groups, but he will push a button, and he will push a button, and he will push a button until he gets a response. And he will play the devil's advocate. He is very much into an individual's own personal development; their own personal journey. And I think that there is a place for that but I don't think that we can do it to the depth that Ian would have liked us to have done here. It is impossible due to our timetable. And also, I felt that we were clipping his wings, and I was frustrated when I was saying that I couldn't give him a whole day with a group of students when that is what he wanted. We got to the point where we just decided we better stop being business partners. We are very good friends and have a lot of time for each other.

I do a lot of work with the Council for Homeopathic Colleges (CHC) and I represent them at the Council of Organisations Registering Homeopaths (CORH). I try to make sure that the students can access the registers and insurance if they want to. A lot of it is alien to Ian Watson's philosophy, and it was getting to the point where we were getting convergent. We just needed to acknowledge and recognise it. I wanted to maintain his involvement and I didn't want him to say, that is it, I am moving on completely. So he will be at graduation, and he will always be there when we need him. Whereas, I think if we had tried to hold on to him when he was ready to move on, then it wouldn't have been as good.

We had a planned a gradual withdrawal where he would do less and less. It was a two year plan that was completed in August of last year because it was really important that the students knew what was going on as well. We are not the kind of place that would just drop sudden changes on people, because it breeds insecurity; so we told them from the beginning.

So now Dave Evans is a director of the Lakeland College and we are trying to involve much more of the staff at a managerial level. London staff meetings now happen on a very regular basis, whereas at one time it was all in the Lakes. Part of my learning is to let go and to stop having such a tight rein on things.

ROWENA: So how many students do you have in London?

ANNE: In London, at the moment, we have one hundred and seven and we have fifty four in the Lakes. We only have twelve in Edinburgh and only two year groups up there; the second and third years. We are pulling out of there at the end of next month when the Edinburgh students graduate. The second year group will travel to the Lakes for their final year. We will make them some sort of concession on travelling and accommodation.

ROWENA: Are there any other colleges in Scotland?

ANNE: Yes, but not in Edinburgh. There is Margaret Roy's Scottish College of Homoeopathy in Glasgow. I have got to know her quite well in the last couple years and have so much admiration for that lady. She had a reputation for being a bit of a dragon but really she is just such a sweetie. She has just written a new first aid book, Homoeopathic Acute Prescribing, a Text for Practitioners, First Aid and Self Help[103], which one of my Edinburgh students has illustrated.

ROWENA: So who influenced you when you were studying?

ANNE: Robin Murphy, Paul Herscu, Ian Watson and Robert Davidson. I think someone should recommend Robert Davidson for an OBE or MBE for his services to homeopathy. I think he is a man who is full of frustrations, and I think it is because he is not acknowledged. I think that homeopathy is in the position that it is in this country because of Robert Davidson; there are others but in my opinion he is the one who has really done it. He can be totally inspiring. David Howell is also an excellent teacher. Tony Southam, who doesn't teach anymore, was also a very good teacher and Philip Bailey, to a certain extent as well.

I am very influenced by our own team; I think that we are lucky with the people we have got. I know that I could start again, on the first weekend of the first year and learn something in every lecture - and really, really benefit from doing it. In fact I think I should just go back to being a first year student and do it all again!

ROWENA: I am learning so much from my process of having all these conversations. It is a wonderful experience and I am learning the whole time. Apart from your own team are there other homeopaths that influence you now?

ANNE: I am still a big fan of Robin Murphy. Outside homeopathy, I am a total groupie of Patrick Holford the nutritionist. I think he is an amazing man and I use his nutritional work and put it through my energetic filter. It gives our students a really good and deep understanding of the subject. Remember I came into this world through nutrition. After that mother turned all the food cupboards out, saying I couldn't feed the children the way that I did, I ran the school completely on additive free, whole food. As a result of the input from this mum, the children were seventy percent vegetarian, and the only meat we had was organic. I would have been sacked as a teacher if local authorities had known what I was doing. I had kids walking down the road making cross signs at McDonalds. If they asked why they could only eat organic free-range eggs, I would take them to a battery farm and ask them whose eggs do you want – those chickens', or those chickens'? I was dreadfully political!

Being careful about what the children ate did make our lives easier. Jamie Oliver has won himself a lot of brownie points these last few months. He has worked very, very hard and stood up for his principles, which I think is incredibly brave. So I don't know who influences me now. It is really hard when you are so involved in training to actually get out and get some training in yourself. I have a lot of time for Ian White who is a homeopath, flower essence practitioner and naturopath and also Steve Johnson who developed Alaskan essences and teaches for us one weekend a year down here in London.

In terms of homeopathy, I think I would walk on hot coals to listen to Robin Murphy speak. I have only heard Paul Herscu twice and I thought he was a fantastic teacher. Nuala Eising is just an amazing woman. When I met her I actually heard her telling someone that her car wouldn't start that morning. She had got so frustrated with it that she had thrown a *Rhus toxicodendron 10M* into the petrol tank, and it started first time after that. So my first contact with her was eavesdropping on that conversation.

ROWENA: That is such a good story.

ANNE: I would like to put Madeline Evans on my list, but she can be quite prescriptive and I think, for me, I am not very good at rules. I like people to say that this is my experience, and your experience may be different. And she killed the goldfish she potentised; I still don't understand why a goldfish had to die. I have an admiration for people who push the boundaries and who do new work.

ROWENA: What about Rajan Sankaran?

ANNE: I love his book, *The Sensation in Homeopathy*[63] but I have never heard him speak but I would like to.

ROWENA: His books are fantastic.

ANNE: I think there are cultural differences. We had a student on one of our courses who came over to this country from India for an arranged marriage. She would say to me that she doesn't understand why homeopaths want to know about a patient's libido. She said to me, you just do it and it is finished. She is completely dismissive of premenstrual tension, for example, so we are working very hard because she almost has an allopathic approach. She sat in with the Indian homeopaths seeing two hundred patients in a day and it is so not like that here. I think it is brilliant that someone like Rajan Sankaran can talk in the way that he does about the spirit and the soul.

ROWENA: So how do you practise?

ANNE: I am a peripatetic homeopath; I don't like clinics and much prefer home visiting. When I first started practising I wanted to work with children and see them in their natural environment where they were relaxed, comfortable and at ease. Where they didn't have to sit still, behave and play with a basket of toys that wasn't of their choice. I live in a rural area, so it lent itself to that. I started by going out and seeing children, which meant that I then picked up a lot of elderly, housebound people, and I suppose the bulk of my practice now is elderly rather than children, although I have got a lot of children on my books. I restrict my caseload to forty at a time, because I just couldn't manage any more. I couldn't do the teaching and run this college with more patients than I have so I have to balance the two.

ROWENA: So, do you sign them off when they are well?

ANNE: I sign them off when they are well, and then every Christmas I send them a card, and say for them to give me a shout if there is anything I can help them with. So I don't push them out completely. And if I am full, I don't take on new patients and just pass them on to somebody else. I need to see the patients to support my teaching. I now have a bunch of menopausal women, because I am at that stage of life myself. I used to see a lot of people in my home, but I now find it quite invasive having to run around, tidying up and straightening the cushions. For me it is much better to go to them. I do offer quite a lot of support to my patients in the early stages, but I am also quite good at eventually putting up boundaries, which I tell them I will do from the very beginning. I say, when we start, I am going to be accessible to you as regularly as I can, but as you start to improve, we are going to change those boundaries.

I had an myalgic encephalomyelitis (ME) patient who, when I first took him on nearly four years now, I spoke to every day for over a year. I now see him once every two months. When I first saw him he was a very sick man, and now he has got an almost normal life. I have got a huge buzz out of being a part of this process. So I can be quite supportive. I love it if a student asks me if they can spend a day with me and I love taking students round to see patients. If people are short of clinical hours, I have got a lot of pet patients who have seen me bring in students time and time again.

I say to the students, you take the case, and I will sit back and watch, and I then usually see a completely different side to the patient. I took a male student in his early fifties to see one of my patients, who was eighty seven and is now eighty nine. She flirted with him. She fluttered her eyelashes and simpered - it was unbelievable! We came out and just looked at each other and we both said *Platinum metallicum.* And I would never have seen that remedy in her, and she did so well on it. I don't think she would still be around if we hadn't discovered that.

ROWENA: So what is the ethos at the Lakeland College? What do you teach?

ANNE: We teach homeopathy philosophy and if you ask me what one of my favourite books is, I will say the *Organon*[4]. But I have been taught to love it by one of our team tutors, Jillian Mitchell; she makes her students fall in love with it as she has a real gift for bringing it to life. But I actually believe Hahnemann was an innovator and an experimenter; he pushed the boundaries, he was brave and years ahead of his time. I really don't feel happy that some people want to restrict homeopathy to the way that it was when Hahnemann practised because if Hahnemann had lived for another hundred years, he would have kept on evolving and developing. He wrote the *Organon*[4] in six editions and I believe he would have kept on learning and moving forward.

So we try to bring into our course not just the traditional Hahnemannian but other methodologies too. If there is one remedy that fits the case, then that is the best way to treat but there are other ways of working too. So, how do we teach? We teach in the way that we think. We want our students to understand that if someone has a physical issue it often started as an energetic problem and so we teach people about the aura, and the chakras, and how the lungs in Chinese Medicine hold grief; the kidneys, fear and the liver, anger. We talk about how if someone is not speaking their truth, their throat chakra may be blocked, and how to open it up and get the energy flowing.

We have an eclectic course with what we hope is a good, sound homeopathic base to it. And we are trying to get the balance between what we call inner and outer work. The outer work comprises the materia medica, philosophy and therapeutics whilst the inner work is the practitioner development, personal growth and self-awareness; the work you need to do on yourself before you can effectively work with other people.

Sometimes it can take us nearly the whole of the three years but we trust that the penny will drop. If it doesn't, then we are quite open with our students, and we say you are just not quite ready. A tutor of ours reads the cases and comes into college every Sunday for the final year students. They have to put their cases in, one at a time and she comes in and sits with them for half an hour each, going through the cases giving individual feedback. They then take that learning and apply it to their next case, so the case process is a real learning experience. It is the only time we ask students to do formal written work and we won't let anybody put in two cases at once. The deadline is the end of May, but no one can come to us mid-May with five cases, it is not acceptable. The cases have to show progression.

ROWENA: What do you think are the qualities that make a good and successful homeopath?

ANNE: A successful homeopath has the ability to listen. A successful homeopath has healing intent and really believes that a case well taken is a case half cured. I struggle with the unprejudiced observer philosophy as I think we are an active participant in the healing process. In Hahnemann's time you would sit behind the desk and you would be very formal; that was the set up then but we don't practise like that nowadays. Homeopaths need to recognise what is going on between them and their patients and be able to set their boundaries and protect themselves. It is about sharing with compassion and empathy. I think it is fine to disclose your stuff to a patient if it helps build empathy, understanding and a relationship.

I have got patients who I have been seeing for years, and as a result I have got to know them very well and some have even become friends. When we are in a consultation though, we are able to put on that particular hat, and work together appropriately. Because I live in a village I learnt that, "How are you?" is a loaded question in a vegetable shop so I now have to be very clear with patients.

ROWENA: So you treat your friends?

ANNE: Definitely. But I do also think that sometimes if you are working with someone really close you cannot see the wood for the trees and it is always good to involve another opinion. So, for example, I often send my own children to the student clinic. I think you can take friends' cases and patients can become friends too. What makes a good homeopath is someone who recognises at which point you cannot push and prod any further; then you have to back off. You need to get permission to go into a particular area; it is not about going through a big, long list and checking things out. It is recognising that you might have a *Natrum muriaticum* sitting in front of you and it may take you six months to go into a particular place. If it is a friend sometimes what you have got to say is just go and see someone else. I don't prescribe for my husband. I will do his acutes but I actually don't want to listen to some of his stuff. I don't want him to talk about the level of frustration he has with the way that I leave the kitchen sometimes. People do benefit from the objective space that somebody outside of their friends and family can offer.

Homeopaths also recognise that they need support. They need to know their limitations and have regular homeopathic treatment. They need to walk their talk. Part of our graduation criteria is that students have to be seeing a homeopath throughout the course. They also need to keep a learning journal. The concept was introduced to the Lakeland College by one of our tutors, Paul Francis, who doesn't tutor for us anymore but runs his own course. We have been doing them now for six or seven years and they are the most fantastic way of getting to know your students and for the students to get to know themselves. They are an absolute gift.

ROWENA: So how are they introduced?

ANNE: We introduce them in the very first weekend. We talk to people about what we want and there is a handout that says what is expected in their learning journals. It is meant to reflect them as an individual. Some of it will be what they have been taught in college, and what they have done with that information. Some of it will be a record of their personal journey. We try not to give too many guidelines because we want it to be very individual. We have a college learning journal, which contains examples of past students' work that we show to the first years to inspire them. We also have sessions twice a year to which the students bring in their learning journals and they share them in a group of four within the classroom. They bounce off and get ideas from each other.

ROWENA: Do they get worried about keeping bits confidential to themselves or do they hide those pages?

ANNE: Yes, sometimes they hide those pages. Sometimes that is not the bit they bring in because they can bring in any part of it. So it could be that they developed a passion for making herbal tinctures, and so they will bring in something that involves their recipes and what they have done and that is part of their process. But usually, by the end of the third year, their level of sharing is very, very deep as the connections they have formed with each other are strong. The tissue boxes go around all the time. On a particular weekend towards the end of the third and final year students will come out of their lectures for an hour long one-to-one session with a member of staff and their learning journal. This is a private and confidential individual sharing.

Two years ago, as her learning journal, a student brought in a big tray filled with soil and in it she had planted grass seeds. She made a mound and planted every remedy that she had been prescribed over the three years in it if they were plants. If they weren't plants, she would put a symbol that represented those remedies. In the Lake District, we are based quite near the Castlerigg Stone Circle and the students at the end of every year go there and do a meditation. In the middle of this tray was a replica of the Stone Circle made out of lakeland slate. As she sat and told her story she illuminated the whole thing with candles. We just had to go and fetch all the students out of their lectures and bring them in to look at it. People sometimes fret and say that they don't like writing a diary and they are not good at art. The learning journal is an individual piece of work and she chose to do this as her personal section. There are so many ways of keeping a diary; it is not necessarily about writing or being artistic.

ROWENA: At our college it was a real problem to get people to do it. You have obviously found a way that works for the individual.

ANNE: Nurturing and nourishing. The people who have the biggest problems are the ones who like to be in control and therefore they need to know what is expected of them, and they need to know what we want them to do. They want prescription and we tell them to do it any way they like it. We just support them through their anxieties.

ROWENA: So your students realise right from the start that they are going to have to develop personally; it is not a hidden agenda.

ANNE: No it is not hidden. It is absolutely out there and even in the prospectus. Some of them don't read it and say they are not going to do that bit. I had a student who came in on the first weekend and said that she had done all that stuff and had been doing it all her life. She put it to me that we could do all that stuff but that she would be a passenger. Three months later she came to me and admitted that she felt like a complete twit. I congratulated her for getting there so quickly!

ROWENA: So did you give her the space to just be a passenger?

ANNE: Yes. It was their first weekend and people need to feel safe and stay in their comfort zone. You need to know when it is ok to give them a little nudge and during their first weekend is not appropriate. We get to know them and if her reluctance had continued, perhaps we would have given her another nudge but in this case she nudged herself first which was great.

ROWENA: Tell me about the shamanic work that you do here at the Lakeland College.

ANNE: The shamanic work is what Lorraine Hart does and she does it extremely well. First of all, we help the student to find their Power Animal and than we do a shamanic journey to introduce the repertory because it can seem very daunting and we want them to make friends with it and feel good about it. The shamanic work grows out of what is going on within the group so we pick up on something that may be happening and we put the shamanic work in as appropriate. We are not unique in working this way. Paul Francis does this on his course as does Yubraj Sharma at the School of Shamanic Homoeopathy. One of the things that we try to do in this college is to extend students' comfort zones. Eventually they will hit the areas where they are stuck and need to develop.

ROWENA: Do you think homeopathy will become dormant again Anne?

ANNE: I think that the public will not let homeopathy slump in the way that it has in the past. But I think that there is a risk from the homeopaths that try to put homeopathy, which is an all embracing, all expansive system of energy medicine, into a straightjacket; that we might end up shooting the profession in the foot.

I think that the CORH is doing some fantastic work but Maggie Wallace, the former independent chair is quite rooted in the NHS. And this entire move towards the single register and all of this, "We want to work within the NHS" is all about the medical profession taking back control because they don't like the fact that individual people are now making decisions for themselves. Maggie is great, but the emphasis on patient safety is coming from a place of fear, and legislation, which is appropriate for pharmaceuticals and doctors should not be the baseline for homeopathy. We belong in a different paradigm. David Reiley is doing great work at the Glasgow Homeopathic Hospital. He is the one that has done the double-blind hay fever trial. I have a lot of time for him and for Brian Kaplan who wrote *The Homeopathic Conversation*[13].

So, what do I think of the future of our profession? I think that if we let this push to bring homeopathy further into the NHS goes forward, the doctors will play the gatekeepers and make all the referrals. They will capture people and say you come and work for us and do it our way. They will restrict homeopathy's availability rather than promote it and as a result, I don't want to work within the NHS. If people cannot afford me then I will find some other way that they can pay me. I had my whole house painted by a patient's husband last year. I looked after her and the family, and they painted the outside of my house.

ROWENA: What a great idea.

ANNE: There are many ways of exchanging energy and we don't have to tie ourselves down to money. Homeopathy has always been available on the NHS, and some of the homeopathy offered as a result is fantastic but I know that if doctors get to play the gatekeeper, then that would be a backward step for our profession. Prince Charles is a very knowledgeable person and I have heard him speak many times about homeopathy and alternative medicine but unfortunately he is listening to all the wrong people. He needs to listen to homeopaths and not to the doctors who say we are dangerous and need legislation. I fundamentally believe that homeopathy is safe. I think you can have unsafe practitioners, but that is different.

ROWENA: I am in agreement with you. I think it is how it is prescribed that can be unsafe.

ANNE: Yes, and it is all about being aware of when you are out of your depth. I might say to a patient that I am stuck and ask them if they would mind if I bring a student with me to the next consultation to get a fresh perspective. I struggled for six months with the patient with Meniere's Disease. All I was doing was palliating; making him better for a few days, and then it came back. Within half an hour of a second year student sitting in with me, she drew a sycamore seed and passed it across to me. I asked her what it was and she told me but I didn't make the connection so she asked me to think about how the sycamore seed falls from the tree. My patient was talking about his dizziness and I thought about the sycamore seed and how it falls and I compared it to Meniere's Disease with its dizziness and I gave him *Sycamore seed 200C*. He cancelled his next appointment and said, "Thank you very much, that was wonderful, I have had no more attacks of Meniere's Disease and no more dizziness, and if I need another appointment I will go and see the student!"

ROWENA: So there is a remedy from the seed?

ANNE: Yes. It is one of the newer ones and I wasn't aware of it either. If you let a student sit in with your patients, you can get fresh insights and because of this student my patient got total and complete freedom from his symptoms. I rung him up six months later to ask him how he was and he replied that he was absolutely fine and I had tried for six months to help him prior to that. We have just got to be open.

ROWENA: Indeed we do. Thank you so much for your time Anne; I have really enjoyed our conversation and you have given me a good insight into the history of the Lakeland College and what it is like to study here.

CHAPTER 22:   REBECCA PRESTON

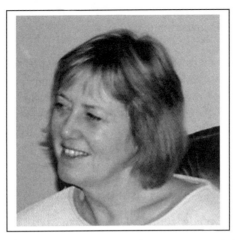

I came across Rebecca Preston at the teachers' seminar in Malvern. Several homeopaths came up to me and said she was an absolute must to interview. She kindly agreed to speak with me but we had to do it by way of the telephone, as Edinburgh was too far for me travel.

"How many times can we honestly say we have given the simillimum? A series of good similar remedies will go a long way."   *Rebecca Preston, June 2005*

"Sometimes you have to do other stuff; for example surgery. In my case, I would have died without it. You cannot treat dead people! In some cases, you have to keep people alive and then work with what is left."   *Rebecca Preston, June 2005*

"I think all the different opinions in homeopathy are just tools for your tool bag. You put some of Jeremy's stuff in your bag, and you put some of Jan's in, and you put some of Rajan's in, and use the bits that work for you and your patients. I also respect George' work. I don't feel that criticising other homeopaths is the way forward."
Rebecca Preston, June 2005

"The more remedies that we have, and the more good provings, the better. But also doing provings is just an amazing way to learn about homeopathy, as well."
Rebecca Preston, June 2005

"The Amethyst proving was very interesting, because it was so heavy and deep. The provers went to hell and back; it was horrendous. But there was really, really deep stuff that came out of it. Sometimes provers can stay in that place, until they can find something that can shift it."   *Rebecca Preston, June 2005*

CHAPTER 22: REBECCA PRESTON

ROWENA: So how did you discover homeopathy Rebecca?

REBECCA: My younger daughter got whooping cough and somebody said I should try homeopathy. This was twenty nine years ago and before that point I had never heard of it. I took her to a homeopath and it cleared up in a day. This was in the Pennines in Cumbria, in a small village, and the local school was shut for two months because everybody had scarred lungs as a result of their whooping cough. My older daughter was given a prophylactic dose and never got it.

ROWENA: So what happened after that?

REBECCA: I thought it was wonderful and I wanted to study it, but I imagined you had to be really holy and pure and I wasn't! And then I started meeting some homeopaths and thought, maybe I can study this after all. So that was it.

ROWENA: So where did you study?

REBECCA: Technically, I studied at the Yorkshire School of Homeopathy, because by then I was living in York, but I joined the Darlington postgraduate collective at the same time, at the beginning of my second year. This was with Jeremy Sherr and was before he had set up the Dynamis School. He had one group in Darlington, one down in Malvern, and one in Norway. He taught us all separately and then he established the Dynamis School and the three groups together became the second year of the first intake. This was in 1990 and by then we had been studying with him for three or four years.

I graduated from the Yorkshire School in 1989. The gap between discovering homeopathy and studying at the Dynamis School was taken up with young babies. We had six between us and I was kind of caught up with other things! I did first aid courses and read a lot about homeopathy before I studied it properly.

ROWENA: Who had the biggest influence on you when you were studying?

REBECCA: Jeremy Sherr, without a doubt; I got my homeopathy from him. He is an excellent teacher and his teaching just resonated totally. His emphasis was mainly philosophy and repertory at that time; he didn't do much materia medica with us. Now I know the new provings better than I know the old remedies and I really rely on the repertory. I use mainly *Isis*, but I have got *Radar* and *MacRepertory*. I have had a computer and used the programmes since I was a student. I worked on *Cara*, I typed in all of *Allen's Key Notes*[104] to get a free programme, so I have always had one. My computer

305

broke down once and I felt like my brain had been sent away when my computer went away to get fixed. It was awful!

I practise in Edinburgh and I also teach, although I have cut it right back as I was very, very ill a few years ago but before that I was away every weekend. Now I just teach in Manchester, Wales and at the Burren School in the West of Ireland, the mob that run the Irish Conference. Nuala Eising is running down the Burren School; next year is the last year. I have been working there for twelve years and I teach mainly casework. Nuala, bless her, just says, come and teach what you do best. Nuala's was residential and the norm was for students to sit around on pillows with duvets, making tea and the teacher would teach what they liked; it worked really well.

Teaching at Manchester is to a timetable; this hour you are teaching this to that group, then the following hour, another subject and another year group. I just teach what I am told but also in consultation. They will ask me what subject I like to teach, what materia medica I have lectures for, what cases have I have got. In Wales it tends to be again, just teach what you want.

ROWENA: Were the weekends more of a process?

REBECCA: Yes, it is what I prefer; teaching one group for a whole weekend in preference to the chopping and changing at Manchester. Wales and Ireland are very similar. You have the same group for two whole days and I go prepared with a whole bunch of stuff, but it can go off on tangents and tangents are often really good. It could be anything. I will be taking a case and somebody will have a case and it brings up something in somebody's case that they are having trouble with, and we might go off at a tangent and work on that, or just follow questions where they go.

ROWENA: What got you into teaching in the beginning?

REBECCA: Oh God, it was awful! The London College of Classical Homeopathy (LCCH) decided that they wanted a repertory curriculum. They went to Jeremy Sherr and asked if he could recommend somebody, and he recommended Dee Maclaughlin and me. I was still in my fourth year at the Yorkshire School, but also studying with Jeremy. We devised a repertory curriculum to be taught over four years and we were hired to teach it. So I started teaching at LCCH in London a month after I graduated. I was absolutely terrified.

ROWENA: Who has the biggest influence on you now?

REBECCA: Now is difficult because I have been really ill. I have really changed my life and I am not eating, sleeping, breathing homeopathy anymore and it is great, to be perfectly honest. It was too much. I basically hardly had a life outside of homeopathy, I was teaching every weekend, working, seeing patients during the week, never getting invited to parties because people assumed I was away, which I was. And now I have got both; I have got a bit of teaching, maybe eight weekends a year, three or four days of patients a week and a life, and I prefer it.

In terms of influence lately, I would definitely say Jan Scholten. I admire his work, his honesty and his vision. I find his ideas very user friendly and I trust him as it comes from a really solid place but he is a visionary at the same time. I have just made an appointment with him actually and I am quite excited about that; so I have to go to Utrecht. He calls his work at the moment the *Secret Lanthanides*[105], the hidden earth elements, and his new book about them is coming out any minute. Basically he is finding these remedies amazing for autoimmune disease and that is what I have.

ROWENA: Had you had good results with homeopathy these conditions before?

REBECCA: No. I have had everybody and their brother prescribing. I have had remedies from Nuala that have changed how I feel, changed my soul, but didn't touch the physical. I honestly don't know why that is. That is why I am going to Holland. I have got great hopes for Jan Scholten.

ROWENA: How does having not so positive experiences with homeopathy affect you and how you practise?

REBECCA: It was quite hard when I first went into hospital; I almost started to question my faith but then getting good results with other people kind of restored it. I have thought for years my remedy hasn't been discovered yet; that is why I got really excited at the seminar with Jan Scholten.

ROWENA: So do you come from the viewpoint that we resonate with one remedy, one Holy Grail?

REBECCA: Not forever, no, but at any one particular time, I think, yes. However, how many times can we honestly say we have given the simillimum? A series of good similar remedies will go a long way.

ROWENA: How do homeopaths get that happy medium where they are earning enough but are not killing themselves in the process? It sounds like homeopaths could be prone to burn out.

REBECCA: It is difficult, to be perfectly honest. When I was teaching I thought, if I give up and stop teaching like this, I will be bankrupt, but now I am actually better off. In fact, there are so many hidden costs with the travelling and it is the travelling, when you are teaching, that is the killer. Just having a more grounded lifestyle now, I am actually better off financially. I was part of a very extensive clinic and I have now left there and mainly work from home. So that means six hundred pounds a month overheads gone, which is great, and the patients prefer it here to the clinic. Patients find me mostly through word of mouth, a few from the Yellow Pages, but that is about it. I have got a website which helps too.

ROWENA: What skills do you think are involved in being a successful homeopath Rebecca?

REBECCA: Perseverance. You have to love it. If you don't, you cannot do it.

ROWENA: Are there books that you recommend when you are teaching?

REBECCA: It depends. If I am teaching, for example, the methodology of provings, I recommend Jeremy Sherr's book *The Dynamics and Methodology of Homoeopathic Provings*[106]. Other than that, I also recommend books of new provings and all of Jan *Scholten's* books.

ROWENA: How do you feel about George Vithoulkas' views?

REBECCA: I don't agree with him. I definitely practise classically; it is how I have been brought up. I have never veered from it. I don't know how to do anything else. George Vithoulkas makes comments like this periodically, it has been going on for years. We all have issues about the future of homeopathy. It doesn't mean he has to disrespect practitioners in other countries.

ROWENA: Do you see homeopathy becoming dormant again?

REBECCA: I don't see homeopathy becoming dormant at all. When I first started practising in 1989, sixteen years ago, patients were all hippies or 'green' people and now they are anybody. I don't see why it shouldn't continue. I definitely don't see it going down. When I was in Ireland a few weeks ago, there was some bad press about a homeopath and my friends were worried about it. They were concerned that it was going to affect their practices and the general consciousness about homeopathy, and I think, rightly so. That kind of press is not helpful.

ROWENA: Why do you think we have the frequent bad press?

REBECCA: Because conventional medicine still holds sway and it is about power tripping; they want to keep the power and people. I definitely don't think it is so much as it used to be - with doctor as God - but it is still around.

ROWENA: I wonder what it would be like if they gave press space to all the mistakes doctors make.

REBECCA: Exactly. It took them seven years to diagnose me and I nearly died in the process. If they had diagnosed it, it would never have come to that point. But, in saying that, homeopathy never helped me at that time either. It kept me going those seven years, but it didn't reverse what was happening.

ROWENA: So it acted palliatively?

REBECCA: I think so yes, it would help with the pain. The remedies were prescribed as curative, though. They were not being prescribed palliatively.

ROWENA: How has that experience affected your practice?

REBECCA: It has opened me up to people and to the fact that sometimes you have to do other stuff; for example surgery. In my case, I would have died without it. You cannot treat dead people! In some cases, you have to keep people alive and then work with what is left.

ROWENA: Are there any other things you would like to mention today?

REBECCA: Yes. I think the whole Bombay School is really, really important. It really got under steam when I was very ill, so I feel like I am behind with all that and I am finding the miasmatic ideas really interesting. I am not finding that the case taking stuff is suiting me at the moment. I have always used some of that stuff, anyway, but having had my case taken the Rajan Sankaran'way, I felt that I was making stuff up. Being asked, "What is the feeling, what is the feeling?" constantly; in the end, I was just saying anything to move on.

Having said that, I know people, whom I really respect, who are finding it amazing and working with it almost exclusively. It really didn't suit me as a patient, but I think all the different methodologies in homeopathy are just tools for your tool bag. You put some of Jeremy's stuff in your bag, and you put some of Jan's in, and you put some of Rajan's in, and use the bits that work for you and your patients. I also respect George's work. I don't feel that criticising other homeopaths is the way forward.

One thing I would like to add is how important I think the new provings are; I think they are the best thing since sliced bread. The more remedies that we have, and the more good provings, the better. But also doing provings is just an amazing way to learn about homeopathy. I have been involved in the provings of *Scorpion (Androctonos amurreuxi hebraeus), Chocolate, Hydrogen, Brassica, Fire (Ignis alchoholis), Eagle (Haliaeetus*

309

leucocephalus) and *Amber*, sometimes as a prover but often as a supervisor. And I have conducted a proving of *Amethyst*.

ROWENA: What was it like doing the *Amethyst* proving?

REBECCA: The *Amethyst* proving was very interesting, because it was so heavy and deep. The provers went to hell and back; it was horrendous. But there was really, really deep stuff that came out of it. Sometimes provers can stay in that place, until they can find something that can shift it. I have got the substance for my next proving already, but I want to publish *Amethyst* before I get started. *Amethyst* is nearly ready; I have presented it at four conferences, and it has been published as an article. I just want to get it out there finally, before I start anything new.

ROWENA: Rebecca, thank you so much for your time today and sharing with me your stories and insights. Good luck with Jan!

CHAPTER 23:   MARTIN MILES

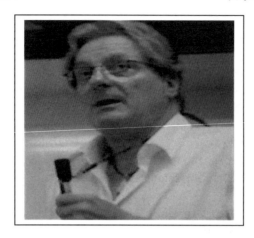

I braved the M25 eastbound through the Dartford Tunnel for my interview with Martin Miles on Monday 27 June 2005. I had made his acquaintance at a postgraduate seminar on cancer, which he presented to the New College of Homeopathy a couple of months earlier. So I was pretty excited to have him all to myself for a few hours, as this is an area in which I specialise. Not only that but he is one of our enigmatic forefathers who was there at the inception of the renaissance of homeopathy in the 1970s and he is a Fellow of the Society of Homeopaths. From reading his book *Homoeopathy and Human Evolution*[75], I knew this was a man whose brain I wanted to pick big time. I perched on a sofa in the front room of his very hippie house, drank herbal tea and revelled in the excitement of having this opportunity.

"I remember asking Thomas Maughan once how many of the old homeopaths were educated in spiritual philosophy. He replied by saying, "All of them who were worth their salt." Homeopathy is a science and an art that grows out of that. It is a form of alchemy and I was conscious right from the beginning of the need to heal; of the need to cure people's ailments, troubles and diseases. I was always conscious that homeopathy was a tool of transformation; you could transform people out of their illnesses and their diseases and out of their miasms."   *Martin Miles, June 2005*

"We teach chakras, endocrine glands and the new remedies. We get other experts in to teach astrology, science and kabbalah etc. It is designed to take students fresh from college. The college experience teaches them to be good technicians who can work with materia medica and the repertory. What we want to do is develop them into healers with knowledge of other things that they may find helpful. The more practitioners understand spiritual philosophy, the more effective they can be as homeopaths; it goes hand in hand. As one learns to see much deeper into one's patients, one is able to do much bigger and better work."   *Martin Miles, June 2005*

CHAPTER 23:   MARTIN MILES

MARTIN: There are as many ways of prescribing homeopathy, as there are homeopaths. You cannot just teach one way, it is far too rigid and it doesn't work. Each finds their own way.

ROWENA: I know. I have to tell you, your book, *Homoeopathy and Human Evolution*[75] had such an impact on me when I was training. It must have been Jerome Whitney that recommended it to me. After that homeopathy started to make sense because it suddenly fitted into the way I already viewed the world.

MARTIN: That was the idea of writing it; to get some kind of sense because up until the time I wrote it, all homeopathy books were more or less the same. They trotted out the same story about Samuel Hahnemann and a single remedy and all that sort of stuff. I thought that there was a need for something else; a different type of understanding. So that was really the reason for writing it.

ROWENA: So tell me your story Martin, how did it all begin for you?

MARTIN: When I was twenty six I got really ill. I considered my life was kind of on hold at the time because I had a deep sense there was something I was going to do but I did not know what it was. I went through a period of wanting to be a doctor but I didn't have the intellect for that and I am rather glad I didn't follow that path. But I got really ill. Not ill in a way that you could put a label on it particularly, and I wouldn't go and see a doctor because I knew it would be a waste of time. And then somebody said to me, "Why don't you go and see this homeopath?"

ROWENA: Thomas Maughan?

MARTIN: Yes. My friend told me to call him straight away so I did. Thomas answered the phone and said come this afternoon at four o'clock. So I did. And that was the beginning of it for me. His cure was quick and dramatic and, of course, I discovered that you didn't just get homeopathy with Thomas; there was a lot of spiritual teaching and philosophy as well.

ROWENA: Did he do that within the consultation?

MARTIN: No. He held classes.

ROWENA: Did he offer those to everyone that came for treatment?

MARTIN: He didn't offer them overtly, but he didn't make it a secret either. It was up to the person to latch onto it.

ROWENA: And you latched?

MARTIN: I did. Yes.

ROWENA: What were you doing workwise before then?

MARTIN: Before then? Oh dear. My father was a very wealthy man and I worked for one of his companies and had done so, other than one other job, since I had left school. Materially it was fantastic - there were a lot of money, fast cars and flash clothes. This was through the sixties and up to about 1973/4. So materially it was a good time but spiritually it was a problem. And I was always very conscious on another level. My father and I were very different; he was a very materialistic man and he was very good at making money. I belonged to that generation that rebelled and he was astonished at my attitude towards life and the world I suppose. He had grown up quite poor in the East End of London so you can understand it from his point of view as well.

ROWENA: Was he a refugee?

MARTIN: I don't think so. I think his family may well have been here for a couple of generations. I used to ask him about his past but he would always fob me off and would never really say anything about the family. It could be that they were refugees from central Europe and settled in the east end. He was a good man but he was very stuck unfortunately.

ROWENA: And your mother?

MARTIN: My mother came from Peckham. She was very different again. My father was a Capricorn and she was a Scorpio and they weren't at all compatible. I am more like my mother than my father and I have a brother who is like my father.

ROWENA: So what sign are you?

MARTIN: Virgo. My father treated my mother really badly. She suffered, became an alcoholic and died of cancer. My brother, a Macmillan nurse and I nursed her through her last ten days. I mention this because it was a crossroads in my life. I met Thomas at that time shortly before my mother died. As soon as I met Thomas my consciousness opened up as to what was going on. I knew straight away what I was going to do. Here was a system of medicine that worked. It wasn't rubbish.

ROWENA: Do you think others are rubbish?

MARTIN: I think drug therapies are rubbish. Mostly they kill people more than they do anything else.

ROWENA: Do you really think there is no place for chemo and radiotherapy?

MARTIN: Yes, I think there are much more sensible ways of treating people. You don't have to treat cancer patients with chemo and radiation. You can treat them exclusively with homeopathy and you can often get the cancers to go away.

ROWENA: I can understand how tumours can grow and how they can go away again but what about leukaemia?

MARTIN: It is difficult but the adult leukaemias are much easier than the adolescent ones. You can get them to go away but the adolescent ones can be very deadly.

ROWENA: So why do you treat cancer with the new remedies?

MARTIN: They are relevant for people today. They have today's energy and they reflect today's issues. Most of the homeopathic materia medicas contain provings from the Victorian times but there has been a social revolution since then and people are completely different now. If you did a proving of *Pulsatilla nigricans* now, do you think it would be exactly the same picture as it was? Of course there would be similarities but people use different language to describe things.

ROWENA: There has been a rise in consciousness so people have changed a lot.

MARTIN: Well it is a completely different consciousness and so the issues in society have changed. One hundred and twenty years ago the great pillars of society were well in place. You had parliament and the law and the church and the aristocracy were in control. People's lives were dictated by a code that was outside them. Society had its laws and you had your place in society and your task was to learn how to be within it.

Then there were two world wars that took the power from the aristocracy and this freed the people up more. Then there was the advent of socialism, which was a tool to try and distribute wealth more fairly. All those things worked together and in the last fifty to sixty years those pillars have broken down. The church doesn't grip people as it used to and the aristocracy doesn't rule the day. You still have vestiges of both but people are largely free to make up their own minds. We still have different types of government control on people but it is time for people to think for themselves and to individualise.

ROWENA: The Age of Aquarius?

MARTIN: Yes. It is time for people to share knowledge and what they have. It is now a hierarchy of ability rather than of the privileged that it used to be. In the past people were appointed to positions because of their parents, which school they went to or club they belonged to. And of course that system doesn't work, as it has been demonstrated many times. You have to live what you believe, and you don't have to believe any more - you have to know. It is no longer about belief - you have to live it and when you live it, it becomes first-hand.

ROWENA: So you weren't expecting to live the life that you did after you were twenty six?

MARTIN: No, I wasn't but I was pleased to wave goodbye to all that materialism because it wasn't what I wanted and it wasn't fulfilling.

ROWENA: But it supported you in those early days?

MARTIN: It did.

ROWENA: Well that is one of the big issues with homeopathy - the struggle financially.

MARTIN: I know it is a problem. I have been most fortunate and have made a living out of homeopathy since I was twenty seven.

ROWENA: Brilliant. How have you managed to do that?

MARTIN: I don't know. I have always had a very busy practice and then I have been teaching as well. I have managed to raise a family on it and still do.

ROWENA: But you are in a minority, so what ingredients do you think you have for being successful?

MARTIN: What you need is a driving determination to make it work. You need a burning belief that this not only is a system of medicine that works, but the real need is huge and the power of homeopathy is far greater than any of us have so far perceived. Our consciousness is limited and our consciousness of it is limited. I keep uncovering layers, more possibilities and new ways of making it work so that the incurable become curable, and that is really worth striving for.

ROWENA: So when did that start for you?

MARTIN: The beginning.

ROWENA: Okay, so go back to those days and tell me more about what it was like then.

MARTIN: I remember asking Thomas once how many of the old homeopaths were educated in spiritual philosophy. He replied by saying, "All of them who were worth their salt." Homeopathy is a science and an art that grows out of that. It is a form of alchemy and I was conscious right from the beginning of the need to heal; of the need to cure people's ailments, troubles and diseases. I was always conscious that homeopathy was a tool of transformation; you could transform people out of their illnesses and their diseases and out of their miasms. You could raise them on other levels, completely. And as Thomas said, you could take people through two or three incarnations in one, which was quite remarkable really. And you could you do it much more efficiently, quicker and deeper with new meditative remedies especially in combination.

ROWENA: Those remedies weren't around though when he was, were they?

MARTIN: No they weren't. They are the product of recent years.

ROWENA: Do you think he would be approving of them or was he not that kind of a person?

MARTIN: I think he is behind them.

ROWENA: Ooooh, tell me more!

MARTIN: Well, Thomas died in 1976. I had spent a lot of time with him as I used to drive him around.

ROWENA: At fast speeds.

MARTIN: At very fast speeds.

ROWENA: Yes, Peter Chappell told me about that too.

MARTIN: He was always pushing to see how far he could go in everything he did. You should speak to Jennifer Maughan, his wife. She is now about sixty two or three; she was young when they were together. Whenever I was with Thomas I knew the time was short and that he wasn't going to be around much longer so I would ask him lots of questions about homeopathy and spiritual philosophy. I know he had been doing homeopathy for about forty years and had worked at the Royal London Homeopathic Hospital. He was a doctor of biochemistry.

He was the original and driving power behind the renaissance in homeopathy and when I knew him he was experimenting with remedies in different ways. He always used them as tools of transformation for his students. Because most of us, by the time we arrived at his front door, for whatever reason, were drugged out hippies – it was quite an achievement to turn us into useful human beings!

ROWENA: So you were there with Robert Davidson?

MARTIN: Yes and Jerome and Kaaren Whitney, Peter Chappell and Mary Titchmarsh.

ROWENA: Is she still around?

MARTIN: Yes, she doesn't practise homeopathy as far as I am aware but she does do NLP (Neuro-Linguistic Programming). Thomas always held his homeopathy classes on a Saturday night, fortnightly. He knew that on Saturday night everybody wanted to go out so he knew only those dedicated enough would come to his class, but I never missed one of them. They continued for between two and three years and then he died in 1976.

ROWENA: He had lung cancer, and...

MARTIN: Yes and his heart was very weak as well.

ROWENA: There seems to be a lot of cancer within the homeopathic community. Have you found that?

MARTIN: It doesn't surprise me. It probably comes about because homeopaths take on a lot of responsibility. Dealing with other peoples' pain is very exhausting and difficult. You have to develop a sense of humour to survive. The deeper you get into the shadow of the valley of death where the illnesses you deal with are dense and severely negative, the bigger the sense of humour and lightness you require. They have a direct relationship.

ROWENA: Is that how you work then?

MARTIN: I try. I try. You have to see the funny side of it all. If you don't then there is an imbalance. If homeopaths don't get that balance right, I can see why they would end up with degenerative diseases.

ROWENA: I better lighten up and get a sense of humour then!

MARTIN: Well, there is a lot that is funny within our profession....

ROWENA: In what way?

MARTIN: In describing remedies to others, for instance, they are pretty funny and peculiar aren't they?

ROWENA: I see your point. Okay, going back to Thomas Maughan, do you want to say anything else about him?

MARTIN: He was like a father to me really. I never had much parenting at all, ever; my parents just weren't there for me. And Thomas knew that, and kind of took over. He was very good, but I must say, since he has died, I have been closer to him.

ROWENA: Okay tell me more about that.

MARTIN: Well, he visits me, I know when he is here because when he was alive and you were near him he had this enormous feeling of power; incredible power that you could feel.

ROWENA: So did he do that with his spirit, unconsciously, or with his people skills?

MARTIN: It was a spiritual quality that he had and that he had developed. When he died there was a time of quiet and then I became aware again of his energy. It was the same but different. While he was here he was locked in a body that was rapidly falling apart. I know that he was in a lot of pain and distress. After he was gone he was able to shed all that, learn more and refine. He didn't have that body, brain and nervous system anymore so when I felt his presence it was a huge refinement of the same energy, which was quite astonishing and extraordinary.

ROWENA: Did he say that he planned on coming back? Did he speak in those terms?

MARTIN: No, I never heard him speak in those terms but we all knew that he could if he wanted to.

ROWENA: So do you think that means that he has not gone into another incarnation?

MARTIN: He hasn't gone into another physical incarnation and he visits in different guises, I have seen him a few times and he comes in a body of light and sometimes as the eagle.

ROWENA: Is this mainly to the meditation groups where you create new remedies?

MARTIN: Yes, he comes into the groups as an eagle or in other forms.

ROWENA: And you can all see or feel him?

MARTIN: Some of us can, yes.

ROWENA: That is wonderful!

MARTIN: It is.

ROWENA: So if he was in a body somewhere, a new physical incarnation, do you think he would be able to do that?

MARTIN: He would probably still be able to do it, but he would be limited.

ROWENA: And do you think it would have to be a conscious intention?

MARTIN: It is always conscious. He comes and goes with awareness. Part of what he was training his students to do was to obtain consciousness outside their bodies, which is quite achievable; you just have to work hard at it. It is difficult to separate yourself enough from the demands of the material world.

ROWENA: But if he was in another life now….

MARTIN: He is in another life but not a physical one. He hasn't been born in another; he hasn't had to be. He has achieved what he came here to do, he doesn't have to incarnate again if he doesn't want to. The rest of us, I am afraid, are tied to the wheel of rebirth, until as such time…

ROWENA: ….that we are enlightened. So where did your path take you after Thomas died?

MARTIN: Our small group - Robert Davidson, Peter Chappell, the Whitneys, and Mary Titchmarsh - we had to do something to secure homeopathy. The torch had been passed to us. We had joined the European common market, and in most of Europe if not all of it, homeopathy was banned. People were not allowed to use it unless they were doctors.

ROWENA: And that had been the case for a long time I imagine?

MARTIN: Yes it had. But we, in the UK, have always had common law, which dates back to ancient times. This means we could practise homeopathy but in actual fact in 1976, very few people did. It was a remnant, really; just a handful of people and they kept a very low profile. So we thought we had to do something, first of all to secure homeopathy, then make it so big that 'they' had to accept it. We wanted to spread it as a healing art.

ROWENA: So how did you do that?

MARTIN: Well we first thought that we should approach the North London Group established by John Damonte. I remember going up there one day, suggesting it and they thought it was a good idea. We used to have regular meetings and from those meetings came the Society of Homeopaths in embryonic form. We established it and then we all took up offices in it. I was the first chairperson. Then Robert Davidson and I started the first school, the College of Homeopathy (COH), which then became Barbara Harwood's organisation before it collapsed completely, and disappeared. We enrolled thirty students in the first year.

ROWENA: So how did you get those students?

MARTIN: We advertised in some rudimentary health magazine something like, "Education in homeopathy, three year course". But it would have also been by word of mouth through all the people who had been treated by Thomas Maughan and John Damonte. It was an idea whose time had come. Given a prod and a dig it would inevitably start to move around. That first intake of students went out and practised, spread the work and then they took over some of the teaching.

ROWENA: These must have been such exciting times!

MARTIN: It was very exciting. By the third or fourth intake Robert Davidson wanted to expand and had decided he was going to invite a hundred people. I thought that this was not a good idea, as I wanted to teach students; I didn't want to stand in front of a class and shout at them. In my opinion, it wasn't really how you do homeopathy and the administration of such a group was a nightmare. Robert wanted to turn it into a big operation and I disagreed. Ever since I had first started prescribing, my practice started to snowball and got bigger and bigger and I found that I was practising all week and then teaching at weekends, which is crazy.

So I had to decide which I was going to do. I couldn't remain in the forefront of COH and run a busy practice; it was just not possible. So we parted company. Robert Davidson took over the college and I threw myself into my practice. I decided also that I wanted more experience practising before I taught further. And that was that.

Meanwhile the Society of Homeopaths grew. With every lot of students that passed out as qualified homeopaths, they joined the Society of Homeopaths or became part of it in some way and, of course, we had a lot of very talented and capable people that we attracted. So they started doing all sorts of things with homeopathic promotion. Of course, over the years it has mushroomed into what it is now.

ROWENA: So tell me about the provings you have done?

MARTIN: For most of them, we sit round in a circle to meditate and we take the remedy. We don't know what it is, but Helios pharmacy have made the remedy.

ROWENA: So how do they make it? If, let us say, it was *Genesis* how would they make that?

MARTIN: They have made one or two remedies like that, but mostly the remedies they have made are just from physical things; plants and stuff like that.

ROWENA: So tell me about the meditative provings? How do you do them?

MARTIN: Well somebody takes charge of the circle and they give instructions on a meditation.

ROWENA: You are talked through it?

MARTIN: A scene is set of a place and you have your guardian angel or wizard with you who comes to visit and gives you something. Each person has their own individual experience around that. If you are trying to invoke some kind of energy or spiritual force, then you would set a meditation around that theme as well.

ROWENA: Then what happens after that; how long does the meditation last?

MARTIN: I suppose about three or four hours.

ROWENA: So is it like a journey?

MARTIN: Yes.

ROWENA: Do people talk in that time?

MARTIN: During the meditation nobody talks because they are meditating. In the group I was in we spent a long time learning to meditate together, as a group; a good two, three years just meditating together before we did any remedies at all. We went through all the chakras so all our centres were opened. We went through many processes together which changed us completely.

ROWENA: I read that you have proved *Lac humanum* meditatively. Is the proving similar to the other proving of it?

MARTIN: I think it is rather different actually.

ROWENA: So how does that work?

MARTIN: If you do a Hahnemannian proving, it takes several weeks and you are doing it with your body consciousness, your brain and your everyday experience in the world. When you meditate you get away from all that and channel universal information. So you get different levels of the same remedy. It doesn't mean that one is right and the other is wrong. It is just fine as it is.

ROWENA: But when you analyse cases do you refer to lots of different books; conventional provings and meditative?

MARTIN: Yes, I do.

ROWENA: Do you find you attract people who need more of these newer remedies though?

MARTIN: I continuously see lots of opportunities to use them, yes.

ROWENA: Why do you think that is? Universally do you think you just attract people in that state?

MARTIN: We are able to sit down, meditate for four hours as a group and channel information on new remedies. That is what we have made ourselves fit to do and we can do that so we attract accordingly. Other people do other things in homeopathy. They investigate other areas, go down different routes and that is fine. They do what they do and they attract accordingly. That is how it works.

ROWENA: Well it makes sense to me but you know it doesn't make sense to everybody in our profession. How do you feel about that?

MARTIN: My view and my experience are that you cannot do a great deal of work with one remedy anymore. You used to be able to when I started homeopathy. You could prescribe one remedy and it would affect people on a really deep, profound level. But those experiences have become less and less frequent as the remedies have got weaker and weaker which is very frustrating.

ROWENA: Why do you think the remedies got weaker?

MARTIN: Well first of all the remedies are not made to quite the same quality as they used to be because they now need to mass produce them. You cannot build in the same dynamic way by machine as you could by hand. And of course everyone is a lot sicker than they used to be. If there was one single issue that you could pull out and say that this is the major reason for the proliferation of so much illness and madness it would be vaccination.

It is not just that though. You have got drugs – allopathic and recreational, food allergies, bad diets and pollution. Radiation from mobile phones is a major cause of illness and will be so in the future as well. You have got all those issues starting with vaccination for most of us. The children get vaccinated soon after they are born, and it ruins them. It wrecks their nervous system, their endocrine system and their brain pushes them out of their body and makes them mad.

There are so many different layers and so much encrusted disease. Diseases are locked in. Nobody is allowed to have an acute. Children have their own issues and their own diseases plus their parents' stuff that hasn't been released. Then they grow up and they have children and their children have their stuff plus their parents and their grandparents. You see what I am getting at here. There is this awful legacy of chronic degenerative disease.

When a woman takes the contraceptive pill there is an instruction to the pituitary gland to shut down. We now have three generations of women that have taken the Pill, so that is three generations of instructions to the pituitary gland to shut down. So when the next generation comes along they find themselves infertile because the pituitary gland doesn't work. If it doesn't work, it doesn't send instructions to the ovaries and therefore the ovaries don't work and the whole system of fertility breaks down.

ROWENA: I have prescribed *Folliculinum* frequently. Do you prescribe that or are there other remedies that you see that work to clear Pill damage?

MARTIN: I do prescribe that a lot and also *Pituitary Gland.* I also prescribe *Sycamore seed* which has a great affinity to the pituitary gland and I suppose the one remedy that clears the pituitary gland, the thyroid gland and to some extent the thymus gland more than any other is *Calcarea carbonica.* That is in everybody because everybody is stuck at that point.

ROWENA: So do you prescribe one remedy sometimes or is it always combinations?

MARTIN: It is always combinations really. You prescribe constitutionally don't you?

ROWENA: Yes. Do you think that people are one remedy in some ways?

MARTIN: In some ways they are, yes, but if you prescribe that one remedy it is not going to work in the way that is needed or maybe in the way you think it would or should work.

ROWENA: Or it did in the past?

MARTIN: Or it did in the past. It is just not going to do it. So you need to prescribe other remedies as well. So I would prescribe constitutionally on one level and then I would prescribe for endocrine glands and chakras depending on which ones are out of balance or lacking.

ROWENA: How do you know when something is out of balance?

MARTIN: When you interview the patient and take the case you find out where the weaknesses, difficulties and problems are. You can tell then which of the chakras and which endocrine glands are malfunctioning and you work on strengthening and correcting those areas. So you prescribe constitutionally and then you prescribe on that level of chakras and endocrinology. Then, of course, you need to give physical organ support, which more than anything else, is usually for the kidneys or for the kidneys and liver. The kidneys in most people are pretty weak so they need to be fortified. I also use nosodes frequently.

ROWENA: Do you have a protocol on using those or does it depend on the person?

MARTIN: Largely it depends on the person but often I prescribe a nosode, then a constitutional remedy, then a nosode and then the next time a constitutional remedy and so on. It really works quite well. If you cannot see what the dominant miasm is then give them a *Carcinosin* 10M or 50M and it will separate the miasms out. So when you see the patient next, you will see the dominant miasm or the first one that comes up. Prescribe for that and then you will see the next one and so on.

ROWENA: Do you get aggravations or over reactions to remedies?

MARTIN: Yes, sometimes you do.

ROWENA: How do you deal with those?

MARTIN: Unless the patient is in danger of losing their life, which is very, very rare, or the patient is in pain, I try and not to prescribe to stop the reaction. It is better not to palliate and just leave them alone. So when the patient phones up and complains bitterly that something dreadful has happened you say very good! You need to read what is going on and reassure them that what is happening is okay, part of a process and what should be going on because that is what homeopathy is. It invites you to take a little journey and sometimes it is a bit bumpy but that is okay. People are so suppressed. You give a homeopathic remedy and it is just a can of worms. The whole lot explodes all over the place and that is good.

ROWENA: So who is in your circle of meditators?

MARTIN: Janice Micallef, Colin Griffith, Jill Wright, Terry Howard, Diane Pitman and Sylvia Treacher.

ROWENA: Do you still see them?

MARTIN: Not officially as that group came to an end but we still do meditative provings. We still gather different people around us, put groups together, and do remedies.

ROWENA: What made you come up with remedies like *Apple?*

MARTIN: Well it is an obvious one to do really isn't it? The fruit trees are said to be really quite refined and advanced in the vegetable kingdom.

ROWENA: So when you start thinking about it there are just endless remedies to prove. Could you tell me more about the meditative provings and what happens during them?

MARTIN: We meditate in silence for an hour to an hour and a half and then we share our experiences.

ROWENA: If people are sharing their experiences how do you avoid being influenced by each other? Or does it not matter? I am just trying to put myself in that space and imagine what it is like.

MARTIN: Well that is part of the training of meditating together. That is part of what you learn to do; to have your own experience of whatever the meditation is. If you are making a repertory you have remedies you put in bold type, remedies you would underline and remedies you would have in plain type. That means that perhaps everybody in the circle might get one or two of the same experience; then half the circle might get a particular experience and then maybe one or two would get something nobody else got and through that you build up a picture of the remedy. If we don't have recording equipment then we have somebody who writes all the reports down using shorthand.

ROWENA: And you don't know what the remedy is before you do it?

MARTIN: No we don't. It is a double-blind meditation. We did a meditative proving of *Latrodectus mactans.* There was already a conventional proving but it didn't have a very big picture. After I took the remedy and went into the meditation, the first thing I got was a spider's web; I was on a spider's web and it was shaking.

ROWENA: That is amazing! Well it is not really amazing as it makes perfect sense but it still is amazing nevertheless! Do you know what I mean?

MARTIN: Yes, I know what you mean and what was extraordinary was, as one side of the spider's web started to shake the other side started to shake as well. Now the spider's web was the size of the universe and it was also the size of a spider's web. It was both. And there was a kind of extraordinary tension and acuteness of the senses. One of the group coughed and I jumped out of my skin. Interestingly spiders have an intolerance of noise and that is what I experienced.

ROWENA: So did you start thinking that it might be a spider or do you stop yourself doing this as part of the training?

MARTIN: You don't start to use your brain to speculate what the remedy is. You keep the brain out of it and you go into the meditation and experience it. What was so interesting about this particular proving was that this was a remedy that illustrated the unity behind all life. We were all on this spider's web, all of us, and the person on one side was connected to someone on the other. When one side started rattling the other side started moving as well. It was quite an extraordinary experience and we realised that *Latrodectus mactans* is a remedy that brings the kind of universal consciousness that all life is one. It is important for people to get that kind of consciousness if they have no concept of the unity of life.

ROWENA: That has brought up a few things for me. I read a book many years ago, *Bridge Across Forever*[107], about that connection that people have, and actually I did see it as a cord, or like part of a web; that once you made a connection with somebody you feel that connection always but also obviously we all have that connectedness. Do you think all homeopaths need to believe in universal connectedness or can they work on a different level?

MARTIN: You can work on whatever level you find it. It is perfectly valid on any level. And it is with patients as well. Patients come for two reasons. They come to have their physical ailments dealt with, whatever they may be, serious or superficial. And then there is another group of people who will come to use homeopathy as an instrument to unfold their own power and their own potential.

ROWENA: So tell me more about the meditation circles.

MARTIN: For six years we have run three two year meditation circles. Janice Micallef runs the meditations and they are really experiential for students and involve them on a very deep level. Then Colin Griffith and I do the class instruction. We teach chakras, endocrine glands and the new remedies. We get other experts in to teach astrology, science and kabbalah etc. It is designed to take students fresh from college. The college experience teaches them to be good technicians who can work with materia medica and the repertory. What we want to do is develop them into healers with knowledge of other things that they may find helpful. The more practitioners understand spiritual philosophy, the more effective they can be as homeopaths; it goes hand in hand. As one learns to see much deeper into one's patients, one is able to do much bigger and better work.

ROWENA: So do you have a course that is running now?

MARTIN: We just did a summer school in Greece.

ROWENA: Was that at the end of a two year training?

MARTIN: No. It was just a one-off for a week. We did it differently this time and took a group of over thirty students. They did two provings and I must say I have never seen a group of people move and change so much in a week; it was astonishing. And of course the little island of Paros is a safe place to be and to open up. There is nothing threatening there as it is like living in England in the 1950s. They loved it and had a wonderful time.

ROWENA: They were postgraduates?

MARTIN: They were all postgraduates and they experienced themselves in a different way that week.

ROWENA: It changed their perception?

MARTIN: Yes. This is the first time we have done a Guild for three or four years as we had closed it down. So now we might open it up again; we will see what happens.

ROWENA: I would imagine there is a demand for it. *Prometheus*[59] the journal, stopped as well, didn't it?

MARTIN: Yes, I am afraid so. That is because the three of us, Janice Micallef, Colin Griffith and myself are so busy that we have no time to organise it.

ROWENA: So going back to how to be a successful homeopath....

MARTIN: Well I think you have to be willing to prescribe in different ways other than classical. If you are just going to prescribe classically it is not going to work. That is on a fundamental level.

ROWENA: Unless you attract those patients that will respond to those remedies, no?

MARTIN: Possibly, I don't know of anybody who would just do well on one single remedy. Others have their own stories and their own ways of using it and attract patients accordingly but for me it does not work.

ROWENA: The concept of the Holy Grail isn't that they only take one dose but that even in an acute, their specific Holy Grail remedy will get them back into balance even if the symptoms of the acute are not in the remedy picture.

MARTIN: Well, sometimes the chronic and the acute are the same remedy and sometimes they are not.

ROWENA: In terms of who has influenced you Martin, obviously Thomas Maughan but what about other homeopaths or spiritual teachers?

MARTIN: Well I am good friends with Janice Micallef and with Colin Griffith and I think we influence and help each other.

ROWENA: When you give remedies in combination, how does the healing work? We were taught that if someone is out of balance, the remedy works as a catalyst to instigate a healing response of the vital force. If they are having different messages from several remedies, how does that work? Are the messages on different levels?

MARTIN: They are not getting different messages that conflict. It is all the same message but from a different point of view. As you say, it is sorting them out on different levels.

ROWENA: Like peeling an onion....

MARTIN: You can peel it from one side and you can peel it from another side and you can then take the next layer off. People come with a legacy of so many different issues. They may have suffered grief some time in their life and their heart has shut down, so you would use remedies like Natrum muriaticum maybe to help the heart open, but at the same time you realise the heart cannot open unless there is some stability in the solar plexus.

ROWENA: So that is the energy centre representing identity?

MARTIN: Yes. So you have to strengthen the solar plexus at the same time as getting the heart to open. The syphilitic miasm has its root in the heart and the thymus gland so you are going to use that to try and help the heart as well. If the person has been vaccinated it will create a blockage, which can be very difficult to break through. I have a patient of my age who has never been vaccinated; I have been treating him for years but there is nothing ever wrong with him. When he came to me he had ulcerative colitis and it cleared up really quickly because he hadn't been vaccinated. He never has any problems that a couple of remedies haven't cured.

ROWENA: I am happy to say that I wasn't vaccinated.

MARTIN: That is wonderful! I suspect you respond very well to homeopathy.

ROWENA: I do.

MARTIN: Well there we are. You might even be able to get a single remedy to work well for you. If you treat children who have been vaccinated you have to use a lot of remedies and repeat them often and that is how you get through it. If you just give one remedy and don't see them for weeks or months, it is just not going to do anything. It just won't because you come up against that barrier of the vaccinations.

ROWENA: But I use LMs with a lot of my patients and they work really well.

MARTIN: Yes, LMs work well.

ROWENA: I always explain homeopathy as a process – that as a result of taking their remedy over a period of time they will experience an unravelling. I especially tell patients this that have cancer or emotional issues. Martin, do you think homeopathy will become dormant again?

MARTIN: The problem we have now is what is happening with regulation; it could stifle homeopathy. In order for our profession to really flourish, it has to be practised with complete freedom. If you try to impose controls about who can prescribe, who cannot prescribe, how they prescribe, in what situations they can prescribe and so on, you are going to kill it off. It is not going to have that bigger freedom that it needs. If you, for instance, say homeopathy has to be taught only in universities then we will only get academics attracted to the profession and not necessarily those with life experience or other skills, for example. I hope it doesn't go that way. If we get under the control of doctors and doctors' practices they will decide what they sell and to whom.

ROWENA: It is very unlikely they are going to refer to a homeopath unless it is one of those heart sink patients that they are just trying to get rid of, don't you think?

MARTIN: Well, yes, that is right. And then when you get those patients they are likely to be taking a range of drugs that they have been prescribed and if you want them to stop taking the drugs you are immediately in conflict with the GPs. It is a hard one but we will see how it reveals itself in time.

ROWENA: Thank you so much Martin for sharing your thoughts and time with me.

CHAPTER 24:   CAROL WISE

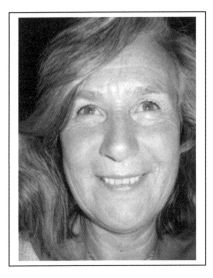

On a sunny Saturday 27 August, the day after I returned from two weeks of writing this book in Spain, Carol Wise came to my house for a conversation on her way back to Yorkshire from a trip to London. Our paths had crossed already a year earlier as the Yorkshire School of Homeopathy was one of the five I liaised with as an education adviser for the Society of Homeopaths. It was good to reconnect and hear her stories. Since the interview Carol has now retired and closed the doors of the Yorkshire School.

"If a person has told you their story and they gain insights from it, that part of their story isn't as important to them as it was before. Having off loaded it, it has already changed. Just because you have got the information doesn't mean that it is still there. It is not fixed."

Carol Wise, August 2005

"Isn't all illness in the mind? Doctors differentiate between what is in the mind and what is in the physical; they fragment us. Illness is in the mind and it manifests physically."

Carol Wise, August 2005

"How can you make a living as a homeopath? By being true to the basic principles - homeopathy speaks for itself. Hahnemann told us how to do provings and the way he described the process makes sense to me. Meditative provings do not."

Carol Wise, August 2005

"Having been around the homeopathy profession for a long time now I feel that there is too much of a wacky element within us at the moment and it is going to undermine us. We need to work together to build a profession that is taken seriously by those making decisions."

Carol Wise, August 2005

CHAPTER 24:   CAROL WISE

ROWENA: Tell me where your story began with homeopathy. That little question!

CAROL: It is quite simple really; in 1979 I met Dorothy Hannon in Hexham. Dorothy was studying with Martin Miles in London and started telling me about homeopathy but in those days, my family was well and I didn't think we needed homeopathy. My son was fine. He had had a natural birth and we were never ill.

ROWENA: There were vaccinations around then though, weren't there?

CAROL: Yes. We hadn't had Tristan vaccinated because there was asthma, eczema and tuberculosis (TB) in the family. He got chicken pox at six months and had two spots, which was fine. I stayed friendly with Dorothy and she gave us some books, Gibson's *First Aid Homoeopathy in Accidents and Ailments*[108] and we did talk homeopathy. When she went down to Martin Miles in London she would come back and tell me all about it. Then when my daughter was about eight months old and Tristan was two and a half they got whooping cough. I asked Dorothy if homeopathy could treat it and she prescribed one dose of *Drosera* 30C each. The doctors had warned me that they were going to be ill for three months. Six weeks coming and six weeks going is the natural course of the disease but three days later they had no symptoms.

ROWENA: How interesting. How long ago was that?

CAROL: About twenty five years ago.

ROWENA: So did someone advise you that you shouldn't vaccinate if you have got that background of health problems?

CAROL: No, but there was bad press about the whooping cough vaccine at the time and I thought, "If we can do without it, we will." So when the whooping cough went with one dose of a remedy I started to wonder what else homeopathy could do. Dorothy told me about a correspondence course in homeopathy and I signed up. I would have liked to have studied with Martin Miles, but with two young children and another one on the way it wasn't practical. Dorothy was quite happy to come back and share what she had learnt, but I needed back up, so I started the Braintree Forest School correspondence course. The correspondence bit was not up to much; they gave me little exercises to do but never marked them and there was no feedback. I cannot remember how long I did it for now, but the main bonus was that they were sending me books like Clarke's *Materia Medica*[28] and Boericke[39].

I started collecting homeopathy books and Dorothy would help me read and understand them and then my husband said, "Isn't it time you did something with all this?"He wanted us both to work part time and share the childcare and housework and I agreed that this was a good idea. I was really excited about starting to treat patients.

I remember my first patient, I went to her house and took her case in a very brief kind of way and charged her two pounds, which seemed like a lot at the time! I said it was to cover the remedy and she got better. Then I got really adventurous and invited someone to come to my house for me to take his case and I remember I was so nervous. I had checklists for everything and I was sweating like crazy as I was absolutely terrified. And he also got better so I thought, "I can do this!" And then Dorothy set up the Northern College in Newcastle and asked me to teach with her but I didn't think I knew enough.

Instead I joined the Northern College as a student in order to get some formal training and I went into the second year. There is always something to learn; you never stop. When I got into the third year the teachers kept on asking me for my advice and I would reply and then I started thinking, "Hang on. I am telling you more than you are telling me and I am paying you!" So I gained my licentiate from the Northern College after two years but I never actually graduated. My studies gave me the confidence to practise, but I still wanted to continue learning so I went to the seminars that Vassilis Ghegas was giving in London for two years.

ROWENA: How often did he lecture?

CAROL: About once every two months for a long weekend but I cannot remember exactly. He was a fantastic teacher; he was totally amazing. I will never forget how he demonstrated the difference between *Belladonna* and *Stramonium* - he did it with a laugh. He laughed *Stramonium* and he laughed *Belladonna* and said, "That is the difference." And there was a tape of coughs. He would say, "This is a *Causticum* cough and this is a *Cuprum metallicum* cough." After a tea break one afternoon we were all chatting and he came and stood by his microphone and waited. Everyone was talking and I said, "Look, he is ready to start." And he coughed, and I said to Roger Morrison, "Just stop them. Shut them up because he is ready to start." And this cough got louder and louder and more frequent and Roger went and got him a glass of water. He drank it and everyone by that time has actually stopped talking, as he looked as if he was about to pass out. And then he said, "What is the remedy?!" I will never forget it was *Cuprum metallicum*. So that is the sort of teacher he was and I loved going to his sessions.

ROWENA: Who were your contemporaries? Who were you studying with then?

CAROL: The late Liz Danciger was a wonderful lady. She was a real extravert and very rebellious. I have got those tendencies but not quite as badly as she did; she was lovely.

Robert Nichols and John Morgan were both around at that time. In 1984, after two years with Vassilis Ghegas I was within the first group to go to Alonissos for a week to study with George Vithoulkas. I can still picture all the people that I studied with but I just cannot remember their names; there were about twenty or thirty of us and mostly from England.

George Vithoulkas was very arrogant and he explained this case that will fix in my mind forever. He told us the case history and then he said, "So what is the remedy?" and I thought, "*Aurum metallicum*, I think it is *Aurum*", and people were offering remedies and nobody said *Aurum*. Every time somebody suggested a remedy he said, "You know why?" and then he shot them down. If I talk about people who have inspired me, he is not on my list. I did not find him to be a good teacher. It went on all day, he would not give way and he wanted everyone to come up with a remedy. In the evening he said, "Sleep on it and come back to me tomorrow."

ROWENA: What stopped you saying *Aurum metallicum*?

CAROL: Terror!

ROWENA: I can imagine.

CAROL: I am just not that confident. I think somebody eventually might have said it and he replied, "Yes" and I thought, "I am just as good as any of these people. I knew the remedy!" But that is pathetic, isn't it? It is this fear of getting it wrong - fear that if you don't get it you are stupid. George Vithoulkas did that to me and I thought, "You are not the sort of teacher I want." Having said that, he came to England and I still went to his seminar. I went to everything. Eizayaga and Candegabe came over from South America and Robin Murphy did lots of seminars, so I went to all of those.

Francis Treuherz and Linda Killick (now Shannon) were making connections at that time. Linda went to India where she met Subrata Banerjea, who was running the Bengal Allen Homeopathic College, and he said, "Why don't you get some students to come across? I will give them a really good time; they can come to all the homeopathic hospitals and we will give them seminars." Francis Treuherz asked me if I wanted to go for six weeks. This was in 1986 and I had three young children, so I put the phone down and said to my husband, "I have always wanted to go back to India and there is this chance, but the children…. " and he said, "Oh you should go, you should go." So I had those six weeks in India. I learned a lot and it was when I came home that I had the culture shock. India felt more authentic and the people/patients seemed more open and straightforward.

ROWENA: I am not surprised!

CAROL: I thought, "What am I doing here? I would rather be in India but I have three young children, I was born here and this is my home. I have got to do what is in front of me." So I carried on doing what I was doing and then it was at the Society of Homeopaths' conference in Warwick that I met Madeline Evans. She bounced up to me and said, "Oh, hi! I have been in London and I am moving to Yorkshire." She had discovered that I was the only homeopath in Yorkshire at that point.

She said that we should keep in touch and when she moved to Yorkshire she said she and her husband wanted to start a college. So this was Dorothy Hannon all over again but this second time it happened I thought, "This is trying to tell me something." But I said, "I'm not a qualified teacher" and Madeline said, "Oh, I am a qualified teacher, so don't worry about that." The idea was to have only one year group going through the four years. We took on twenty five students and Richard, her husband, did all the PR administration and we were just there to team-teach.

After the first year, we had twenty one students who all wanted to go on and train as homeopaths. We thought that we were obviously going to keep on going but Richard said, "We really need to take students on every year. If you get a hundred students in, I can do the office work. We will do a foundation course for the first year and then the ones that want to be serious practitioners will go on." And I said, "I am not going to teach a hundred students for anything or for anyone and I am not a lecturer. This small group is about sharing, talking and discussion like an apprenticeship".

This is what Madeline and I wanted so instead of me backing out and leaving them to it, Richard left. We took on a second group after the four years, so we did it for two groups over eight years. Later on when Madeline decided not to be involved anymore, we had to reinvent the College and called it the Yorkshire School of Homeopathy. Also when Madeline left I had to look for other people to come and teach with me so I invited some of our graduates, Rebecca Preston and Christine Millum.

ROWENA: I haven't heard of her.

CAROL: Oh, you never knew Christine? She was gorgeous. She got killed in a car accident. She was coming back from a dance class a few weeks after our last college weekend of the academic year in July. She was halfway through marking the students' exam papers. She taught philosophy and she was one of our first student graduates. She would walk into the teaching room and the students would go silent, and then they would hear her loud authoritarian voice. She would ask people questions at exactly the right level that they could answer. She was an excellent teacher and you don't get many of those; she was wonderful. We missed her a lot.

ROWENA: And she just taught one year?

CAROL: No, no, I don't know how many years she was teaching with us, I lost count.

ROWENA: That is really tragic, it must have really knocked you. The Yorkshire School is a classical college isn't it?

CAROL: It depends what you mean by classical. How can you make a living as a homeopath? By being true to the basic principles - homeopathy speaks for itself. Hahnemann told us how to do provings and the way he described the process makes sense to me. Meditative provings do not. There are loopholes, of course, because nobody is completely healthy and you are supposed to be healthy when you take your remedy for the proving.

I did a proving with Jeremy Sherr and I got symptoms to the point where my supervisor guessed what the remedy was on the first day that we had taken it. We talked over the phone and she said, "I think I know what the remedy is." And I said, "You cannot possibly, this is the first day." And she told me what she thought it was and three months later when we did the extraction and gathering together she was proved right.

ROWENA: How did she know?

CAROL: Because of the way I was talking." There was no way she could have known what it was as it was a brand new proving.

ROWENA: Wow.

CAROL: If you think that is wow, wait for it; I was taking placebo.

ROWENA: Fascinating. What remedy was that?

CAROL: Diamond (Adamas).

ROWENA: That is funny, because *Diamond* came into my mind as you were speaking and I had forgotten that it was one of Jeremy Sherr's remedies.

CAROL: It blew my mind that I had actually taken placebo. And I thought, "What the hell is this all about?" It was a classical Hahnemannian proving, and we knew that someone had been given a placebo, but you just never think it is going to be you. And particularly when you start to get symptoms and they are the same as everyone else's.

ROWENA: So what do you think that is about?

CAROL: This gets us into the wacky side of homeopathy. I know that you can send a remedy down the telephone or write the name of a remedy on a piece of paper, put a glass of water over it and take it as if it were a pill. I can give you examples.

ROWENA: Oh, please do.

CAROL: A friend's partner had absolutely furious rage and was litigating for other people. I think you get the job that suits you and that you need to do until you don't need to do it anymore and then you move on. I told his partner on the telephone, "He needs *Nitricum acidum*, have you got any?" and she said, "No", so I said, "Write it on a piece of paper" and she said, "Can you not just send it down the phone?" So I said, "I have got a bottle here, I will just take the top off. Here you are."

ROWENA: How did she then transfer it to him?

CAROL: I don't know. Maybe she had a bottle and caught it. I don't know! Anyway, he did really well on it. And another time, I was in a pub and a woman had a really sharp, stabbing pain in her chest. After making various suggestions eventually I said, "Would you like a homeopathic remedy?" and she said, "Oh, yes please." So I replied, "I haven't got any remedies on me, but I can do this." I went to the bar and said, "A glass of water please" and I wrote on a piece of paper *Bryonia* 200C. I took the paper and the glass back to the lady, put them on the table, put the glass of water over the paper and said, "There you are, drink that." And she said, "It is OK now, the pain has just gone." I feel that a lot of what we do is about intervention and the focusing of energy. If you know the shape of the energy that you need to heal someone with and can focus that energy, the person will be able to take it in.

ROWENA: Do you need the intention of the specific remedy?

CAROL: If you want to use homeopathy, it helps to know the name of the remedy so that you can focus it in your mind, but you don't actually have to take the remedy. This is how Rae machines work; they make the remedy out of thin air just by focusing the energy and clicking a dial. I don't understand it, but I know people who make their remedies that way.

ROWENA: Carol, who inspired you and who inspires you now?

CAROL: Dorothy Hannon. Do you want to know what happened to her? She went to work in London and practised quantum homeopathy. She was working in the business world, and found that the principles in the office were not holistic. She was trying to make the people in the office have a more caring attitude towards their fellow workers. For Dorothy, it wasn't just about getting their work done; they were real people with real lives and if they were happy, she felt, they worked better. But then she realised that she could actually apply these principles to homeopathy, which led her on to look at homeopathy in the quantum sense rather than the linear.

The question for her was no longer, "What is the remedy?" but more like, "In the here and now, in this space, what do we see? What energy is moving around?" You can take a case today, work on it the next day and then send the person the remedy, at which point they have probably moved on. You have to look at energy in terms of how it is shifting around and Dorothy Hannon did that in a more holistic sense. She examined the mind, the emotions, the physicals and the miasms in a shifting energy field to see where it needed help.

ROWENA: So how would she prescribe with that approach?

CAROL: It is about valuing the information that you have got in a different way. If a person has told you their story and they gain insights from it, that part of their story isn't as important to them as it was before. Having off loaded it, it has already changed. Just because you have got the information doesn't mean that it is still there. It is not fixed. I remember a wonderful case of a young girl who had panic attacks. She came to me and she told me that she panicked and panicked and the only thing that made her feel more comfortable was playing the piano, but she didn't play the piano any more. I asked the obvious question, "Why don't you play the piano?" and she burst into tears and said that her piano teacher sexually abused her when she was five. Somehow she had not thought about it, locked it away and never made that connection. So somewhere in that space something I said just loosened it up a little bit and the prescription came through as an insight. She felt she had worked out her own healing and therefore she no longer needed a remedy to help her.

ROWENA: I guess you know a big article[109] came out in *The Lancet*[110] yesterday saying homeopathy is all in the mind.

CAROL: Isn't all illness in the mind? Doctors differentiate between what is in the mind and what is in the physical; they fragment us. Illness is in the mind and it manifests physically.

So back to your question, the teachers who inspired me were the ones that were authentic; the ones who didn't make it up as they were going along. Jeremy Sherr is a good homeopath and he is a very inspiring teacher. When he gave us a lecture on the periodic table it was absolutely mind blowing.

ROWENA: Were you a Dynamis School student?

CAROL: Yes. Through one of his lectures I suddenly realised that the periodic table is a spiral, it is not a table at all. Spiral energy, spiral knowledge, the elements, the pattern of life, and the esoteric - suddenly it clicked for me that everything is a spiral. It was just a wonderful lecture. I have learned a lot from all my teachers but if I had to pick one that has inspired me the most I would probably say Vassilis Ghegas.

ROWENA: What do you consider to be the most important qualities of a homeopath?

CAROL: Passion and integrity. Having been around the homeopathy profession for a long time now I feel that there is too much of a wacky element within us at the moment and it is going to undermine us. We need to work together to build a profession that is taken seriously by those making decisions.

ROWENA: Carol, thank you so much for sparing the time to come and see me on your way back to Yorkshire. It was lovely to spend time with you again and I wish you a safe journey home!

CHAPTER 25:   LINDA RAZZELL

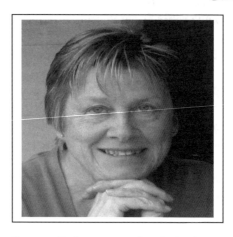

I interviewed Linda Razzell, one of the principals of the New College of Homeopathy (New College), on the telephone on Tuesday 13 September 2005. I had watched her charismatic lectures on the bowel nosode programme twice earlier in the year for the Society of Homeopaths' Continuous Professional Development group in North London and the Alliance of Registered Homeopaths' (ARH) Spring Conference. I had also attended two postgraduate seminars at the New College at the University of Greenwich in the summer - Mike Bridger and Martin Miles. Unfortunately the New College has closed its doors since the interview.

"We hold a mirror up to our patients and they see themselves in it and what they see is a different future and a different possibility. And people stop believing in the medical model! They stop hearing, "There's nothing we can do for you." Many people's attitude now will be, "Well, I'll see about that!" And then they will go and look for something. Great if they find homeopathy. Great if they find reflexology. Whatever they find, it is because their mind changed."
Linda Razzell, September 2005

"Offer yourself as someone's practice assistant; open the doors, make their appointments, ask if you can sit in on complicated cases, and you will learn an awful lot!"
Linda Razzell, September 2005

"I am very, very shocked and dismayed at the lack of business acumen among homeopaths, and that it doesn't appear on the curriculum of many colleges. It doesn't even appear on the European Guidelines for Homeopathic Education, unless they have changed it radically. I am not quite sure what homeopaths think is going to happen to them when they set up in practice. Is the world going to suddenly smile at them and pay out good money? Why would that happen in any other business?"
Linda Razzell, September 2005

CHAPTER 25:   LINDA RAZZELL

ROWENA: What kind of students do you think you attract at the New College?

LINDA: Well, this will surprise you! Do you know that more than half of our intake is men?

ROWENA: Really?

LINDA: Yes.

ROWENA: That is fascinating. Why do you think that is?

LINDA: I don't know and I would love to know, because it has always been a great sadness to me that classes have been ninety eight percent women and two percent men. It simply unbalances the whole dynamic and I feel sorry for them because they stick out a mile from the others, because they are isolated and it takes them a long while sometimes to meld down with the women. It is a shame, isn't it? But this is not what is happening to us! We actually have slightly more men than women. We are promoting the use of technology perhaps more than other people do, so maybe that is why. It would be a shame if that were the reason but I think it might be.

ROWENA: So do you put this in your advertisements?

LINDA: What we talk about is bringing the subject into the twenty first century and the good use of technology because that is what we do. I have to be honest.

ROWENA: Tell me more about what you do.

LINDA: We are trying to teach materia medica in the way that it makes sense. We are trying to get people to get a grasp of the remedy in terms of themes and kingdoms. I know that this isn't new now, but it was when we started. And we believe in finding out how students learn and what their unique learning pattern is. Whether they are kinaesthetic, visual or auditory – so we actually run psychological tests and things like that to help them. And then when we have worked out our students needs, we can use all sorts of media to help them learn. The majority of what we use in the classroom is multimedia.

ROWENA: And the New College was the idea of Charles Wansbrough?

LINDA: Yes.

ROWENA: I saw his system when I interviewed him. It was just amazing.

LINDA: I realised when I was studying materia medica with the class that I was completely visual and that if I could just sit at the back of the class, chill out and watch what they give out without taking notes it would go in. I was amazed that this happened because like many people, learning materia medica was a struggle for me. I admired those doctors in India who would get up at four in the morning just to study their materia medica for hours and hours. I thought that that was what you have to do, but that I could not do it.

ROWENA: So, how do you do it? How does it work for you? Do you see it and you get it?

LINDA: I see it and I get it. Yes. So Charles Wansbrough's work is in picture form and I see the birds, for example, and I get it. Then I get the slight difference there are in the characteristics of the different birds and I get that too. There is a bird theme like there is a Natrum theme. Suddenly I just see and then, of course, instead of learning one remedy you have learnt a dozen in one day.

ROWENA: So how did you meet Charles Wansbrough?

LINDA: It was Valerie Probert, the other principal, who introduced me to Charles Wansbrough. I had known about him for many years because of *Prometheus*[59] but basically I couldn't understand a word he said in his writing. I told him this and he knows it is true. And I hope I helped him to be a bit more accessible, because like many geniuses, he knows what he is saying, but it is not always true that everybody else does. So, for him to have to come down to our level of teaching has been very good for him and it has been very good for us to try to go up to his level of thought too.

ROWENA: So, tell me how you got into homeopathy in the beginning. You have been around for a while, I know.

LINDA: Yes, I have. Like most people do, by having health problems that it didn't seem that anything else could solve. I had quite a dramatic life changing event, a car accident in 1979 and after a while I realised that I wasn't going to get better by the conventional methods, because I was being told, "There is nothing we can do for you, you won't walk again."

ROWENA: Oh, really, THAT dramatic?

LINDA: Oh, yeah. But it didn't seem to me that I should just sit and do nothing. I thought that there must be something I could do so I started my exploration of alternative medicine.

ROWENA: And how did you come across homeopathy?

LINDA: That was quite interesting. My youngest son was quite little and had been ill since birth, with coughs, infections and tonsillitis treated by antibiotics. He then got gastroenteritis and had to go into hospital. Finally a very old doctor in Wales said to me, "Look, Madam, if you keep doing this, he will keep being like this. What you have to do is stop treating him!" I said, "What? Stop giving him his medicine?" And he said, "Yes, if you stop, then you give the body a chance to get better by itself; and you could try homeopathy." So, that was it. From that day on my son has never had anything else and he is now thirty five.

ROWENA: It is great, isn't it?

LINDA: Yes, it is. And then I thought, "Maybe this could be something for me." Eventually, a yoga friend of mine said, "You should go and see my friend Tony; he is a homeopathy student."

ROWENA: So this is Tony Hurley?

LINDA: Who in those days was a hippie with big hair and bare feet! He used to sit on the examination couch cross-legged. He gave me my first remedy and it was like my life again changed. Everything changed and I suddenly saw the light.

ROWENA: And was it the homeopathy that got you walking again?

LINDA: No, it wasn't. It was a wonderful osteopath.

ROWENA: I would have been surprised if homeopathy did. I am sure it is capable of most things but...

LINDA: Well, I don't know, you see, what happened is that my attitude changed. There was something inside me that said, "You don't want to believe this. There are people out there that believe you can do anything!" You know, I think that is what actually did it. And then finding the homeopathy reinforced that, because with homeopathy you discover that almost anything is possible. It is a mindset. We get lots of patients, don't we, who have been told there is nothing that can be done. It is so wrong to say that to people.

We hold a mirror up to our patients and they see themselves in it and what they see is a different future and a different possibility. And people stop believing in the medical model! They stop hearing, "There's nothing we can do for you." Many people's attitude now will be, "Well, I'll see about that!" And then they will go and look for something. Great if they find homeopathy. Great if they find reflexology. Whatever they find, it is because their mind changed.

Then something quite amazing happened. I was looking for a class to study meditation or flower arranging for a bit of relaxation and I went to the City Lit, a great old place, and blow me down, the flower arranging class was full and the receptionist said, "How about homeopathy?" I climbed the stairs to the classroom, which was very difficult with my gammy leg still trailing along behind me and there was Margaret Roy, our teacher, sitting with a class of about thirty people. She looked at me and said, "Sorry but I am full" but she must have seen my face and how disappointed I looked and changed her mind and said, "Come on in." That was it and I studied with Margaret for three years. After the evening class, she took a few of us on privately and it was very hard work. You had to see maybe six to eight patients with her on Friday nights and Saturdays and then you had to turn up on the Sunday with the cases worked out.

ROWENA: Oh, I didn't know about this part of our history.

LINDA: This was when she was in practice in London. She had left the College of Homeopathy (COH) and there wasn't really a progressive class to go to after the course at City Lit, so she just took a group of us on privately, at home.

ROWENA: And what year was this?

LINDA: This must have been 1981.

ROWENA: I thought you studied at COH?

LINDA: Yes I did. One day Tony Hurley said to me, "Look, you know, Margaret Roy is leaving, why don't you go to college?" And I asked him, "Where is there to go?" So he said, "Well, there is COH." And that was the first I had heard of it.

ROWENA: And it would have been going for three years or so by then.

LINDA: And there were a hundred and twenty people in my first year. Can you imagine? We were divided into two classes with Robert Davidson and Sheilagh Creasy.

ROWENA: An interesting mix. And who else was in your year?

LINDA: Oh, lots of people; Keith Smeaton, Lorraine Hart, Sonyo (Julia) Peters, Joel Jaffey and Hilery Dorrian. Francis Treuherz, John Morgan, Lesley Gregerson, Nicky Pool, Linda Shannon, Mike Bridger and Anthony Bickley were a year above and Barbara Harwood was two years above, to name but a few. Many became heads of schools. When I look down the Society of Homeopaths' register, I think most of my class are in there.

ROWENA: It must have been an amazing experience for you.

LINDA: Yes, it was. Unlike me though, many of them were already in practice at that point and we were told not to prescribe. On the whole, we were obedient; we did what we were told.

ROWENA: That is quite tough if you have already been seeing patients, to then put your practice on hold.

LINDA: Yes, but it was a very good thing because I realised, after a while, that I only knew what I was doing up to a point and I didn't know what any of these remedies were apart from *Thuja occidentalis* and *Sulphur*. I didn't have a clue what they were, really. However Margaret Roy had taught us very, very well; we had a brilliant grounding in philosophy by the end of the first year and then we watched her cases, which I still believe is the best way to learn.

ROWENA: Yes. So is that what you do in the New College?

LINDA: As much as we can. We try to teach everything via the cases, because that is what homeopaths do, isn't it?

ROWENA: Yes.

LINDA: Certainly our assessments are all done through cases.

ROWENA: So, does it feel like your students are apprentices?

LINDA: Yes, apprentices; that is a good word. And I wish there was more room for people to be apprentices. When I was a student we did an awful lot of sitting in and observing. In my third year at COH, I sat in for five hundred hours and I am sorry that we cannot get everyone to do that now. The requirement was only a hundred, but I found Sylvia Treacher, bless her, and she let me sit in every week and I learnt so much from just being there; from being the fly on the wall. That is all you have to do.

ROWENA: Absolutely. I think that it is a real shame that we don't have that facility.

LINDA: Of course, one of the ways that we used to teach at COH, on the full time course anyway, was to have the whole class watching the clinic. And obviously that is a very good thing to do because you can start that right from the first year.

ROWENA: We did that from our first year in the London College of Classical Homeopathy (LCCH).

LINDA: Yes, I recall that; it was in the big hall, in the chapel in the Russian Embassy.

ROWENA: Yes, that is right. Oh, how I miss those days!

LINDA: Yes, me too! I used to love doing the clinic in the chapel. It is a very, very valid way for people to learn and it is a different kind of observation. OK, the role model may not be so perfect, but you are still seeing the cut and thrust of what they used to call 'the messy reality' of daily life in practice; people come, people don't come, they are happy with you, they are not happy with you, etc, etc. There is a lot more to it than just giving remedies.

I remember being in that chapel for the whole day, from nine in the morning until nine at night and the evening patients were astounding as they were always *Nux vomica* workaholics who wouldn't allow themselves to come during the day. I do think that is a good way to learn and I think apprenticeship should very much be recommended. I would say to any graduate, offer yourself as someone's practice assistant; open the doors, make their appointments and ask if you can sit in on complicated cases. You will learn an awful lot and you will understand how to run a business, which is of course another important skill.

ROWENA: I agree and did that myself for a year working for Michelle Shine, and I learned many things from her. She definitely had a big influence on me. So, what do you think are the ingredients of a successful homeopath; one that can actually earn a living?

LINDA: Well, for a start, having the awareness that that is what you are supposed to be doing. I am very, very shocked and dismayed at the lack of business acumen among homeopaths, and that it doesn't appear on the curriculum of many colleges. It doesn't even appear on the European Guidelines for Homeopathic Education, unless they have changed it radically. I am not quite sure what homeopaths think is going to happen to them when they set up in practice. Is the world going to suddenly smile at them and pay out good money? Why would that happen in any other business?

That is one of the principles of the New College because it is my business and I wouldn't be doing it if I didn't think that people could make a living out of it. I think it is very sad, that if someone mentions at the seminar that we are running a business here, everyone looks very shocked! It is only because you are doing something that is good and worthwhile that you think you shouldn't somehow be earning money. It is just a sheer lack of professionalism.

ROWENA: But it is a big part of society, isn't it?

LINDA: Like nurses, we are supposed to put up with low pay because of the fact that the job satisfaction is so great? Well, that is rubbish. This will change only when we believe in ourselves but it is up to us; based upon what we teach our graduates. There is huge poverty consciousness in the profession. You hear people talking about there not being enough people to treat.

ROWENA: What about the impact of the recent negative press?

LINDA: Sometimes we are a bit naïve and we underestimate the weight of the drug companies' lobby. That was what was in the papers recently, nothing else. Who do the scientists work for? I don't think most people, especially many patients, take any notice of that. It happens regularly. It happens about once every couple of years and it has been going on forever. That is when you know they are running scared and that is why they make completely illogical statements. On the one hand it is a placebo, but on the other hand our patients could end up in hospital on an overdose of *Echinacea*. The public aren't naïve; people see through statements like this.

ROWENA: And then there was the article in the Daily Mail, *Killed by Homeopathy* [111].

LINDA: Oh yes, that one. For fifteen years she had breast cancer, but homeopathy killed her.

ROWENA: Do you specialise in any particular area?

LINDA: It seems to be fertility.

ROWENA: How did you get into that?

LINDA: I wish I knew. It just happened. I suppose I partly got interested because my son's partner seemed to have a problem conceiving, and yet they were very young. And then they conceived the night that they set the wedding date and I thought, "There is something interesting going on and there is more to this than meets the eye." The next person that came with a fertility problem happened to be a forty five year old, and she had a reversed sterilisation. She didn't think there was any hope and then at the next meeting, she came back and said, "I think I am menopausal now, because I haven't had a period." And I thought, "Aha!"

ROWENA: And this is just with constitutional prescribing?

LINDA: No. Certainly not. Constitutional prescribing doesn't work for this.

ROWENA: So what does?

LINDA: Looking at why they are not getting pregnant. In that woman's case it was a simple matter of really undoing the damage that had been done to her via sterilisation. At forty five she was pregnant! She was my first one and it was so easy.

ROWENA: So, how did you undo that?

LINDA: Well, I looked at it from the homeopathic point of view. What is sterilisation? It is suppression. So that was the line I took. *Kali carbonicum* is my great remedy for infertility; all fertility problems. It is like the *Sulphur* of obstetrics; it can undo almost any damage or interruptions to the female cycle.

ROWENA: That is interesting.

LINDA: Yes. Most people don't get taught that in college so, if you ask me who has influenced me the most, I would have to say, my patients. If you trace back the timeline in patient's lives, you will usually find something or a collection of things that have caused this problem and then you can work systematically back through it.

ROWENA: I have been working with a lady for the last year or so, and we have progressed, but she is still not pregnant.

LINDA: In my practice, the average time from start of treatment to pregnancy is a year. The main thing is not to give up but try looking at it from a different way. Go back and examine all the 'obstacles to cure.'

ROWENA: I have been clearing her use of the Pill and IVF hormones.

LINDA: You see, those two things stack up the odds rather heavily.

ROWENA: I know and she has had a lot of IVF.

LINDA: You will need to really get rid of that.

ROWENA: Are there any remedies that are specific for doing that?

LINDA: Well, *Kali carbonicum* would be where I would start but I usually end up with the bowel nosode programme. Most of them don't get even half way through it before they get pregnant.

ROWENA: So how did you discover their use in fertility?

LINDA: I am always intrigued by anything different. I attended a very enthusiastic lecture on the bowel nosodes but I was right at the back of the room, as an organiser, and I could neither hear nor see properly so I didn't really think much of it. And then, it was a little while later, probably after a month, something clicked in my mind. I had a very complex case, and you know when you feel, "I don't know where to start"?

ROWENA: Yes, I do.

LINDA: Well I REALLY didn't know where to start and suddenly felt that maybe I should give the bowel nosodes a whirl and realised that I didn't have to worry where to start, I just had to start at the beginning. I think at that time I had been reading Hahnemann's later cases and I had been thinking very hard about giving everybody *Sulphur*, because he said you must get rid of the psoric miasm first and so it led on from that.

ROWENA: So do you think that everyone could benefit from going through the bowel nosode programme?

LINDA: I think if you had to choose one solution or one method that would be the one I would choose.

ROWENA: So do you think it addresses the way we live our lives at the moment?

LINDA: I put it together with a notion of treating what the ancients called the chakras and what we call the endocrine system, which has a knock-on effect on the rest of the body. So we start from the base, the bowel and elimination and work upwards.

ROWENA: Do you find that you prescribe more with the bowel nosodes than with anything else now?

LINDA: Yes. Certainly if I ever get that feeling that I don't know where to start, that is what I would do and certainly for fertility problems. Emma, my practice assistant and apprentice and I have got statistics; it is the best thing we do here. That is the one that usually sorts it out, so now we would probably do it first rather than last for a patient with fertility problems and then prescribe *Kali carbonicum* or *Folliculinum*.

ROWENA: And when you give *Kali carbonicum*, is there a particular potency that you go for?

LINDA: 1M or higher.

ROWENA: As one dose?

LINDA: Usually two or three. I get quite classical at that point. They would have all taken the Pill as I have never had anyone come to me with these problems that hasn't.

ROWENA: So it would be *Folliculinum* 1M as well?

LINDA: I may give that lower; I might give that actually to induce ovulation, which is of course a homeopathic trick, which I expect you know. I like to give *Folliculinum* 30C on days eight, nine and ten of their cycle and then they nearly always ovulate but unfortunately it takes more than just ovulation to conceive. Any homeopath can make a woman ovulate, but the rest is a lot trickier.

ROWENA: So, tell me Linda, what do you think holds those homeopaths back that are not making enough money?

LINDA: It can only be about self-development. Homeopaths need to believe in homeopathy and themselves and have the courage to take the jump. I don't actually think you can do it when you have a full-time job and you are trying to fit building a practice around that. So I think somehow you have got to make a big leap. Personally, I was pushed because I was made redundant half way through college. I just had to be brave and when you are bringing up two kids on your own, and you are paying the mortgage, your business has just got to work.

I think homeopaths are born, and not made and I think what we do at the New College is just assist people through their self-development. When we started college they said to those who had already been in practice, you have to stop, because they knew that we were not yet self-developed in that way and I do agree with that. Robert Davidson and Barbara had a huge influence on me and this was partly due to the fact that I learned there was more than one way to do it. I think psychologically, I would never have been happy believing there was only one way to do anything.

Through my study of the *Organon*[4], I could see that you can justify almost any course of action homeopathically. If you read the *Organon*[4], you will come up with perhaps a hundred different methods, including giving two remedies at once. Read *Chronic Diseases*[76] and you will see. It was a revelation for me, that right from the start I was taught there were many ways to do this that could be appropriate to the patient. As Robert Davidson said, "Appropriopathy". One must be patient centred not practitioner centred.

Sheilagh Creasy had a great impact on me, and I am very glad that I learned bog-standard classical principles of homeopathy from her. That meant that I was at my leisure to disagree with them but at least I knew what they were.

ROWENA: So did you disagree with them?

349

LINDA: Yes, there were some that I did disagree with, and the single remedy never made sense to me.

ROWENA: Is it sometimes OK with you?

LINDA: Sometimes it is appropriate but it can be a challenge to people's belief systems, so I think you have to watch out for that and explain.

ROWENA: So how do you explain?

LINDA: I actually say to them, "I realise that this challenges what you understand about medicine but sometimes we do only give one remedy, and this is why, and other times we give three a day. It just depends." Thomas Maughan was another homeopath who had a great influence on me. When you don't know what to do, you can usually find one of his combination remedies to sort it out. That is what I heard from him. Remedies can work on different levels and contrary to what is taught in classical colleges, it has not been my experience that the case gets confused. Combination remedies are very special and they become a simillimum, the three of them, together.

All I teach students is that there are many, many methods that will work. Your first criteria for judging a method is, does it work and does it get good results? But your second criteria has got to be, is there a rationale? You look at these two elements and you make your judgement.

I am not against formulae, when appropriate, but I am against the entire use of formulaic methods, and I find that students who have been taught that way cannot then make a decision in other cases. That is the danger. You need to know everything. You need to know every which way to do it, and then be able to select. It is like a toolbox and we are like DIY enthusiasts. You know the screwdrivers that are star shape at the end? If you try to go through a flat head screw with those, you will just conk it out and I think it is the same with patients. The screwdriver's OK, but the head has got to be right.

ROWENA: And you need to be taught all of that in college?

LINDA: You do. And even more than that, you need to be taught to take it further yourself. As Hahnemann said to us - experiment! And that is what he would be doing; I am sure of it. Homeopathy is a lifelong learning.

ROWENA: And that is what appeals to me about it.

LINDA: It is unique like that and I think we are very lucky.

ROWENA: I think we are very lucky too.

LINDA: There is another person that I mustn't miss out - Martin Miles. He is my homeopath and I have probably learned more from him than from anyone else because I am the recipient of what the remedy does. I find it hard to quantify what Martin does; he does something very special.

ROWENA: Go on.

LINDA: I don't know how to explain it; the way he practises is mystical. I guess it comes from his deep belief system but I think Martin Miles manages to give more love with his homeopathy than anybody I have ever seen which is not an easy thing to do if you have got a big practice and you try to have a life as well. It must be very tiring, but he never looks weary.

ROWENA: I spent an afternoon at his house recently interviewing him, and he was very relaxed, and I very much enjoyed being in his space.

LINDA: He is a very good advert for what he does. He keeps you happy and relaxed. I used to work with Martin Miles; I was his receptionist for a brief time and the miracles I saw come in. There was a woman with liver cancer and she was vomiting into a bucket when she first came. She used to bring it with her and within a year she was a cured woman.

ROWENA: Was this mainly on his new remedies?

LINDA: No, this was a very long time ago but I admire his pioneering attitude to the new remedies so much because I think it took such courage. We did a proving last year and it half killed me. I don't want to discourage people from doing provings but I learned what it was like to suffer, and not realise that it was the remedy. It was extraordinary. So, I was back to realising that this is the power of symptoms; they are all in the mind. It is all about metaphor. I did not have those symptoms before I took the remedy; the proving made me feel as though I did. So I think everybody who wants to prescribe should do a proving.

ROWENA: I love your enthusiasm Linda; I could listen to you for hours and hours. You must get that feedback quite a lot. There is something special about you.

LINDA: A friend of mine says I am charismatic. I don't really know what he means but I guess he means I am enthusiastic. I have got lots of energy; perhaps that is what it is.

ROWENA: Thank you so much Linda. I am looking forward to more of your postgraduate lectures at the University of Greenwich, because besides the fact that I love the place, I can take my breaks in Greenwich Market!

CHAPTER 26:   NICKY POOL

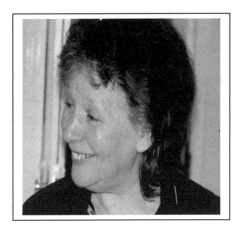

I snatched a quick half hour's interview on Thursday 29 September 2005 with Nicky Pool, the former principal of the Purton House Homeopathic Centre (Purton House), in our lunch break. We were both teaching all day. I work at Purton House, which is now housed in the Slough campus of Thames Valley University, as module leader and lecturer for practitioner development. This is a role I am slowly taking on from Nicky, year by year, as she gently steps back from college life to focus on her retreat and personal development workshops. Since completing this interview Purton House have had their course validated as a degree by Thames Valley University.

The invisible and intangible in life has always held a fascination for me. That is why I love
homeopathy. *Nicky Pool, September 2005*

"I believe that we do now need the degree course. I would never have thought it, but the
way the mood of the general public is going, people want to make sure that the
practitioners they go to have recognition and what they recognise these days are degrees.
My fear is that homeopathy will lose its heart in the same way that nursing did."
Nicky Pool, September 2005

"Jeremy Sherr explained how Hahnemann talked about the spirit of life and this
encouraged me to include even more personal and practitioner development at Purton
House. Hahnemann and Jung would have seen eye to eye in many things!"
Nicky Pool, September 2005

"Sometimes we give the simillimum and the person is not ready and we have to honour that
and not take it upon ourselves that we have failed - as long as we have done our very best.
If we consider that we have failed, the flip side of that coin is that we are the ones who
are getting people better and if that is the case we are putting ourselves in God's seat. I
am not a miracle curer and I don't profess to be." *Nicky Pool, September 2005*

CHAPTER 26: NICKY POOL

ROWENA: The first thing I want to ask you Nicky, is how you got into homeopathy in the first place?

NICKY: It was when I was in South Africa and my kids kept going down with high fevers. After repeated antibiotics I thought, "This is absolutely ridiculous!" A friend then said to me, "I know someone you ought to go and see." On her recommendation, I booked an appointment with an anthroposophical doctor who practised homeopathy. The kids were prescribed one remedy each, which I later learnt was *Tuberculinum bovinum*, and that was the end of their sore throats.

I had always been interested in holistic medicine and while I was in South Africa in the early 1970s I started to explore shamanism, witch doctors and the concept of an interconnected species. For as long as I can remember I had been searching for my purpose in life and the idea that we are cells within the greater body of God Life. This is a concept I gleaned from *The Soul of the White Ant* by Eugene Marais[112]. But there I was in psychiatric and general nursing where we were told off for talking to our patients! Instead we had to go and clean linen cupboards and sluices. The mindset was that it was a waste of time listening to patients. Ponder on the symbology behind 'cleaning the linen' and 'dealing with the shit'! When I worked in a private psychiatric unit I started looking at the food that the patients were given so I went to the head psychiatrist and asked, "Have you ever thought of the patients' nutritional needs?" I had been reading about how diet, nutrition and vitamin supplements can help mental states. "Rubbish", he said. This was in the early 1960s, so a long time ago.

The invisible and intangible in life has always held a fascination for me. That is why I love homeopathy. When I came back to England in 1972 I made enquiries into studying homeopathy but I discovered that you had to be an medical doctor before you could do that professionally. As a nurse I would have had to complete a two year training to become a doctor and then I would have been eligible to study homeopathy. That was the only option but I had two young children and a baby, so it was not a viable option for me then.

Instead I worked in an acupuncture and osteopathic clinic where they did nutrition and I met a man there whose wife had just begun studying at the College of Homeopathy (COH) in its first year in 1978. In 1981 when my youngest son was old enough, I went and found out about it and enrolled. It was their third intake in a large class of about eighty students but we whittled right down to the upper twenties as the years went on; there was a high drop out rate. The classes were very impersonal, and of course, the teachers were doing it by the seat of their pants as many of them had only just learnt homeopathy themselves and were only a few steps ahead of us.

ROWENA: Who were your contemporaries?

NICKY: Francis Treuherz, Jeremy Sherr, John Morgan, Susan Curtis, Stella Berg, Ernest Roberts, Lesley Gregerson, Anthony Bickley and Rob Barker. At that stage, when I finished my first year, COH started a parallel year for those who had medical training in some way or another. This is when John, who was a pharmacist and Jeremy, who was an acupuncturist joined but I decided to stay with my original year as both groups joined together quite regularly.

I remember that Francis Treuherz used to fall asleep on my shoulder in class and I would have to wake him. Because the group was so large, unless you were pushy, you could go through your whole studies and not be known by any of the tutors but Francis was impossible to ignore – even when asleep! Lectures were only an hour at a time so we couldn't get into the nitty-gritty and there was no real time for discussion. When I think about it now, we were thrown out into the community with hardly any practise of case taking. One could almost go through one's entire training without having a real grasp of repertorisation. Exams have never been a problem for me; my problem was that I would forget it all two days later! Other people knew far more than I did and failed because they went to pieces in exams. That is why we have continual assessment at Purton House.

Sheilagh Creasy came to teach us and she was a breath of fresh air. George Vithoulkas was also around in England at that time and Joseph Reves from Israel. They were exciting times and in a way, it was much more fun than it is now - or was it because I was the student and not the teacher?! We worked bloody hard. Students talk about working hard now but many of them lack the self-motivation that we had. Sometimes they seem to think that the assessments are hurdles imposed upon them rather than part of the joy of the learning process that they willingly embarked upon.

George Vithoulkas and Sheilagh Creasy would have us go through the entire repertory to study a remedy and write down all the rubrics. It would take us hours if not days, but they said that was the only way we would get to know our remedies and our repertory, and it was. It was hard work. But we were motivated to do that. Now it is so clear-cut, and there is little room for the individuality of the student. Compare that to the teaching methods of the East as explained by Gary Zukav in *The Dancing Wu Li Masters*[113].

I believe that we do now need the degree course. I would never have thought it, but the way the mood of the general public is going, people want to make sure that the practitioners they visit have recognition and what they recognise these days are degrees. My fear is that homeopathy will lose its heart in the same way that nursing did. Nurses are now managerial people rather than carers. The whole art of nursing, including clearing out linen cupboards and cleaning sluices, has been lost. I trained at University College Hospital in London and we were accused, at the time, of being second rate doctors instead of being praised as first class nurses.

ROWENA: Who inspired you the most? Are there a few characters about which you think, yes, they really did it for me?

NICKY: When they were on form, they were all individually inspiring. Misha Norland was amazing and has a very special place in my heart. I learnt a tremendous amount from Joseph Reves. He didn't teach at COH, but we used to go to his different groups. I have a lot of time for him, as he is a great thinker. Sheilagh Creasy also lives in my heart. Later Rajan Sankaran joined the ranks and, like Misha, his teachings resonated at soul level, as did Jeremy Sherr's in 1990. Tony Hurley, who is in my heart and soul as well. Martin Miles and Robert Davidson also inspired me. Robert had this lovely art of being at the vanguard and then when everyone else joined ranks he would go off and find something else to do which was equally enthralling. He used to really make us sit up and take notice.

Then Sheilagh Creasy came along, and she was quite fantastic. I had been working at the osteopath's clinic in Hampton, the one I mentioned earlier, throughout my studies and when I graduated they wanted me to be their homeopath and expand the practice, which already offered nutrition, acupuncture and osteopathy. As my experience progressed I had a growing number of patients who wanted to know more about homeopathy and they asked me to run a small group teaching acute remedies. I thought about it and replied that I would not teach acute prescribing without the homeopathy philosophy to back it up.

I also talked to the different colleges established at the time and proposed to them that if I were to run my course for a year, would they consider accepting the students on their courses for the second year. They agreed and Sheilagh Creasy came to teach with me, as did Tony Hurley and many of the others a little later. It was a small group of ten but at the end of the first year they said that they didn't want to go to a big college and wanted to stick with the small group and asked if I could get some more lecturers to come along. This was 1985.

ROWENA: And that is how it all started. So why did you call your school Purton House?

NICKY: Because that is the name of my home. We ran the school from there for a while but when the school became too large for Purton House we began our wanderings - we did move around a lot! At one point we ended up at a Buffalo Lodge; a pub with buffalo heads all over the walls and I think it also housed a secret society. The students would put in their orders for lunch and go on to the pub afterwards. From there we went to a very swanky Golf Club, until they put the rent up and then to the John North Centre, followed by the Community Centre in High Wycombe.

Next we had the blessing of the late Kay Samuel' lovely home at Penley Grange in Stokenchurch with the red kites wheeling overhead. She and her sister, Daphne Creer and I were aiming towards creating a retreat where we could integrate homeopathy and other holistic therapies. Much earlier in 1983 Ian Gordon-Brown from the Transpersonal Psychology Centre had inspired me at the first Society of Homeopaths' Conference. He had talked about how certain aspects of our inner self needed to break through the now imprisoning walls of our once protective cocoon in order to fulfil our potential (*Aphorism 9*[4]) butterfly (psyche or soul) nature, and that the way to understand what needed to change was to listen to the language of symptoms. Symptoms are not our enemy; they are trying to tell us symbolically how we can help our body get back into harmony. To me, that was perfect – I had come home!

Nursing was all about the body and psychiatric nursing was all about the mind. I would see psychiatric patients in the general hospital who should have been in the psychiatric unit, and people in the psychiatric unit who should have been in the general unit. There was no communication between the two but homeopathy brought together mind, emotions and the physical body.

It wasn't until I started to train as a transpersonal therapist that I really found the tools with which to explore the soul. I asked myself again, why do we want good health? Joseph Reves taught, quoting our friend Sam that it is for the higher purpose of our existence. Jeremy Sherr has picked up and enlarged upon a lot of what Joseph said so I learned much more of this at the Dynamis School. They both would open up the *Organon*[4] and it would come to life. This was not experienced at my training college when we considered the *Organon*[4] to be awfully longwinded and quite laborious. Jeremy explained how Hahnemann talked about the spirit of life and this encouraged me to include even more personal and practitioner development at Purton House. Hahnemann and Jung would have seen eye to eye in many things!

ROWENA: When I was studying, I heard that Purton House was the college where it was all touchy-feely and where everyone was into therapy.

NICKY: Which is a shame, as it has also got a very strong academic background with Sheilagh Creasy's and the late Janet Meldrum's input. However, I also believe with every fibre of my being that if we are to understand others we must first learn more about ourselves. I am, after all, influenced by the sixties, know thyself, and a lover of Shakespeare, "To thine own self be true, and it must follow, as the night the day, thou canst not then be false to any man.[114]"

ROWENA: That may also be true, but I was also at a very academic school and the difference that I was told about between the London College of Classical Homeopathy (LCCH) and Purton House, was that your focus was on the personal development side of things. As you say, Purton House is also very academic, and you are now moving forward with degree status.

NICKY: There is a large part of me which hopes that we as homeopaths have enough integrity not to let it lose its heart as a result of the degree status.

This has been one of the biggest lessons of my life; to stick to something longer than I really wanted to. Janet Meldrum, a beloved friend and colleague, was going to take over Purton House a long time ago when I wanted to step back because Kay Samuel, Daphne Creer and I were talking about having the college and a retreat within the same premises. The idea was to encourage our students to see homeopathy and what we offered at the retreat, as preventative medicine, as well as a healing process. I am not one of those people who think that if we do everything right we will never get ill because I have been in touch with the darker side of life, and I know that the dark side is valid and real and we have to embrace it. There is a belief that if we do it right, we will not get punished. It is very biblical.

ROWENA: Seeing ill health as a punishment?

NICKY: Lots of people do. We talk about some of the people with cancer being the nicest around and really not deserving of the affliction. We say that it is not fair that it should happen to them. But the soul is demanding a totality of experience; I believe it needs more than love and life because it is nourished by experience. And I believe that disease is part of health, as long as we listen to its message. Sometimes we gain our healing through death, be that the final death or one of our smaller deaths, like severe illness, divorce or redundancy. As homeopaths we have already embraced cause and effect; we cannot stop that. It is not what happens to us that is important; it is the way that we deal with it.

You know how naïve you are when you first start out in homeopathy? You think you can cure anything and everybody. It was only when I went deeper into transpersonal psychology that I understood the viewpoint that some souls have chosen to experience the path of being seriously ill; being in angst, being insane or being depressed. And who are we, with our very limited view of the greater totality, to say what is right and wrong? As homeopaths, a lot of our work is dealing with people in these dark places, helping them to come to terms with that and to find their way through. If they get 'better' that it is great. But I do not think it is we as homeopaths that get them better. What we have done is to walk alongside, having given them a mirror in the simillimum, but they are the ones who have got themselves better, or not, and that is their soul's journey. However, we do need to support and encourage them through the process.

I see too many homeopaths taking credit for getting people better, but people get themselves better. The homeopathic remedy might indeed help. Talk to Murray Feldman, another inspiring homeopath, about this. We can give them a great remedy, the simillimum even, and it cannot help but have an effect, but if they are not ready to make the change and are not encouraged to make those changes, then they may not run with it. It is like a relay race. We can give them the baton, but they may drop it again after a short while. This is seldom a conscious decision however.

I could tell you a story about a psychiatric patient.

ROWENA: Oh, please do Nicky.

NICKY: This guy came to me and I did not totally listen to what he asked to be cured. He was on Lithium and he wanted to be treated for the side effects; a dry mouth and symptoms like that. He was a poet and an artist and I saw him three times. I asked him to bring some of his work; it was amazing and it was so 'transpersonal.' He was talking in archetypal images. So much of what we call insanity is that people are on a different or altered level of consciousness, and because we do not understand them, we label them as mad. As homeopaths we say that we don't label people as disease states, but we do label them as remedies. The disease and the remedy are the same thing. And then we pat ourselves on the shoulder and say we don't call them diseases – *Syphilinum* or the syphilitic state, or whatever. It is the same judgement call!

So this psychiatric patient and I talked a lot and he got many insights into what his pictures and poetry meant, and this helped me find remedies for him as well. And then he came a third time, and this is why I really admire him, for he said, "I am not going to come and see you again because I know that if I do, I will get better." And he added, "I don't think I want to." What courage, what responsibility for his choice!

When my husband left me I was distraught because there had been a lot of abandonment in my childhood as well. But it was very difficult for me to admit that I was getting over it and was starting to enjoy myself. Lots of our patients are in that place; they will get better in their own time, when they no longer need their symptoms as a crutch or as a message. These so called 'miracle cures' that many of the 'great ones' tell us about; they don't take into account that some of these patients are just ready to get better. If we think of the consultation as a point along the time line between life and death, and take into account that they have already invisibly done a lot of healing work behind the scenes, then it makes sense that when we give them the remedy, they make that final leap from dis-ease into at ease. We are just there at the right time with a boost of similar energy in the form of the little magic white pill.

Sometimes we give the simillimum and the person is not ready and we have to honour that and not take it upon ourselves that we have failed - as long as we have done our very best. If we consider that we have failed, the flip side of that coin is that we are the ones who are getting people better and if that is the case we are putting ourselves in God's seat. I am not a miracle curer and I don't profess to be, but I do love my work as a healer guide and magic pill dispenser!

ROWENA: Thank you so much for spending your lunch break chatting with me Nicky. It is really interesting to hear how Purton House first began and I feel I have got to know you a bit better. Now back to teaching!

CHAPTER 27: LESLEY GREGERSON

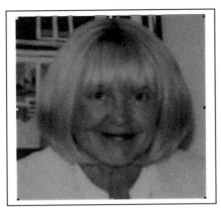

Lesley Gregerson invited me to the offices of the London School of Classical Homoeopathy (LSCH) in Winchmore Hill, North London on Thursday 13 October 2005. She sat at her large desk and I relaxed into her stories of the past. This was the first time I had actually met her but we had spoken several times before on the phone and subsequent to the interview, I have taught for her at LSCH. Since the interview she has now retired from her role as principal.

"Altruistically, you can give so much and help so many with homeopathy. It is also possible to earn a good living. You can stretch your mind and never stop learning. So it covers just about everything."
                                                            Lesley Gregerson, October 2005

"I started by running tutorials in my home in Mill Hill with Sheilagh Creasy for four or five people but over time upwards of thirty people would attend. They would study with us on a Saturday and I would feed them with lasagne and quiches that I had cooked the night before. It was like Fred's café on a Friday in my house."   *Lesley Gregerson, October 2005*

"A lot of people think that if you practise classically, you give a remedy and your patient doesn't come back for a month. If somebody is having a heart attack, you are not going to say, "Well, this is the remedy that I have worked out for you because your grandmother had such and such miasm.""
                                                            Lesley Gregerson, October 2005

"When I started in practice I had already done an awful lot of work in school clinics. So where we say now that our students have to do a minimum of fifty hours a year, I must have done hundreds. It was what I wanted to do and I do get a bit distressed when a student says, "Well, you know, I have only got three hours left, do I have to come for the whole day?" And I say, "Well, it is for your benefit. Do you actually want to be a homeopath?" The more experience you have, the better you are prepared in practice. I know I found my school clinic experience invaluable in my practice and was very pleased I put in the extra time."
                                                            Lesley Gregerson, October 2005

CHAPTER 27: LESLEY GREGERSON

ROWENA: I know you have been around for a while in our profession Lesley. Tell me how it all began for you.

LESLEY: Ever since I was three years old, I can remember being fascinated by natural things. I always really, really loved animals and had a passion for plants and herbs. When I was a little girl I used to put leaves on my dog if he had a scrape; I was always putting things on to try and make him feel better. I would just place them on him and say a little prayer, "I hope that you are going to feel better." I used to look after snails and worms if I thought they were going to go into the path or on the road. I would carefully pick them up and put them somewhere safe. I still do. I must be mad!

ROWENA: I once saved a hedgehog. I was in Corsica with a friend and we stopped all the traffic in the road so we could pick it up and take it so safety, so I know what you mean.

LESLEY: Yes, I have done that many times as well with ducks and foxes and I guess people probably thought you were a bit mad too! Anyway, that is what I used to do and I can remember at seven reading about some Sioux Indians and how they used natural medicine and that really fascinated me. Then I can remember reading a book on hypnotherapy and various other things and this went on. My love for herbs grew and grew and eventually I went to see a herbalist and I said that if he would teach me about herbs, I would work for him free of charge in the office or do whatever sort of work he needed me to do.

ROWENA: How old were you when you took on that job?

LESLEY: Oh I had children of my own, so it was later on. And he said, my dispenser has just moved on, so I will teach you to be a herbal dispenser. It was really good timing.

ROWENA: Brilliant.

LESLEY: And that is how it all really started. It was something I had wanted to do and I read about it non-stop; it was such a love and passion of mine. Even when my children were tiny, I was desperate to continue reading and learning about natural medicine. So I went to work with him and I started training to be a herbal dispenser. I went first to Edgware and then over to Wimbledon where I would make up herbal remedies. However I found that I was so incredibly busy making up the tinctures and remedies that I wasn't learning as much as I wanted to do, so I decided to go to college to study herbs properly. I applied and was accepted onto the course.

While I was studying I met a student homeopath, and she introduced me to homeopathy philosophy and it was just literally like a huge electric shock. I can remember this 'zing';

absolutely everything felt right for me. As a result I turned from herbalism, much to the disgust of my colleagues, to homeopathy, and I have been madly keen ever since. It just took over my life. Homeopathy is wonderful because it sort of covers everything, doesn't it? It is a science and art and if you want to participate, socially there is always something going on too. And also, altruistically, you can give so much and help so many with homeopathy. It is also possible to earn a good living. You can stretch your mind and never stop learning. So it covers just about everything.

ROWENA: I feel the same way, actually.

LESLEY: And I have been passionate about it ever since, and still am.

ROWENA: Where did you study?

LESLEY: At the College of Homeopathy (COH) when it was at the YWCA in Great Russell Street. I think I was in the second intake. Barbara Harwood, Robert Davidson, Misha Norland and David Mundy were my teachers.

ROWENA: Do you remember who was actually in your year of study?

LESLEY: I sat sometimes next to Francis Treuherz and became good friends with Barbara Winton and a lovely lady called Dianne whose last name unfortunately I am unable to remember. We had a lot of fun together and were very busy scribbling down every word that was said. I can see the whole class so clearly in my mind but one of my problems is that I have a dreadful memory for names. I have a memory for faces that I never ever forget and I tend to give people adopted names, which they have for the rest of their life and is nothing to do with their name at all.

ROWENA: So who influenced you the most back in those days?

LESLEY: Well, I became very close with Sheilagh Creasy very quickly.

ROWENA: She still teaches here doesn't she?

LESLEY: Yes and we have worked together for many years, and I have to say that she was my biggest influence. I was also very fond of both Martin Miles and David Mundy and I loved their work. They have both gone a little bit in a different direction to me, especially Martin, but nevertheless I have great respect for his work and he certainly knew his stuff inside out. He was a fascinating lecturer; always lots of fun and he brought things to life. David was hilarious. He used to come into the class and act remedies out and read poems to us. He was great.

But, as I said, my very biggest influence and inspiration was Sheilagh Creasy and remains so; it was wonderful when she came to lecture for us. I immediately knew that this was somebody that I had quite a strong connection with and we went on then to form a relationship very quickly. Together we helped to write the first education curriculum for the Society of Homeopaths years ago along with Ian Townsend and Bob Fordham.

ROWENA: I didn't realise you were all involved with that.

LESLEY: It caused quite a stir at the time, as at subsequent meetings, every time a decision was made, if someone wasn't present at that meeting, when they attended the next time they wouldn't agree with any of it and this went on and on and on. We would take three steps forward and then two steps backward or so it seemed then.

ROWENA: Approximately when was this?

LESLEY: Oh, it must be getting on for twenty years ago I suppose. It used to drive me to distraction. But yes, we did write the first curriculum and if I have left anybody out, please forgive me. You know what I said about my memory. We all worked very hard and then I taught at other colleges, before I set up my own originally with Anthony Bickley. In the beginning I started by running tutorials in my home in Mill Hill with Sheilagh Creasy for four or five people but over time upwards of thirty people would attend. They would study with us on a Saturday and I would feed them with lasagne and quiches that I had cooked the night before. It was like Fred's café on a Friday in my house.

ROWENA: Do you remember roughly when this was?

LESLEY: Well, it was before LSCH so it has got to be twenty odd years ago, because LSCH has been going since 1987. I had three small kids at the time and I had four very busy practices. I was inundated with work and I was seeing God knows how many people a week. I had practices in Wimbledon, Covent Garden, Mill Hill and Barnet.

ROWENA: How did you have the time to do all that?

LESLEY: Pure determination, I gave up on almost everything, including a social life, but my children always came first.

ROWENA: And I was just thinking that you must have had a very supportive husband!

LESLEY: It was actually when I got divorced that I really decided that now I had the opportunity to follow my dream and went to see the herbalist. So my life was very busy and still is but I said to the students who wanted me to open a school that I couldn't possibly do so as I had all these other commitments. I can remember there was an eleven month period where I worked every single day of the week including weekends, because I was teaching and I didn't have a day off and I was looking after the children.

I care desperately about homeopathy. I can remember when I went for my interview with Robert Davidson and his wife at the time and them saying to me, "How can you possibly do your course, when you have got three small children and you are on your own with little income"? I thought, "Oh my God!" and I was so scared, but I replied, "Well, my children will always come first – always – but homeopathy will be second. I am prepared to give up all my social life and everything for this because it is a dream that I have had all these years. And no, I am not incredibly educated and no, I am not wealthy either, but I can finance it and will."

And it has been my life really, since then. Eventually I got talked into opening a school, so I sat down with Anthony Bickley at the time and we decided to go ahead. I never dreamed then, what a huge journey and learning curve it would be.

ROWENA: I didn't realise Anthony was involved in LSCH.

LESLEY: Yes, he was. We initially decided we would open a school that was solely for educating people to a very high standard. We wanted to go back to the basics in homeopathic education, because we felt that people were possibly being given too many different concepts at once and were being sort of left to sink or swim without quite understanding how to follow their cases through.

ROWENA: Was there a classical college at the time?

LESLEY: Yes, Anne Larkin's London College of Classical Homeopathy (LCCH). A lot of people think that if you practise classically, you give a remedy and your patient doesn't come back for a month. If somebody is having a heart attack, you are not going to say, "Well, this is the remedy that I have worked out for you because your grandmother had such and such miasm."

We hope that at LSCH, by the time people have graduated they are both competent and confident to practise. Everything is included, from business studies to the medical sciences. It is important now to have quite a strong medical science knowledge, because more often now people come to see us first, rather than coming to us as a last resort after they have been to see everybody else. You need to recognise what you don't know and when to refer to another homeopath or for tests or something like that. We don't have an in-house hospital as part of our practice, even though there are some homeopathic hospitals. If somebody comes to you with pancreatitis and needs to have nil by mouth for four days, you have got to send them into hospital. You cannot say, "Here is the tablet, go away and don't eat or drink for four days". They will die of dehydration!

I find it extraordinary and a bit sad that when prospective new students come here, they are terrified because other colleges have told them that classical homeopathy is old-fashioned and it cannot deal with this, that and the other. I find it disheartening because people don't necessarily know what we do and without putting down other courses, which I don't ever want to get into, I can only explain what we do, really. I am proud of LSCH; it has done really well. We have had some excellent graduates and it is wonderful to see.

ROWENA: And this is all out of the building in Hampstead?

LESLEY: Yes.

ROWENA: But you were working from another building before?

LESLEY: Yes. We were just around the corner with the British School of Osteopathy and Naturopathy, which is now called BCOM. We might actually continue doing some work with BCOM because we are looking into gaining degree status.

ROWENA: Are you?

LESLEY: Well, I don't think we need it for homeopathy but a lot of people who don't know much about education; their eyes light up when they hear the word degree. The reason I haven't done it before is because I won't if it is at the expense of my homeopathic course. We believe in continuing to learn and we are always ready to learn. We learn from our students. We learn from anybody that gives us something good to learn about. But we won't spoil the integrity of our course for the sake of teaching something like biochemistry, for instance.

ROWENA: What do you think are important lessons for homeopaths to learn?

LESLEY: I know I can be a bit of a mummy; I always want to help so much. I say to my students, "Be careful what advice you give to you patients." For example, if you know they are having a terrible marriage, you cannot say, "Look, why don't you get a divorce?" You have always got to be aware that your patients might not actually be able to deal with the consequences of the advice you give them. You have to be very, very careful that you don't open people up and then just leave them to deal with the consequences if they are not ready or prepared to. People have to come to their own decisions in their own time and patients really can take you in. I know it is difficult sometimes to be an unprejudiced observer. I would say we should never take on cases that are too difficult or complex and we should know when to refer and have supervision.

ROWENA: It is about knowing oneself, isn't it?

LESLEY: Yes. That is why we only take in a small amount of people, so that we can actually give them the supervision that we want to and that they need. If we had a very big school, then I don't feel that we could give them that personal attention. I think all our tutors have given a very big commitment to LSCH; they are wonderful. The team here has been consistently loyal and understanding and have always given that bit more. I am eternally grateful to them. I just don't think we could do that if we had masses of students. Not that there are masses of students at the moment anyway. A lot of schools have said to me that there is a very poor intake this year, which is a shame.

When I started in practice I had already done an awful lot of work in school clinics. So where we say now that our students have to do a minimum of fifty hours a year, I must have done hundreds. It was what I wanted to do and I do get a bit distressed when a student says, "Well, you know, I have only got three hours left, do I have to come for the whole day?" And I say, "Well, it is for your benefit. Do you actually want to be a homeopath?" The more experience you have, the better you are prepared in practice. I know I found my school clinic experience invaluable in my practice and was very pleased I put in the extra time.

I think that students should be doing masses of cases. Some of them moan about having to find ten cases to complete the course. Well, how are they going to be homeopaths? How are they going to make a living? I worry about it. I tell my students that I still work out every one of my cases to a conclusion and a justification. This way when you look back you can see clearly why you made your choice. Good case management is so important and imperative to a busy and successful practice.

I have met so many interesting people along the way both here and abroad and have learned something special from all of them. For instance, I have been studying local herbs and cures in a small island in the Caribbean and I am looking forward to continuing this work when I return there hopefully very soon. This is the wonder of homeopathy; while fundamental principles remain the same, you can always learn something new and always have something to be excited about.

ROWENA: Lesley thanks for your time and sharing your thoughts with me today; it has been really interesting.

CHAPTER 28:   SUE STERNBERG

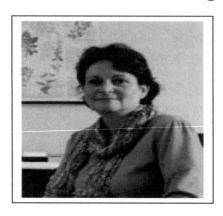

I went to see Sue Sternberg at University of Westminster on Thursday 20 October 2005. She is co-leader of the degree course along with Julie Smith. I had been to visit the University of Westminster earlier in the year when I spent time with Annette Gamblin, who is part of the degree teaching team. It is familiar ground for me anyway as my course at the London College of Classical Homeopathy (LCCH) was still affiliated to University of Westminster during my studies. For the last two years of my licentiate my class amalgamated, for all our homeopathy modules, with the much larger class studying for the degree. As a result, I attended a few lectures at this campus as well as my original interview back in 1998. My visit with Sue brought back fond memories. There was a real buzz from the students and a multicultural atmosphere that I couldn't help but notice as I sat in the foyer for my appointment. The energy and enthusiasm of the students was quite infectious.

"I have never been able to understand how you can give several remedies at the same time and how they can all be similar. It doesn't make sense to me."Sue Sternberg October 2005

"I am a classical homeopath and I make absolutely no apology for it whatsoever. It is what makes sense to me. It is what works for me. It is what I understand. It is the basis of everything else. I had a patient say to me recently, "I don't really know what homeopathy is because I come here and I get one tablet but at my last place I was taking three different liquids; I don't understand what homeopathy is."   *Sue Sternberg, October 2005*

"I think a lot of our graduates go on to practise, because there is something about studying full time; it becomes your life and then they go on to practise full time. A weekend part-time course is great; it is how I did it, but it can stay weekend and part time. It can create a hobby attitude. This is what I do half a day a week when my kids are at school, all of that. You come and do a full-time course and homeopathy becomes your life from day one and you want to carry on with that life."   *Sue Sternberg, October 2005*

CHAPTER 28:   SUE STERNBERG

ROWENA: So how did you come across homeopathy in the first place?

SUE: Like with many others, I came across homeopathy because of a health problem with my son. When he was born twenty five years ago, he had a kidney problem - nephrotic syndrome – and he was put on steroids when he was a year old. We were told that he would have to stay on them until he was fifteen or even longer. I had never really been ill or thought about health much but realised that there had to be another way. I read about Prednisolone and saw that one of the long-term side effects was that it destroys your kidneys, so if he had been on it for fifteen years he would probably have been on dialysis soon after. I didn't know anything about medicine, but this didn't make any sense at all.

I remember asking the paediatrician, "How do you know that this is going to solve this problem? What is the evidence? What are the trials?" And he replied, "Steroids like Prednisolone work for all sorts of things, and we have just found that it is really effective for this particular condition." So even all that time ago, the answer I got was "it worked." Interestingly, these are the questions that homeopaths are now asked all the time. "How do you know it works?" and "What is your evidence base?" My eighteen month old baby on Prednisolone, "because it works."

I read a lot and chose homeopathy for him. It took a year for my GP to refer him to the Royal London Homeopathic Hospital because he thought I was a lunatic. We would go every month or two and he would be given one tablet to take once a day, another tablet for his kidneys to take three times a day, and if the protein in his urine went up, you would have to swap to another tablet. Literally, for our month's supply I would have five or six different bottles of homeopathic remedies to give him. So basically it was constitutional treatment with organ specific treatment on top of that.

ROWENA: So they took his case and gave a specific constitutional remedy?

SUE: Very briefly. I think it was more a case of immunity boosting than what we would call constitutional treatment. This was a long time ago and even from the brief research I had done, I thought if 'like cures like', how can all these remedies be the most similar? It wasn't possible. With this treatment, he stopped going down into these terrible relapses where he would end up in hospital but I couldn't get him off the Prednisolone completely. I thought, "Well, at least it is doing something", but I had looked at all these books telling me that this wasn't the way to prescribe and I became more and more interested in classical homeopathy.

I started doing courses locally and eventually took him to a classical homeopath, not a medical homeopath, and it was the miracle story that brings everybody into homeopathy.

He had a constitutional remedy at the age of three and he only relapsed once during puberty, at fifteen, and that was it. I am not saying he had one tablet – he had regular visits to his homeopath and doses of his remedy to keep him in balance.

This is why I am so passionate about classical homeopathy; it does make sense and it does fit with the first few aphorisms of the *Organon*[4]. I have never been able to understand how you can give several remedies at the same time and how they can all be similar. It doesn't make sense to me.

ROWENA: The doctors at that time were not prescribing classically, but there are doctor homeopaths now that are classical

SUE: There are some very good classical prescribers among the medical homeopaths.

ROWENA: I think they take their training beyond what the Faculty used to do. Even though we have a longer grounding, homeopathy is one of those professions for which you study for the rest of your life anyway. OK, so carry on with your journey Sue. You were blown away by how your son responded to homeopathy. What happened after that?

SUE: Well, I just went to every local course that I could lay my hands on and was by then really interested. I had another child and my children were being treated homeopathically and so was I. I wanted to know more so I went to Anthony Bickley's British School of Homeopathy. Julie Smith and I were in his first intake. This was in 1985 and in those days it was based in Swindon.

I cannot imagine how many applicants I have interviewed over ten years for the University of Westminster; perhaps hundreds but I have heard similar stories over and over again. They might say that they were travelling in India and dealt with their symptoms with their little homeopathic kit. Everyone in homeopathy has some story like that, but the question is, is that enough to make a homeopath? I have no idea, but I do think there is something in the profession where we think, "I could do that. Anyone could do this." Because you have experienced a miracle with homeopathy, it doesn't make you a homeopath, and I think that is an area that as a profession we need to be very careful about.

One of the wonderful things about homeopathy is that it can be practised on so many different levels. On one level, it is so simple. I have patients coming to see me with a little first aid book from their chemist in their hand. They proudly say they have matched up their five year old son to a remedy picture, for example, *Lycopodium* and low and behold he is not nervous anymore and he is going to school happily. They have done all of that by reading half a chapter and buying some tablets over the counter in Boots. And to me, this is where we go wrong. We all get those successes because homeopathy is just so brilliant, but the mistake we make is thinking that we are all brilliant and that we can all be brilliant homeopaths.

To be a homeopath and to take it beyond that level of the *Lycopodium* for the little boy who doesn't want to go to school, to dealing with complicated health issues in a professional and respected way is a whole other story. I wouldn't think that just because I had taken some medication that worked, I could be a doctor. It is a ridiculous notion, which is why I think we need homeopathic selection onto our courses. Very few courses have any selection at all, so anyone can train as a homeopath. Then you get the question, "Why aren't I making a living at it?"

ROWENA: I think that is a good point. I applied to the University of Westminster for the degree and I was selected and I remember it was a really tough selection process. I felt very anxious and that I had really achieved something by getting in.

SUE: Well, there is a sense of achievement, isn't there? People think we select because we are a university and if you haven't got your Grade C in Biology, we are not going to have you. This has to be true for students under twenty one but older than that you are considered a mature student, and then we select on life experience. We are looking for people who we think will make good homeopaths. They have to have a bit of health science knowledge and they have to have GCSE English so they can write essays.

ROWENA: Do you observe them?

SUE: They have to write about what brought them here to want to study homeopathy; a reflective piece so we can see if there is potential.

ROWENA: And what if English isn't their first language and it is difficult to understand what they have written?

SUE: There is an English requirement and that is the other reason why we have the written reflection - to assess the English of the many international students that are here. There is a certain basic level they have to reach before they can come but we are also looking for why they want to be homeopaths as well. We do turn people down if we feel that they are not ready for that journey.

ROWENA: Do you have a certain number that you have to have on the course?

SUE: All of that is much easier here because we are not a private college, and I accept that. There are six courses in the Department of Complementary Therapies, so what tends to happen is one year we might have a bit of a dip but another course will have a few extra, so it balances out. We have one hundred and twenty first years across herbs, acupuncture, nutrition, complementary therapies, homeopathy and bodywork. With six courses you are going to get a balance. We remain pretty steady, although the competition gets more and more every year.

We have a target of twenty five students in a group and it is a good number because you always get some who drop out in the first year, however careful you are with selection. There are people who come along who just realise they have made a mistake and it is not for them. The courses receive higher education funding and the cost is the same as you would pay for any other university course.

ROWENA: And do people get grants for that, as well?

SUE: The way it works at the moment is you get a student loan to cover fees and living expenses. Nothing is paid at the point of delivery and you don't have to pay it back until you are earning over fifteen thousand pounds per year.

ROWENA: Fifteen thousand pounds from homeopathy?

SUE: From any work and that is true of any degree course. The minute you start earning fifteen thousand pounds, the government deducts the debt on a monthly basis. This financial structure is available to any student from the European Union so we have many European students.

ROWENA: So why do they prefer to study here and not in their own countries?

SUE: Well, part of why they want to do this course is because it gives them a degree and a degree is internationally recognised. They feel they are more likely to be able to work if they have got a BSc honours degree.

ROWENA: In Italy I thought it was that you had to be a doctor.

SUE: Well, we have got graduates working in Italy; I think it is because they have got degrees. We are also getting people now from Eastern European countries, such as Poland and the Czech Republic. It is very interesting. In terms of selection, yes, we are hitting a target like everybody else. We take gambles and risks but we do always look for some background in homeopathy when we are selecting. People may come on a Complementary Therapy course and then decide that they want to do homeopathy. We are looking for people who have got some basic health sciences, English skills good enough to perform at higher education level, and a passion for homeopathy. You need passion. That is what keeps you going. If you didn't have a passion for homeopathy, you wouldn't do it.

ROWENA: What else do you think makes a good homeopath post-qualification? What do you think makes a successful homeopath and one who can earn money?

SUE: One that could earn money? I don't know. I am not the best person to answer that, because I had a background in education anyway, so I have been involved in homeopathic education, in some way, ever since I started.

ROWENA: How did you come to be here?

SUE: Julie Smith and I were in the same year, as I mentioned earlier, and we qualified together. In those days, Lesley Gregerson of the London School of Classical Homoeopathy (LSCH) used to have an apprentice working alongside her and Julie took on that position and started being very involved in the organisation of the course at LSCH. At that time, I started practising as a homeopath and working at the National Extension College in Cambridge writing open learning materials. As I said, I am a qualified teacher anyway. Lesley was very interested in having a distance learning course, which I think she is still using. The whole team contributed to it and I co-ordinated it and got involved with LSCH and started teaching there as a result.

As part of my training at the British School of Homeopathy we had to do ten supervised cases. When I started, a friend of mine in East London said to me, "There are loads of people around here who want homeopathy. Why don't you come over once a month and see them here, rather than taking the cases of your friends?" This was a good decision because by the time I had finished my ten cases, I had easily a day a month in East London.

I also got an opening in a GP practice in Ely, which is near where I live. I cannot remember what it was called in those days, but GP practices were beginning to become their own budget managers and their forward-thinking practice manager had this idea of getting in complementary medicine practitioners. I was given a room rent-free and on the very first day I had six new patients and that just carried on. I only gave the practice up when I went to the London College of Classical Homeopathy (LCCH), because I didn't have enough days left in the week to do everything. By this time it was 1996 and I was practising three to four days a week; one in Bury, one in Ely, I practised from home and I was keeping my East London connection going as well.

ROWENA: So you had the passion and the enthusiasm. Do you think it helped that there were not as many homeopaths around then too?

SUE: When I started out there were only two homeopaths in the whole of East Anglia; Stephen Gordon, Sue Crump and maybe a couple of others. Now there are five or six in every town and we all work completely differently. It is really confusing for the general public and, in my view it is a mess.

372

ROWENA: What can be done about that, do you think?

SUE: I really don't know. I am a classical homeopath and I make absolutely no apology for it whatsoever. It is what makes sense to me. It is what works for me. It is what I understand. It is the basis of everything else. This story must be common to everybody - a patient goes to see one homeopath and gets tested on a machine or has their hair sent away and is given a remedy and a Bush flower remedy or a flower remedy and something else. And then they stop doing that for whatever reason and they come to see me and are given one tablet. I had a patient say to me recently, "I don't really know what homeopathy is because I come here and I get one tablet but at my last place I was taking three different liquids."

I don't have a problem with how anybody works. Anybody can work however they want, but how does that make us look? Because to be honest, I think there are as many different methods out there as there are homeopaths. Homeopathy is all about being individual. We are all very individual. We all believe in individual medicine and not mass medicine, otherwise we wouldn't be here doing this. But for people out there to be unable to understand what homeopathy is because the methodology from everyone they have seen is so different, is ridiculous.

ROWENA: So how do you feel about us all being on a single register?

SUE: I don't know what the answer is. To me, accreditation is a big part of it; we have got to have some standards. I am not saying this is the only way; this is one way. This is what we offer here. People can do what they like but we do need some standards. When that patient comes in and says to me, "I don't really understand what homeopathy is," what can I answer? I know the homeopath down the road would answer differently. What image are we trying to put out there? We are not helping ourselves at all. We all think we are brilliant. Have you ever heard a homeopath say that they are not very good. We are a really egocentric bunch of people. We all get fantastic results and the way we work is the best. That is not just true of classical, it is true of everyone out there working and there is something very immature about a profession that sees itself like that. We are like fledglings.

ROWENA: I wonder what we can do differently, though.

SUE: Well, accreditation would at least agree some standards across the board.

ROWENA: What about the work the Society of Homeopaths has done?

SUE: When a graduate leaves college, what level does their standard of homeopathic education have to be in order to practise?

ROWENA: They need to have completed a three year full-time or four year part-time course that covers a certain amount of modules.

SUE: We have full-time and part-time courses and we know we cannot get enough homeopathy into them. We would love to do four years full-time but students cannot get funding for the extra year. We have thirteen homeopathy modules, which is fifty hours of contact time per module plus three hundred logged hours in the Polyclinic, which I think is the highest number of clinical hours anywhere, although we are always being criticised for being too academic. The big question is how do we assess the level of homeopathic competency when students graduate? I think the single register has to come. It is one of the bottom lines from the *House of Lords report*[115].

ROWENA: It has been five years since then.

SUE: Exactly. It is bottom line stuff that we have a single register. But as I say, there are as many methods in our profession as there are homeopaths.

ROWENA: I thought the Society of Homeopaths specified a minimum amount of clinical hours?

SUE: I don't think there is any specification but I am not sure. Also, we have never agreed what is a 'clinical hour'. Some places give clinic hours for a case in a classroom. I feel despairing of the profession, but I still feel really passionate and excited about homeopathy.

ROWENA: Will it go dormant again, do you think?

SUE: I don't think it will go dormant at the moment. They say these things go in waves and seven year cycles are a good way of looking at it. According to recent research published in the *Smallwood Report*[116], half of all NHS referrals for complementary therapy were for homeopathy. Without understanding how it works, without any solid research about efficacy (of course this is a debatable point as we do have a lot of research but that is one of the criticisms levied against us); people are turning to complementary medicine and to homeopathy in particular. *The Prince's Foundation for Integrated Health Response*[117] suggests that homeopathy does not need to be state regulated and will therefore join with reflexology and aromatherapy and all of those. Personally, I think the National Occupational Standards (NOS)[96] guidelines are not doing us any favours.

ROWENA: In what way?

SUE: Well, NOS[96] is for vocational training and it works well for short courses. When the House of Lords created the different groupings for complementary therapies and placed us in Group one, I remember the other four decided they would definitely not go along the NVQ/NOS[96] route. Remedial Therapies such as aromatherapy and reflexology were interested in that route and some of us argued from the very beginning that this would shoot us in the foot.

Homeopaths are interested in education at a higher level and I think everyone agrees with that. Homeopathy is a complete system of medicine so how do you deliver it? It is not just training somebody how to practise; it is a whole philosophy, a whole medical system in its own right. Many of us tried very hard to say that NOS[96] was inadequate for homeopathy at the time and we are still saying that to the Council of Organisations Registering Homeopaths (CORH). The other four of the Big Five did not go down a competency based outcome route, which is what we are doing.

ROWENA: There are so many different perspectives on this subject aren't there?

SUE: You were an education adviser for the Society of Homeopaths; I am very interested to know your perspective on this because you must be interviewing far more people who don't practise in a classical way than do. We are in a tiny minority and getting smaller, and you were trained and educated in quite a classical way. What do you make of all of that?

ROWENA: I met Ellen Kramer of the College of Practical Homeopathy (CPH) in Finchley, London, earlier in the year and my mind was completely blown away. I met her quite a few times and I sat for a day in their clinic. It was a completely different experience to me from my training here, but they also seem to be getting results. They also work with integrity. I cannot get my head around it. It doesn't make sense to the way that I learned homeopathy, it doesn't fit with my paradigm, but I trust CPH that they are getting the results that they say they are.

SUE: It helps because homeopathy is so brilliant and the simillimum, or something close to the simillimum, is in there somewhere. But in terms of being respected as a profession, in terms of putting down on paper what it is that we do….

ROWENA: That does make it terribly complicated and that does come through. I don't think one can compare the way they practise homeopathy with the way we do; there are no similarities and it is a different way of thinking. I heard a case while I was in clinic where *Nux vomica* and *Carcinosin* were prescribed combined in the morning and *Cortisone* was given in the evening.

SUE: But that is not even homeopathy, is it? That is isopathy.

ROWENA: They call it tautopathy. On another subject, I wonder why there are so few schools for studying chiropractic, acupuncture and osteopathy but with homeopathy there are so many. Why do you think that is?   ·

SUE: It is so easy to set them up; anybody can set up a homeopathy college.

ROWENA: And chiropractors cannot? You don't think it attracts a different type of person – one who is more creative and innovative, maybe? I don't know.

SUE: Anyone can be a homeopath; not everyone can be an osteopath. Law now protects the titles 'osteopath' and 'chiropractor'; you can only use these titles if you have attended a registered, accredited course.

ROWENA: I think less people want to be an osteopath or a chiropractor, maybe. I don't know. What do you think?

SUE: They have all been accredited for years; that is the difference. It is all to do with accreditation, isn't it? Standards have been set in those four disciplines for a long time. That is also why they are making a better living than homeopaths.

ROWENA: So when they became popular, they went straight into accreditation and we did not. I do not know when they did become popular. Do you?

SUE: All of this starts to happen in the late 1980s.

ROWENA: So do you think chiropractic and osteopathy had resurgence at the same time as homeopathy?

SUE: I am not sure about those, but acupuncture and herbalism did. In order to set up a medical herbal college even ten years ago, you had to meet accreditation whereas you could set up a homeopathy college tomorrow. We are not doing ourselves any favours. The medical homeopaths are very together; they engage with research, have some excellent Continuous Professional Development programmes going and look at what David Riley has done at the Glasgow Homeopathic Hospital.

Who do we think we are, really? For a profession that looks at spiritual ways of being, we have got the biggest egos. What is all this guru business? What is it? We have tried really hard on our course at the University of Westminster to deliver a curriculum that is consistent, sound, and professionally taught by a dedicated, stable team.

ROWENA: How do you feel about the criticism levied at classical colleges, that they produce fearful homeopaths?

SUE: Fearful of what? Is it classical in particular? Fearful of getting it wrong; not getting the right remedy? You have been through our training; you tell me.

ROWENA: I am not fearful, but I am cautious. I don't lack confidence. When I am working with cancer patients, I research thoroughly and I don't prescribe unless I am sure. Sometimes it takes two consultations before I prescribe. Often they are crying so much during the first of the two that it takes a second to get the full case. I explain what I am doing and they are fine with that.

SUE: Well, that is good. It is nice to hear you saying that having done this course that you are thorough, you work with integrity, and you will do your homework until you are sure that you feel happy about prescribing. I am proud of you, if that means anything to you!

ROWENA: Yes, of course it does. You were there on my first day. In fact, I remember calling you up and asking you whether I should do the full-time degree or the licentiate.

SUE: Fearful? No sort of medicine should be based in fear, should it? That is what is wrong with Western medicine. I think a lot of our graduates go on to practise, because there is something about studying full time; it becomes your life and then they go on to practise full time. A weekend part-time course is great; it is how I did it, but it can stay weekend and part time. It can create a hobby attitude. This is what I do half a day a week when my kids are at school, all of that. You come and do a full-time course and homeopathy becomes your life from day one and you want to carry on with that life. So cautiously and with integrity, prepared to do my homework and think about a case - that is still how I work. I wouldn't want to work any other way. I wouldn't want to dish remedies out that I am not sure about.

ROWENA: And I wouldn't want to go to a homeopath that pulled things out of the air without thinking about it, either.

SUE: If a patient asks you, "How have you come to a decision about my remedy? Why have you given this to me? Why this remedy? Why this potency?" They have got every right to ask those questions and to know what the answers are. I have to work in a way that makes sense to me and I have to know why I am doing something.

To be honest, I think our students are pretty confident by the time they leave here. What they do in our Polyclinic is going to be far harder than what they do in their private practices because in the clinic they have got two or three people sitting in with them, and a supervisor. Demographically we get a huge range of patients in the Polyclinic, because it is subsidised and costs twenty pounds for a first consultation, which is very cheap for central London. Our graduates are not going to see a lot of those people in private practice, either. By the time the third years leave, they can cope with private practice whatever it is like.

We do stop students at the end of year two if necessary and we use a trial case to assess them. It is only fair. Nobody wants to do a tough three year course and then fail at the end of it. It is much better to do whatever you need to do earlier on and to take more time.

We have developed graduate diplomas, so anyone who has done a degree here in any of the disciplines can come back as a graduate and do another discipline properly and get the licence to practise it. So you could finish the homeopathy course and do herbal modules and get the licence to practise herbalism.

ROWENA: Obviously what you provide for your students here is quite unique. It is good to be back. Thanks so much for your insights and time today Sue. It has been really interesting and is most appreciated.

CHAPTER 29: LIONEL MILGROM

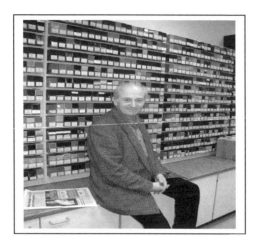

Friday 28 October 2005 took me back to Nelsons Homeopathic Pharmacy in Duke Street, Mayfair, London this time to meet with Lionel Milgrom, a director of the Society of Homeopaths and a regular contributor to the Society's intranet system, *First Class Mail*[118]. I had been following his passionate views for about a year so when he agreed to our interview I was rather excited as to what I might find. I knew he would be challenging but he was different to what I had imagined. He was much younger and fitter than I had perceived him on line and his strong opinions, passion and depth of thought I found endearing. Like with other geniuses in our field, sometimes we can get a little lost in his process but I feel he has a lot to offer the profession and we are lucky to have him on board.

"As a chemist I am wedded to the idea of substance, atoms and molecules therefore if you dilute something to nothing, how can it do something? There was the challenge and that, I do believe, is basically what most people find so obnoxious about homeopathy. It flies in the face of everything that you have taken for granted."   Lionel Milgrom, October 2005

"It is fascinating, becoming a homeopath and looking back at conventional medicine and how scientists have completely missed that whole area of individual susceptibility."
        Lionel Milgrom, October 2005

"I actually think the randomised control trial methodology destroys the very thing that it is trying to investigate in this context and therefore it is the wrong tool. You don't use a spanner when you need a hammer."   *Lionel Milgrom, October 2005*

CHAPTER 29:   LIONEL MILGROM

ROWENA: So tell me how you got into homeopathy Lionel?

LIONEL: Basically, when my partner and I moved down to London from Liverpool, we signed up with a GP, Geoffrey Douch, who in fact was also a homeopath. My background is in hard science but when we moved back down here I had already taken some time out and had been working as a musician for six or seven years.

ROWENA: In what way were you a musician?

LIONEL: I was a bass player but I did all sorts of things. I played rock and funk and worked in a theatre for a year or two. It was great. I wouldn't do it again but I do miss gigging. That is why I like standing up and giving talks; it is the same kind of thing. Anyway, I decided that I would get back into hard science again, so we moved down to London and I took up another PHD.

My partner – we are both quite enthusiastic smokers as you can probably tell - would periodically get bronchitis. After our first kid she came down with some quite bad pneumonia, at which point she had been through about three courses of antibiotics and they had just bounced off her. So our doctor said, "I want you to try some homeopathy." As a result she started getting better. Then he said, "What you need to do now is eurythmy" and she has been doing it now for the last twenty odd years.

Eurythmy is a series of movements, which actually represent letters, so as you move you are actually spelling out a language. That is putting it at its most simplistic but it is also about a form of harnessing energy. Clearly it has worked on my partner, because she is still an enthusiastic smoker and she practises eurythmy once a week with this wonderful old lady and she has never had bronchitis or any chest infections since.

ROWENA: Wow that is very impressive.

LIONEL: So I then asked the doctor what was in those pills and he told me, "Nothing." And that is where it all started, because as far as I was concerned, this was an affront. As a chemist I am wedded to the idea of substance, atoms and molecules therefore if you dilute something to nothing, how can it do something? There was the challenge and that, I do believe, is basically what most people find so obnoxious about homeopathy. It flies in the face of everything that you have taken for granted, especially if you are trained in any kind of 'hard' (as opposed to 'softer' subjects like the humanities, etc) science, for example a chemist or biochemist. One can see things on a molecular level, so how can nothing do something? That is the challenge that homeopathy has to rise to and that was the challenge that I rose to. Clearly this doctor was getting results, so I wanted to find out what was going on. Instead of just going down the usual route of testing it out, I decided I would become a homeopath and go to college! I wanted to walk the walk and talk the talk. So here we are today.

ROWENA: So how long ago was this?

LIONEL: I started training in 1995.

ROWENA: Where?

LIONEL: The College of Homeopathy (COH) in London, sadly now defunct.

ROWENA: Who was in your year group?

LIONEL: Ros Abbott – I don't know if you know her. She practises in West London. She is probably the only person I still have regular contact with.

ROWENA: And do you think the others are practising?

LIONEL: I hope so, but we started off a group of about sixty in the first year and by the time the final year came we were barely twenty.

ROWENA: That is a big fall out. I started in 1998 at the London College of Classical Homeopathy (LCCH).

LIONEL: LCCH, oh right. They merged with COH in 1999. So you are a classical homeopath? Ooh. Spooky.

ROWENA: So who inspired you the most?

LIONEL: Definitely Mike Bridger.

ROWENA: He is quite classical, isn't he?

LIONEL: Yes, he is. I have got nothing against the classical way of practising homeopathy. I just think that what is important is the patient sitting in front of you.

ROWENA: Yes, of course, but I think classical homeopaths would say that too, no? How do you practise?

LIONEL: How do I practise? Off the top of my head for most of the time. It is a good question.

ROWENA: If you had a cancer patient, how would you treat them?

LIONEL: If I had a cancer patient? That is a tough one because again I am still in touch with my hard science background. In fact, I actually started a company from Imperial College with a brand new anticancer therapy called Photodynamic Therapy which is a much more gentle way of treating cancer conventionally than the usual treatments.

ROWENA: A company?

LIONEL: Yes, the company is just about still in existence but I am not running it anymore, thank God. So I do straddle the two; practising as a homeopath but still working with biochemists and a few medical people. I think working with allopaths you get to have a different perspective on cancer. I think cancer is basically civil war within the body. Certainly when you look at cancer from the point of view of what is actually happening at the cellular level, you begin to see that something very strange is going on. Homeopaths talk about the vital force and everything working together in a hierarchical manner and so when you look at a cell, when it is produced, right at the very beginning, it is completely undifferentiated.

The cell doesn't have a purpose yet and then at some point after that, quite quickly it becomes what it is supposed to be – a nerve cell, skin cell or blood cell, but there is a moment before that when it is undifferentiated. When you look at most tumours, the cells making up the tumours are in that undifferentiated state; they haven't yet been told what to do. That gives you some sort of feeling for where the breakdown is and I have got this weird idea that cancer is essentially about a divided vital force. It is at war with itself. It is like a civil war within the same state between rival factions, only the bit that is still in overall charge, as it were, cannot recognise 'the rebels' because everyone has the same DNA and produces the same 'markers' (antibodies) on the outside. So 'the rebels' (tumours) expand and grow unrecognised. They even hijack some of the bodies transport system in order to propagate themselves. However, when a tumour dies, it releases special chemicals called cytokines that the body recognises and immediately sends in the clean up squad, the phagocytes.

Where you have to be very careful here of course is that there are carcinogenic substances. That doesn't mean that everyone who takes carcinogenic substances is going to get cancer. I smoke, for example. As far as I know, I might well have cancer; I don't know.

ROWENA: Don't you think you would know?

LIONEL: That is a whole different ball game. And there is of course the issue of whether I would care or not, but anyway, it all comes down to the idea that there are disease causing agents and there are susceptibilities and we are of course far more interested in the susceptibilities. It is fascinating, becoming a homeopath and looking back at conventional medicine and how scientists have completely missed that whole area of individual susceptibility. But this business of carcinogenicity and health and safety in the work place is actually making the teaching of chemistry so damned difficult these days. Of course everything you touch is carcinogenic, so all the solvents we used to have at school, we don't have anymore. Consequently chemistry as a science is actually dying because people are so damn scared of the material.

ROWENA: So they don't burn phosphorus in class anymore?

LIONEL: I used to work with kids on Saturdays and I did some experiments. I nicked some sodium and potassium from the lab and took the potassium out from under the oil and took the sodium and put it into water and it skidded across the water and burst into flames. I then threw the potassium in (from a safe distance, of course!) and it exploded. The kids just loved it but they don't teach chemistry like that and they don't like people taking risks. So the subject is dying and science I think is dying too. A lot of people are antiscientific now and science, to a certain extent, is to blame for that because it is seen as the handmaiden of politicians, the military, and big business. Nobody trusts the pharmaceutical companies. It is seen very much as being in hock to vested government, military and commercial interests whereas forty or fifty years ago, scientists were seen as saviours.

ROWENA: Do you think that school children feel that?

LIONEL: Absolutely, we have got statistical evidence showing that without exception everywhere in the developed world, Europe, the USA, Japan, Australia, etc kids are turned off science between the ages of nine and sixteen; absolutely turned off it. However, in the developing world, the same stats show that people want to become scientists. It is still seen as a good profession, as something that can benefit people, like it used to be in the West fifty to sixty years ago. But now it is uncool and certainly it does worry me that maybe people who come in to homeopathy seem to be so antiscientific. And if there is anything that is truly scientific, it is homeopathy. And it does worry me because we have got some real fruitcakes flying around in our profession. It also bothers me that there is such an imbalance of female to male in homeopathy in this country and probably elsewhere as well.

ROWENA: Why do you think that is?

LIONEL: I would have thought it is fairly obvious.

ROWENA: I discussed this with Sue Sternberg at University of Westminster the other week and she said homeopathy looks so easy, especially at that level of treating children that the mothers all think, "Hey, I can do this."

LIONEL: It is not just "Hey, I can do this." I have got a lot of respect and time for what I call mature students. They know why they are at college and want to learn. I taught at a polytechnic for some years and then at a so-called lower class university, and the mature students were always the ones who asked the most interesting and penetrating questions and who really paid attention. That is another interesting thing that is happening on the British academic scene. Because we have now got these new universities and because they are competing with the conventional universities for the student pool, they have to offer something that the conventional universities wouldn't touch with a bargepole, and so what is that going to be? It is going to be Complementary and Alternative Medicine.

What worries me is that we are now churning out possibly too many students for the actual therapeutic 'cake' that is out there - the number of available people who want treatment. Until we can actually guarantee the supply of patients into Complementary and Alternative Medicines and homeopathy in particular, I am worried that we may be producing too many practitioners. On the other hand, I wouldn't want to turn anyone away. But if you think you are going to earn a living out of it, think again; it barely pays the bills. I have got to do lots of other stuff like writing and teaching though I wouldn't call myself a homeopathy teacher. I am a nutcase who likes to inflict my ideas on people; if they want to listen to them, that is fine with me. If they are even dafter and want to pay me for them, that is even better, but I wouldn't call myself a teacher.

ROWENA: But you are inspiring.

LIONEL: Am I? Oh, good. I do enjoy it. I enjoy standing up in front of people and spouting and I hope I am good at it, but as I say, part of that is due to years of having to teach people stuff that they didn't want to learn. So how do you put it across in a way that they will want to learn? There is a lovely saying in the *Talmud*[119], "A lesson taught with humour is a lesson learned." So jokes are absolutely de rigueur, not that I try hard to make people laugh or that I am recommending one goes off and learns a joke book. It is just about being yourself, I suppose, whoever that is….

ROWENA: So where do you think homeopathy is going?

LIONEL: Down the tubes if it is not very careful, because I think certain people are beginning to wake up to what they consider a threat. I think the whole sceptic thing now has taken off quite a bit, especially since *The Lancet Article*[109] and I would like to see the Society of Homeopaths being far more proactive rather than reactive in its approach. It did, however, respond very well to the whole brouhaha over that.

When you start doing trials, you look at all the trials' data and it strikes me that you can either believe them or you can disbelieve them. There are not enough definitive trials that say one thing or the other. I have my theories about that, obviously. I actually think the randomised control trial methodology destroys the very thing that it is trying to investigate in this context and therefore it is the wrong tool. You don't use a spanner when you need a hammer. The fact that sometimes you do see effects, well, that is all to do with this whole business of entanglement that I have gone on about for years. And unfortunately examining systems that are entangled is incredibly difficult. And also the biomedical community is not ready to take on quantum physics ideas.

What is so interesting about the whole quantum physics thing is when you actually look at the way quantum physics is taught philosophically, it does raise huge questions about the nature of reality and our relationship to it. And precisely because of that, there is this wonderful phrase in physics for when people start asking these very difficult philosophical, ontological questions, they just turn around and say, "Shut up and calculate", because quantum physics calculations give us things like computers and electronics and all of that. Homeopathy in my view is all about quantum physics and it does make us ask some very cogent questions about what we are and what this reality is. When you come back down to it, what you are actually seeing is the clash of two essentially opposing philosophical paradigms.

There is the atomistic view of the universe which starts with people like Leucippus and Democritus back in ancient Greek times and was carried forward by Newton, Descartes and all those sorts of people and this is where modern science really started from. And then you have this other philosophical view, which was instigated by Hindu and Buddhist philosophers in the East, and Heraclitus and Plato in the West. Their theories actually became the philosophical basis for Christianity, which is the idea that the universe as we see it is an illusion. There is a famous saying from Plato about the shadows on the cave wall and how life is going on somewhere behind; what we perceive is not necessarily what things are.

ROWENA: How does that fit in with Christianity?

LIONEL: The notion that this earthly life is not all there is. The Christians took on board some of the philosophy of Plato and also some of the philosophy of Aristotle. Each was a different school and where they differed was on the nature of reality. It was Heraclitus who said, "You cannot put your foot in the same river twice." We can sum it up in terms of questions such as, "Does a tree crashing in the forest make a sound if there is nobody there to hear? That is essentially it. The reductionist Cartesian would say, "Of course it does", whereas if there is nobody there to partake of that reality, does that reality actually exist? In other words, is it right to consider ourselves as separate from the reality we inhabit? Are observer and observed, knower and known, really separate ontologically? It is a fascinating question and these questions come to a head in quantum theory.

It is interesting that science has developed over hundreds of years and gets to this pinnacle where the very thing that it was flying from actually begins to undermine its reductionist nature, and that is what so many scientists cannot take on board. You also have to realise that science is not a homogeneous thing. It is actually a bit like London; a bunch of villages loosely connected by a very bad (and incredibly expensive!) communication system. So there is no reason, for example, why biochemists should take on board ideas of quantum theory. Actually, they do so without knowing it, because all the equipment that they use like electron microscopes are the result of quantum theory.

And the point is, in the chemical sciences, the belief in atoms and molecules, which goes back thousands of years, is perfectly OK because it works. But there are certain situations, which most chemists and biochemists don't actually come across, where the notion of atoms and molecules actually breaks down. Biochemists use quantum theory to actually bolster their ideas of atoms and molecules. What they don't realise is that in order for quantum theory to give you atoms and molecules, you have to make approximations.

There are two famous approximations; one called the Born-Oppenheimer approximation (after the guy who led the research on the atomic bomb project) and the other, the Orbital approximation. As soon as you make those two approximations to quantum theory, atoms and molecules fall out of it like Pandora's box. Unless you make those approximations you've got zilch. All you have are fields. Behind this comforting idea of atoms and molecules that are bolstered by years of work, there is actually something much more mysterious; an all encompassing field which has of course been written about.

ROWENA: So you have read Lynn McTaggart's *The Field*[20]?

LIONEL: I reviewed it. She is a journalist so she goes around garnering ideas from people and putting it together in a readable form, which is great. So there is this thing that we are part of which connects us all together and that is essentially where my entanglement ideas come from. This is where I turn green, curl up into something small, and in my best Yoda voice say, "A Jedi's strength flows from the Force!"

I think that essentially what goes on between the patient and practitioner with a remedy is a form of entanglement. You can consider that entanglement mathematically because mathematics is a language; a very sophisticated language, but it is a way of talking about something. What I have found is that the discourse of quantum theory, when you really get down to the nuts and bolts, is very similar to the discourse in homeopathy and that has been a real eye-opener for me in the last couple of years. If there is that similarity of discourses then we would be able to use the same sort of concepts as the quantum physicists. A lot of them get rather cheesed off by this because they think that we are robbing their territory.

There was a wonderful experience I had in Germany a few years ago. I was attending a private conference and there were a couple of German physicists there and I was talking to them over dinner the night before. They were very pleasant and we had a nice dinner and good conversation. The following day I got up and gave my talk and I could see them getting more and more annoyed and one of them asked a very dismissive question at the end of my session. This was just before the break, and we went out for tea and coffee and you know what? They just turned their backs and ignored me as if I had taken a dump in the middle of the room. A bit shocked, I asked the conference organiser why he thought they were behaving that way and he replied, "This is what academics do in Germany when they think you are trying to invade their territory." It was so funny, but very revealing. They were actually outraged by what I was suggesting.

And here is something else. A dear friend of mine's father is an ex-Astronomer Royal. You know, a top of the range head honcho don't mess with me I am a physicist type of physicist. Well this friend showed her dad some of my entanglement stuff, and do you know what he said? "This man is dangerous!" Get that! Little me! Dangerous, for God's sake! Just for suggesting that perhaps we can take some of the ideas from quantum physics and apply them to what many scientists believe are 'The Whacky Races'. I think that is one of the best compliments I have ever been paid....

ROWENA: But in terms of entanglement, even if a remedy is not prescribed there is entanglement, isn't there?

LIONEL: The remedy is part of the entanglement. So what does it mean to prescribe a remedy? Is it the pills or is it the process? Or is it some combination of both? And what, after all, IS the remedy? Is it the pills, or the process, or some combination of both? And are we mistaken if we think the process and the pills are indeed separate? Maybe it is the whole shebang - process, prescription, the giving and the taking of the remedy....try plugging that little lot into a double-blind randomised controlled trial! Do you see what I am getting at? Because before there are remedies, before there is even homeopathy, there are just two people; one who (hopefully!) can heal, and one who wants to be healed. Everything starts from there, and it is as true of conventional medicine as it is of homeopathy. As Shakespeare once wrote[121], "We are such stuff. As dreams are made on....", but I think I detect your eyes are beginning to glaze over....

So, homeopathy is supposed to work well even with young children and animals. How do you explain that? Of course you don't get the case from the animal; you get the case from the owner, unless of course you live in *Narnia*[122]....

ROWENA: But is that always the case? Some homeopathic vets will just observe the animal.

LIONEL: That is right but I cannot see the owner remaining silent throughout; there has to be some exchange between them. If that is the case, then perhaps you have to consider the owner and the animal as an entangled entity. Ergo if you gave the remedy to the owner, would it have the same effect? I was giving a talk down in the South West recently and apparently there is a vet down there who works in that way, which I find absolutely fascinating. I would love to talk to that person. Obviously this is anecdotal. I have no idea how you would test it. And that really is one of the big problems with this whole entanglement way of trying to describe Complementary and Alternative Medicine. I think we are getting there and I am not the only one working in this area.

ROWENA: That would be like if I took all the remedies that my kids need. I can understand that when kids are very small and one is breastfeeding, for example, but when they are twelve and fourteen? It doesn't really make sense to me.

LIONEL: Yes, you and me both! Entanglement is presumably going on all the time. And why does it have to make sense? If you walk around thinking and believing what your senses appear to be yelling at you, that you are isolated, on your own, the centre of your own little universe, then none of this makes any sense. But then what does it take to experience a sense of oneness with the world that at least one could refer back to? You cannot just manufacture it, although there are and always have been certain pharmaceuticals that are supposed to deliver short cuts to such a state....

ROWENA: Have you ever tried such 'short cuts'?

LIONEL: Weren't you going to ask me about my kids?

ROWENA: How old are your kids?

LIONEL: I have got one of twenty seven, one of twenty two and one coming up to twenty one.

ROWENA: So they are pretty separate from you. Even at twelve and fourteen my boys are pretty separate from me.

LIONEL: Maybe, I don't know. I consider myself extremely fortunate to have the kids I do. In our relationships, the only thing they have to worry about is when I will need to be sectioned..... But seriously, I don't know what the boundaries of this are yet and what it means to be entangled with the patient. Does it have anything to do with intention? I don't know yet. Can I wish to become entangled? I suppose all I know is what we all know - that sometimes, something clicks and you are there. At other times - brick wall, zilch. I don't think I can put my hand on my heart and say I intended either result.

ROWENA: Every question that you ask in a consultation meshes you together with the patient.

LIONEL: I come back to what I said earlier - before anything, there are just two people sitting in front of each other but when it clicks then its like being on a trail. You can sense the remedy and I suppose I start to ask questions around my understanding of the remedy picture. On quite a few occasions the patient has broken down as a question seems to have gone right to their heart. The feeling then can be quite overpowering; on the one hand a sense of confirmation, yet on the other a sense of humility and privilege to be allowed in to share something with the patient. It gets really emotional.... But then even Kent said that sometimes with the best intention and the best homeopathic prescribing, the remedy doesn't work - so what is going on? Entanglement is a much more subtle thing than just intention. I don't quite know what it means yet.

ROWENA: In terms of how you practise, who has inspired you to practise in the way that you do?

LIONEL: I don't know that I practise in any particular method. I am not a follower of any 'guru'; I just listen to what people say and see what comes up. I should probably do far more casework than I do. I usually prescribe on the spot and not necessarily one remedy. I wouldn't say I was the world's expert on prescribing.

ROWENA: How would you decide if a person needed more than one remedy?

LIONEL: There is so much coming in on all levels and I usually like to use organ support if that too is indicated. We must not forget the material level of existence even if all that I have said would seem to contradict that! I find I tend to use *Carcinosin* a lot as the miasmatic remedy behind the indicated remedy. I am also increasingly a fan of LMs.

ROWENA: Sheilagh Creasy says *Carcinosin* is a much over-prescribed remedy; what do you think?

LIONEL: I prescribe it a lot, because that is what I see. Monkey see, monkey do. I think Sheilagh Creasy's point is that it is lazy prescribing but she is coming from, in my view, a certain authoritarian stance; this is right and this is wrong, this is black and this is white. I cannot stand it in men and I really cannot stand it in women.

ROWENA: Even more so?

LIONEL: Yes.

ROWENA: Why?

LIONEL: I don't know. It must have something to do with my background. My mother was quite a little toughie. My father was as well but they did it in different ways. It is a fair cop, guv, but my parents are to blame.....

ROWENA: Do you think you recognise *Carcinosin* easily?

LIONEL: Yes. It is one of those remedies I seem to resonate with.

ROWENA: It is fascinating isn't it? What skills do you think a practitioner needs to have to be a successful homeopath?

LIONEL: I just wonder to what extent people are practising on a daily basis and making a working living on homeopathy alone. I think very few, because everyone has got some other angle on it, either setting up a course or their own college. How many people are so busy at homeopathy that they don't have any time for anything else? So what is a successful homeopath? When you actually see someone come back into your practice and say, "I took the remedy and this and this changed, and thank you." That to me is being a successful homeopath.

ROWENA: I agree. So what do you think keeps people at it? I ask because so many give up and go back and do something else.

LIONEL: Well, I suspect that financial pressure has a lot to do with that. I think for me, it would have to be something incredibly emotional to turn me off it. It would be something probably around homeopathy that has upset me in some way. I can put up with the, it shouldn't work therefore it cannot work, that sort of attitude. In fact, that keeps me going to a certain extent, because that is the nature of the cussed individual that I am. If they say, "No", then I will say, "Yes". And that explains my attitude to some of these characters I have mentioned in homeopathy. As soon as somebody is there laying down the law, I don't want to know. They really piss me off and it is not jealousy. It is just that the idea that there is a right and a wrong way and there is only one path; it really hacks me off and it tunes into something very deep in me about being told what to do.

ROWENA: People who see there being a right and a wrong way see it as George Vithoulkas does; that we are destroying homeopathy; that we are making it less potent and making it confusing for patients to be told one thing and then something else. There is that lack of security in the profession.

LIONEL: Maybe he is right, I don't know. But I don't think we are alone in being confusing to our patients. Have you been to a conventional doctor recently?

ROWENA: We are all pretty individual characters. If we all did the same to a certain extent, then patients would know what homeopathy was but patients don't. A lot of patients think that homeopathy is having their tarot cards read or the use of aromatherapy oils.

LIONEL: You can argue this from two points. George Vithoulkas is saying we need something that is presentable to the outside world and I am saying, "Why?" What you are doing then is presenting a limitation. We have got all this stuff coming in and actually fructifying the whole brew as it were, and we might have to wait for a bit before something can be distilled out of it. I think you have obviously got to have some guidelines but to actually lay down the law about how you are going to practise, I think, is limiting and a mistake. If the patients are confused, then we haven't done our job properly as homeopaths in the first place.

In any case, patients don't come in to find out about homeopathy; they come in to be healed. That means they have expectations. As I said before, the bottom line is that at the very beginning and from my perspective, there are just two people in a room. Where we go from after that is anybody's guess and is all part of the wonderful process. Obviously, with me, they are going to get an earful about homeopathy if I decide such exegesis is appropriate. But don't worry, I am not so daft that I don't know when to keep my trap shut. I gave up long ago worrying about whether I have got the right remedy or whether I have 'connected' with the patient. Not that I am supremely confident in my abilities, it is just that life is too short – especially at my age.....

ROWENA: How do you think we are going to stop homeopathy becoming dormant again Lionel?

LIONEL: I think we have to somehow try and get more people involved in trials; we have to redesign the trials processes. We need to get more and more research done, certainly, but that costs money. The Society of Homeopaths' Research Committee is getting people more interested in research and I think we have desperately got to get more research done. We have got to start questioning the conventional research methodologies and develop our own. I certainly think we have got to become united as a profession; there has got to be some kind of unification. I would also like to see more integration with the medical homeopaths, as well.

Medical homeopaths are doctors suffer more from all this debate over homeopathy than we do. They get it in the neck from their medical colleagues and also from the British Medical Association so they are actually our vanguard, in that sense. I am hoping that we can actually unify. We always form the wagons into a circle and fire inwards; it is what we are very good at and I suppose I am just as guilty as anyone else because I have my very strong likes and dislikes.

ROWENA: What are your views on voluntary versus statutory regulation?

LIONEL: I think at some point we are going to have to go for statutory regulation, as long as we have a very large say in the statutory process.

ROWENA: Finally, on another subject entirely, Lionel, would you like to expound on life, the universe and everything?

LIONEL: Yes, why not. I don't think creation is a done deal; I think it is happening all the time. This is not me being religious because I don't know if there is a God or not, but creation is a process that is going on and where does that put us? Where are we in that? I think where we are is right on the edge, because there is the created and there is the uncreated and if you look at creation as being kind of like a wave that moves into the uncreated zone as it were, we are on that edge. Therefore shit happens because you are on that edge between the created and the uncreated, between order and disorder. Shit happens. Not all the time, but that is what life is like on the frontier. Things are going to go on that you don't like or cannot understand. We are on the edge precisely because we are part of the creative process. That, in my humble opinion, is possibly why we are here - to be creative and to actually assist the process along - if one wants to deal in such Pythonesque absolutes. If we are not doing that then we are not doing what we are here for, and are worse than a waste of space. Perhaps that is why there are so many of us clogging up the works......

ROWENA: And you are talking about homeopaths or human beings?

LIONEL: I am talking about human beings being creative. If you do it through homeopathy, fine, if you choose to do it through physics, fine, if you choose to do it through washing dishes, climbing mountains, or playing pinball, fine. As long as you know what it is you are doing and you do it with all your heart and soul. If you read the *Bhagavad Gita*[123] it is all about war and killing people but there is also something highly spiritual in it. How does that work? Well, it only works, as far as I am concerned, within that context of being part of the creative process and allowing it to work through you, and that requires being. It requires being here and now and also being out of the way; so it seems very complicated. But when you are in it, it is like riding a bike. Are we in contact with that most of the time? No. If you are lucky, you get a burst of it every once in a while. It informs you, hopefully for the rest of your life, but it is so big and we are so not here and now. As The Beatles sang,"And to see you're really only very small and life flows on within and without you." ....[124] At least, I know that is true for me.

But there is one other thing. A lot of people talk about intention being part of the healing package. I think I am beginning to disagree with that. Intention is much overrated. After all, if we really had even a tiny fraction of the intention we think we have, then war would have been outlawed aeons ago. The unpalatable truth is that real intention, as we are, is way beyond us. Real intention means that we have the power to do, and with us, things just happen. This is tough to listen to and take on board. On the other hand we can exercise ATTENTION. We can listen and feel and sense, both outwardly and inwardly. And the more we practise that, I am beginning to realise, the finer attention becomes. Then we are better placed to entangle with the universe around us, including our sentient breathing fellow humanoids, and perhaps be those beings capable of partaking of and helping with the creative process. And if there is one sure-fire way of stopping the universe running down, then this has got to be it! Now, could it also just be that this is also where healing comes from? It is worth taking a look, don't you think?

ROWENA: From reading all your contributions on First Class Mail[118], I knew you would blow my mind Lionel, and you have not disappointed. Thanks so much for sharing your time and thoughts with me.

CHAPTER 30:   BARBARA HARWOOD

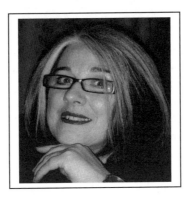

I first met Barbara Harwood back in 1999 when the College of Homeopathy (COH) bought the London College of Classical Homeopathy (LCCH) from Mary Hood incorporating the two colleges as the Combined Colleges of Homeopathy (CCH). She moved into our building on Welbeck Street and came to introduce herself during one of our materia medica lectures. People around me said that she was a legend; that she was famous for her fabulous lectures where she had made remedies come to life as she acted them out. We had discussed my teaching at CCH when I graduated but soon after, CCH disbanded, and our paths didn't cross again until Thursday 3 November 2005 when I had a very long chat with her in the conservatory of her home in Brondesbury, near Kilburn. Afterwards she took me around each room so I could see the pharaonic scenes painted on the walls. Her home was as creatively decorated, as you would expect from a character with such a colourful life story - in true congruence with who she is. What a fascinating lady.

"Eventually, I came across Thomas Maughan, and that was it really. He was an amazing person. He lined us all up at one point, a whole load of straggly hippies and he marched up and down saying, "You are going to wish you had joined the Army by the time I have finished with you! You lot are going to learn to get disciplined in your minds and learn how to think and use your brains.""
Barbara Harwood, November 2005

"Even when I had started college, I had never intended to practise. Basically, I was an ex-hippie punk who had used drugs, been a groupie and political activist and was into esoteric pursuits; I wasn't exactly the kind of person who would make a good image for homeopathy. People like Robert Nichols and Stephen Gordon who were in the class with me when I started in college, still remember meeting me for the first time. Robert Nichols says he recalls me coming to class with green punky hair, dressed in bin liners and see through fluorescent T-shirts, camouflage trousers and sexshop stilettos. My hair was green one minute, pink another and blonde the next, and I wore heavy punk make-up. When I started actually seeing patients I had to totally change. I had my head almost totally shaved at that point and the little hair that was left, I dyed black and I wore a dark red suit in clinic."
Barbara Harwood, November 2005

CHAPTER 30:   BARBARA HARWOOD

BARBARA: Underneath the surface, everyone wants to make a difference. One of the reasons I got involved in college rather than in practise is that I actually prefer students. I do understand logically that when you are with a patient, the benefits of the interaction spread beyond just the patient; they will go and tell all their friends if they feel better. But the immediacy of a whole bunch of students, being inspired in a lecture and then going out spreading the word is more satisfying for me. The mindset of students is different from most patients. So many patients come to homeopathy in a powerless mode and without any sense of involvement. It is as if some divine meat axe has dropped out of the sky and made them ill. They don't take responsibility and there is no sense of how their health and illness relates to them as a whole person. The teacher in me found it frustrating dealing with patients.

ROWENA: Were you a teacher before?

BARBARA: No, no.

ROWENA: Tell me how it all started for you.

BARBARA: I was quite a deep thinking child.

ROWENA: Where were you brought up?

BARBARA: All over the place. My father was in the Air Force and was posted to Germany after the war, when I was born. As a kid, I lived near areas that were devastated by the bombings and it was a huge issue of contention. I had screaming rows with my father when I was ten about what the English had done to Germany. It really affected me and I became very concerned about war and what made people tick. Neither of my parents were religious and I found the concepts of Christianity stupid.

I was heavily into sports, especially horse riding and swimming; I rode and dived all the time. We had a very privileged lifestyle in the Forces with great sports facilities. The horses were kept at the Berlin Olympic Stadium where there were swimming pools and an amazing amount of leisure facilities. I competed in events on horseback, in the pool and also track and field, especially when I went to boarding school in Germany for a while. Our dressage teacher there had been at the Spanish riding school in Vienna and I was the youngest person in Germany ever to win a bronze medal for dressage while I was at school. My army riding teacher taught me at Spandau barracks where Hess was kept in prison; the riding stables were underneath the barracks tower. In 1961 we moved to Cyprus and it was there that I had my first teaching experience when I taught riding to young airmen at the Saddle Club.

Between Germany and Cyprus we came back to England and moved to York in 1958 where I started having a secret life. My parents were very strict and I used to sneak out when they thought I was in bed. I went to art school at the weekends and I liked the whole bohemian crowd. Everybody was into smoking dope and there was a whole beatnik thing going on which was exciting for me as a thirteen, fourteen year old. I used to go on nuclear disarmament marches, much to my parents' horror. Unfortunately, we were sent to Cyprus in 1961 and there was no subculture so again I spent my time horse riding and swimming.

My father was a bomber pilot and after the war he worked in air traffic as a controller. His work environment in Cyprus was not a healthy one and he and his colleagues would get sick quite a lot. They worked under glass all day in great heat and then in the evening, the temperature would drop suddenly and it would get cold. The Americans and the Russians were flying regularly over Cyprus at that time and one day there was a near miss between two of the fighters. My father was in control of the tower and air space that day so there was an investigation and if it was discovered that he had been at fault that would have been the end of his career. He became very stressed as a result and unwell with flu and gallstone colic. He was flown by helicopter to hospital and after surgery, the day he was due to come home, someone from the local library turned up at our house to tell my mum that he had died of a pulmonary embolism. He was forty two. This was April 1963 and after that my mother, sister and I were sent home to Devon, England.

I was right in the middle of extra O and A Levels but the school in Devon was studying a different syllabus from Cyprus so when we came back to England, I completed the exams I could and moved to London where I went to business and secretarial college. I was seventeen and 'Swinging London' was buzzing with influences like Christine Keeler and Mary Quant and I threw myself into it. At first, I lived in Hampstead for a few months and then I moved in with some West Indians in Shepherds Bush. I lived with musicians and artists and for a while I lived in the Kings Road with a lesbian couple, one of whom was reputedly an ex-girlfriend of Frank Sinatra's. I did temporary secretarial work and I just moved around.

Also, I worked for the administrator of some riding stables in North London. Everybody who was anybody stabled their horses there, for example, Terence Stamp and Jean Shrimpton, who were two of the darlings of the time. Terence Stamp had to learn to ride for *Far from the Madding Crowd*[125], which he starred in alongside Julie Christie. Jean Shrimpton, who was then the model, just before Twiggy, gave him a horse called Modesty, because he had just finished filming *Modesty Blaise*[126]. If celebrities wanted to ride or had horses in London, they often used our stables.

Socially, I mixed with intriguing groups of people who I had got to know partly through these stables and also through polo in Richmond. I moved into a flat with a girl who lived between London and Ibiza and through her I started to mix with yet more interesting people; it was all sex, drugs and rock n' roll. I worked in clubs and for Jackie Collins' husband, Oscar Lerman. Jackie and Joan Collins were frequently at his club. I remember I gave Jackie Collins' fur coat to someone by mistake once and had to get it back. The London club scene at that point, was an amazing cross section of people: the Saudi royal family, rich Jewish people, aristocrats, models, movie stars and of course musicians, like James Brown, who used to come to the club when he was in London.

I used to go to George Raft's place, the Colony Club. He was a black-and-white movie actor who used to play gangsters with Humphrey Bogart and he had a club in London on Berkeley Square. I was going out with a guy called Eddie Slim who was a Lebanese gambler and we used to go for late night coffee with George Raft. Telly Savalas, and all those American gangster type actors, and genuine international gangsters frequented and would play blackjack there. This was in 1965-66 while I also worked for a while in a shop that was selling Palestinian goods to support Palestine.

I was involved with the jazz club scene and people who worked in Ronnie Scott's and the Flamingo. When the clubs closed and we finished work, we used to meet people who had been playing or working in the other clubs. I would go to China Town where there are all-night Chinese restaurants, with people like Coleman Hawkins. At four in the morning we would be sitting with a bunch of jazz musicians chatting away. Basically, through this whole subculture and alternative lifestyle I gradually turned into a real hippy. I was also something of a groupie as I was around a lot of musicians. One night when I was clubbing, one part of the evening I spent with the Krays and the other part with Jimi Hendrix; those were exciting times.

By 1966-67, I was living in Notting Hill in a house that was owned by Chris Blackwell, who founded Island Records and introduced Bob Marley to the world. We lived over the ground floor record shop. A few doors away was one of London's Black Power centres. Australian Vytas Serelis, who lived with us and is now a popular artist at home, painted our and next door's shopfront. We were a very active multicultural alternative community and by that time I was into alternative everything, which is when I started getting interested in natural medicine. I was excited by mysticism, occultism and that whole alternative, hippie lifestyle. I was macrobiotic for a while, vegetarian for a while and into alternative technology such as wind pumps, water and solar power. I had friends who wrote books on those subjects which I helped work on.

I was incredibly ethnic in my dress. The first thing I did when I came to London was start growing my hair, something my mother would never let me do, so as a hippie I had very, very long hair. I had always been the tomboy. My sister was the girl, who was allowed to wear pink, grow her hair long and pull it back with Alice bands. I had everything blue and had my hair cut in the barber's when I was a kid. I was supposed to have been a boy and interestingly I was going to be called Robert so they called me Barbara so that they could shorten it to Bobby.

When I first came to London, I dyed my hair black and started growing it in that Cleopatra/Mary Quant style; it was very London - black hair with a fringe and big eye make-up. By 1966-67 my hair was long and I used to wear Palestinian wedding dresses, with all this heavy duty embroidery and bangles up my arms and those painted on eyelashes of the 1960s, bare feet, and bells around my ankles. And I used to walk around London like that. I didn't live anywhere for a while; I was on the street most of the time. I used to sleep on Hampstead Heath sometimes and I was mostly off my head. My belongings were all over the place. I ended up wherever I ended the evening, for the night.

ROWENA: It sounds like a lot of fun.

BARBARA: For a couple of years it was, yes. That is how we lived. Even when I changed peer groups in the sense of moving out of the Swinging London set into a hippie lifestyle, it was still the same in many ways. We knew the club owners and the doormen. We would just arrive and it was, "Hiya", whereas other people were queuing to pay to go in. I just moved in and out of it. I was backstage when The Doors and Jefferson Airplane played at the Roundhouse. I have spent time with Jim Morrison. Many of the people in my life at the time are legends now.

ROWENA: And you swapped all that for homeopathy?

BARBARA: No, I didn't swap it at the time. What happened was that people started to die or get committed because they had taken too much LSD. As I said earlier, I had got into the occult, UFOs, mysticism, philosophy and Transcendental Meditation and I went to all sorts of meditation groups, started looking at Buddhism and then tried to work out who were the teachers.

Eventually, I came across Thomas Maughan, and that was it really. He was an amazing person. He lined us all up at one point, a whole load of straggly hippies and he marched up and down saying, "You are going to wish you had joined the Army by the time I have finished with you! You lot are going to learn to get disciplined in your minds and learn how to think and use your brains."

ROWENA: Who was part of the group when you joined?

BARBARA: The only person whose whereabouts I know now is Jennifer Maughan, who was his partner. After Thomas died, she got into a relationship with Peter Firebrace, who became principal of one of the acupuncture colleges. She and Peter are still together. Later on, other people came. The next person whom I still know is Jerome Whitney; he joined with his wife Kaaren Whitney. I was already quite well entrenched by then and this was still in the late 1960s. I attended Thomas' meditation classes and my primary interest was in his attitude and what he said but additionally he gave us meditation instruction; we were learning how to meditate and how to become disciplined and the other thing was that he was heavily anti-drugs.

The last time that I took serious mind-altering drugs was at the Rolling Stones concert in Hyde Park; I was on mescaline. After that I didn't take any more LSD, mescaline, psilocybin or any of the other psychedelic drugs for which the 1960s were famous. I stopped on that day because of Thomas. He said it was all very well to have an insight into altered states but that you need to get there through your own work; that was very much his creed. He used to say to us, if we were too airy-fairy in our discussions and not walking our talk, then we would be better off cleaning the toilets. He said it was a complete waste of energy because nothing would change.

Thomas' patients would start arriving at about nine in the morning and he would see them throughout the day and by seven o'clock his students would arrive. He taught homeopathy fortnightly on a Saturday and also on Monday evenings in north London. John Damonte, who taught Misha Norland and some other homeopaths, was in the same classes as I was. John and I would invariably stay late and then drive home. When I lived in Norfolk, I used to hitch to London and I used to stay on a camp bed in Thomas' house. Watching him I started to realise the insanity of his life. At the end of the evening, he would go up to his print shop on the top floor and print all the brochures for his classes. He often used to watch the sun rise, go and get some sleep, and be up for his patients at nine. He was a phenomenon.

ROWENA: And this was in south London?

BARBARA: Yes, in Dulwich. Although he also used to come north of the river but eventually he stopped travelling and John Damonte took some of Thomas' north London classes.

ROWENA: Do you know who inspired Thomas Maughan?

BARBARA: A mix but I don't really know. Thomas was quite secretive about his past. Thomas and John Damonte had a past together, a past that supposedly went back to the war. People used to say all kinds of things about Thomas' past; he used to twinkle and you never quite knew what was legend and what was real. Someone said that he and John had met because they had both been, not exactly spies, but something to do with the secret service.

Another part of the legend was that when he was really young, he was involved in the strikes in Scotland and the marches on Downing Street out of which the Labour Party was born. My understanding was that he had quite a strong political agenda when he was young.

I remember him saying, "What did they then do as soon as they got into Downing Street? All they learned was which side of the plate to put their knives and forks on. They forgot their principles."

But the thing that really grabbed me about Thomas was that he had this thing that the West had a job to do. It was fine to be into the concept of nirvana and to sit contemplating our navels in the lotus position; that was mysticism and had its place in the energies of the world. But also we had a duty in the West to make it real. People were starting to make it real - physicists, geneticists; people were starting to understand the idea that when something material disintegrated, the vital field or the electromagnetic field, which contained all the blue prints and the information, never disappeared.

Thomas taught us that in medicine it is all very well treating the body like machinery taking into account the chemistry and the material elements, but what actually formed the body, what influenced it and what created its health, was its energy field. The electricity, the information and the blueprints were all held in the vital force. He opened up the whole nature-nurture debate - are people a product of their genetics and nature or is it a result of the way they are brought up and their psychology? We had to learn all sorts of things including basic Hebrew, for example, in order to understand *the Bible*[27]. He talked about *the Bible*[27] as metaphor; that each letter of the old Hebrew alphabet meant something.

ROWENA: I remember Jerome Whitney mentioning this to us at college. Do you know who influenced Thomas with that part of his teaching?

BARBARA: He came from a long line of teachers one of which was Robert MacGregor Reid, the Chief of the Ancient Order of Druids, who had been influenced by William Blake, William Butler Yeats and D H Lawrence. There had been a whole tradition of teaching from people who had been into esotericism, the Druids, occultism and so forth. Also he drove overland to Australia, certainly to India, and I think this is true and not a myth in terms of the Thomas legend. He taught classes in India and he studied as well. He also philosophised with people in the East. He talked to us about how he was seriously ill in Africa and was treated by the local witch woman with folk medicine and he had an interest in Native Americans too.

ROWENA: Did you think you were going to be a homeopath?

BARBARA: No, I never intended to. Homeopathy was one of the many classes I attended but I got really obsessed and went to Thomas' every night for a while. I became very obnoxious and I tried to get all my friends to stop taking drugs. Everybody used to turn into little Thomases, except that they weren't like him. Everybody grew beards, and they would open their mouths and you would hear Thomas coming out! But it was not real Thomas. The same used to happen with George Vithoulkas. Disciples are often more righteous, narrow-minded and rigid than their masters. I used to think I had a bit of an advantage around Thomas, being a woman, because I didn't have to be him. The men got this need to emulate him; the beards and everything.

ROWENA: So who grew beards?

BARBARA: Everybody – Jerome Whitney, Peter Chappell, Robert Davidson, Martin Miles, they all grew beards. At face value, Thomas could be quite Victorian and chauvinistic. He used to say to us, "I am a Victorian, chauvinistic Scot. It is part of my training and upbringing but don't copy that; it is just my shell." We believed he was capable of quite amazing things. He used to talk to us about how you had to go into the psychic vital force level in order to alter anything that was in the material world. So he talked to us about how ritual magic worked. Part of that related to homeopathy; how you move in that energy to affect change in the material. That is part of the way that remedies worked.

ROWENA: So when did you decide to become a homeopath?

BARBARA: Several things coincided. I freaked out one day and an American girl who was staying with us, Joan Sokolov, shoved me in a taxi and phoned Thomas and said, "I am bringing Barbara; she has totally freaked out." She took me down to Thomas and waited in his front room while he took me into his consulting room. He took my case history and I was in there for hours with him. I always remember him looking at me with his dark beady eyes, white beard and hair, quizzical eyebrows and shaking his head in disbelief saying, "Whatever are you trying to do to yourself?"

He prescribed for me and I suspect he might have given me *Ignatia amara* and maybe *Medorrhinum*, when I think about the state I was in, and the wildness. Because I used to drive home with John Damonte all the time, he also started giving me remedies. I had a history, as well as the drugs, of sexually transmitted infections and hence gynaecological problems and John started treating me, giving me remedies to clear me out. Then I started having treatment with Thomas every month so I became a patient as well as going to classes. I had been told I might not be able to have children by the orthodox doctors and I repeated this to Thomas who asked, "You haven't had anything out, have you?" I replied, "No" and he said, "Well, that is nonsense then!" He just prescribed and prescribed and under his treatment, I really changed. I became so much more together; I got clearer and my body got together and I became healthy. He treated me through both my pregnancies in 1971 and 1972 and treated the kids when they were babies.

I had moved to Norfolk and self-sufficient country life at the end of 1970 and also spent a little time travelling with gypsies and also going round fairs and festivals but eventually things drew me back to London. I still knew a lot of musicians and activists and I moved down to World's End. One of my close friends was the late Nicholas Carr-Saunders who wrote the books *Alternative London*[127] and *Alternative England and Wales*[128]. He had the most amazing flat and the toilet system was a fish tank. Another friend of mine was Nick Albery, who had started a charity called Roof and he was involved in Shelter as well. We set up a charity called CAT – Child Aid Trust – to support single parents and a group of us with our children lived together down at World's End at the end of the King's Road. There was a lot of action and we were out on the street all the time. At this point, I knew homeopath David Curtin's now wife, Dee Maclaughlin. She and I shared a house together, in 1974-75; it was so funny that she eventually got into homeopathy.

When I came back to London, Thomas was still my homeopath and I was still going to his classes. The London life drew me back in and I had a spell of being into the 1970s cocaine drug scene. I was running around with various musician friends. Sharing a house with a bunch of single parents gave me a lot of freedom because we took it in turns to look after the kids. I did that for years and I was into community politics as well as organising squats.

I was very friendly with Heathcote Williams. He was a playwright and he has been in a couple of movies as well. He wrote a poem called *Whale Nation*[129] and that is one of the things he is famous for. Heathcote and Nick Albery were best friends and they took Thames Valley Police to court over the Reading Valley Festival. They were two of the first people ever to legally challenge putting lead in petrol and they also co-founded Frestonia, an independent state in the Westway development area west of Ladbroke Grove. I learned quickly that it tends to be middle class liberals who want social change.

Most people who are at genuine poverty levels, who are struggling to make ends meet, think middle class people like me are a bit mad. All they want is a car, a job, a house and nice clothes. I had to learn that. You had people like Nick Albery, Heathcote and Nicholas Carr-Saunders who were from upper middle class, aristocratic backgrounds, who had gone to public schools and who were totally brilliant and also hippies. Because of their families and their background, they had the resources to do things like write books and campaign to organise things differently. They were all well-educated, philosophising and quite fascinating people to be around and often seriously alternative.

Heathcote started the Ruff Tuff Creampuff Estate Agency, which was an estate agency for squatters. We ran leaflets around Notting Hill and other areas offering property for squatting. I started community transport networks and went to councils to get support from people who were influential. I got the backing of Brent Trades Council, the head of the trade unions, and Brent Law Society. We went to the councils to challenge them on all their empty properties. On one level, I was involved daily in the local community and alternative politics. I had a renewed interest in the clubbing scene but this time by association with punk. That is what got me into homeopathy in the end.

I became a lay practitioner in the 1960s when I had taken classes with Thomas and I used to self-prescribe and prescribe for friends. I remember there was a dog that was bleeding and bleeding after she had her puppies and the vet didn't think she would last the night. I just couldn't handle it so I rang Thomas who said, "*Crotalus horridus*". I had never heard of rattlesnake venom at that point. He was always at the end of the phone for me.

When he died, I suddenly didn't have anyone to phone anymore. I had to resort to some of my old classmates who had always been much more disciplined in their studies than I was. It had always been a bit of a dilettante thing for me; I never saw myself as a practitioner. Whereas, when Robert Davidson joined Thomas' classes in the early 1970s, he became a very serious scholar. He really worked and was very dedicated. One day, when I called him for help, he said to me, "I want to start a college." I said, "If you start a college, I will sign up. I need to get more involved and I need to become more efficient with my homeopathy."

What did it finally for me was Sid Vicious. I drove the Sex Pistols on tour and I was very involved with the Heartbreakers and The Slits as well. People used to meet in the Roebuck down at World's End, just a few doors away from Malcolm McLaren and Vivienne Westwood's shop. Up until that point things had started to become boring in the early 1970s except for David Bowie, Mark Bolan and the New York Dolls. From then on in I got very into punk. The whole liberation of marching around the streets in leather, chains and safety pins, swaggering around in Doc Martins and fishnet tights was totally liberating. I started getting assertive and self-confident.

Thomas had always nagged me about the numerology of my birth date, what it meant and what I should be doing with my life. He said that there were a lot of assertive qualities in my birth date and would regularly ask me, "What are you Barbara, a lion or a mouse?" He used to tell me that I had to learn to be powerful. He used to put us in his seat to run classes and be in charge of the room and he often wanted me to do it. Peter Chappell, Robert Davidson and others used to compete for that position and when I saw him looking at me to do it I would run and hide in the loo.

One day I opened the toilet door, and he was standing outside and he said to me, "Whenever I want to put you in the position of authority, you disappear. I will tell you my opinion; you are so righteous about it. You think all these people fighting for power and authority are wrong and you are so proud of the fact that you don't. Let me tell you that what you do is exactly the same thing but just on the other end of the polarity. The avoidance of it is just the same behaviour. It is almost worse because you are not learning to do it. You really need to learn to have authority and express it quietly. You need to have the self-confidence to be able to assert yourself instead of this erratic way that you either over-assert or under-assert yourself and be apologetic about it. You have got to learn about power."

Around 1977 I was living with Steve Strange, one of the icons of the 1980s New Romantics. We had a big house in Alperton, near Wembley and he was one of the people who lived there. People often used to meet in our house to go into London clubbing. We often used to hitch home, in pairs, so we didn't frighten everybody. Steve and I used to do a lot of hitching together. Sid Vicious was often wrecked because of his heroin addiction. Malcolm McLaren and the band were trying to keep Sid away from Nancy Spungen because she was such a bad influence on him. We were trying to get him straight enough to just stand up and play and Nancy and her whole heroin habit kept getting him into trouble. When we were on tour, I was with Sid virtually twenty four hours a day to make sure he was ok. Even when they were on stage I was often sitting on the floor behind his speaker. In the breaks, part of what I had to do was to stop him disappearing into the crowd to try and find someone to get him a fix.

One night we were in Plymouth, and Sid and I were in our hotel room. He said to me, "Barbara, why aren't you doing your homeopathy? Why are you doing this and not your homeopathy?" I said, "Oh well, ..." and he demanded, "Why don't you get me healthy!" I replied, "Sid, it would be really bad for your image! You are becoming a living legend now, like James Dean; you are part of living mythology. What will it do to your image to be healthy?" I didn't have the ability, homeopathically, to take on a case as difficult as Sid's.

ROWENA: He is not alive anymore is he?

BARBARA: No, no. He died. His death is what flipped me into homeopathy. I had started thinking about using my homeopathy more seriously after that flippant conversation with Sid. Then I rang up Robert Davidson because someone else wanted treatment for something and this coincided with the start of his college COH, which I joined that September in 1978. Malcolm McLaren, Sid Vicious and Jamie Reid basically paid for my college fees.

I was living with Jamie Reid by then; we were a couple. Jamie used to be Malcolm's best friend. Coincidentally, Jamie is the great grandnephew of Robert MacGregor Reid whom I mentioned earlier taught Thomas Maughan. But my association with Jamie was through punk. Jamie is a brilliant artist and he has had a couple of exhibitions this year. Robert Davidson's fees were very cheap for the first year and we did classes at the YWCA in Great Russell Street.

ROWENA: And then did you treat your punk rocker friends?

BARBARA: Yes, our families and friends. The year I started college we had been making the film, *The Great Rock 'n Roll Swindle*[130], a film about the Sex Pistols. The brothel scenes were filmed in my house! Sid went off to the USA with Nancy Spungen and he was living in the legendary Chelsea Hotel in New York. Then Sid was arrested for killing Nancy, in the hotel. There was never a trial because he died when he was out on bail.

ROWENA: How old was he?

BARBARA: Twenty one. He lived fast and died young. He always said he would be dead by the time he was twenty one, and he was.

ROWENA: How old were you?

BARBARA: Thirty two, thirty three. He died on 6 February 1979 from an overdose. The truth about what happened to Nancy Spungen never came out. There are all kinds of stories about Sid's drink being spiked at the party on the night he came out of jail. I went to college that weekend and sat in the back of the class with tears just pouring down my face. It was just Robert Davidson and Martin Miles teaching at the time. They had no syllabus; they decided what to do the next weekend out of the questions we asked. It was real organic teaching.

When Thomas died, my understanding is that he left his patients to Martin Miles and his students to Robert Davidson. Martin had what it took to be a practitioner but Robert was more leaning towards being a teacher. Thomas had tried a couple of times in the 1970s to found a society of homeopaths in his lifetime, but without real success. When he died, his students got very active. There was a sense of urgency to try and put into practise some of what he stood for. Teaching homeopathy, trying to make homeopathy widespread, having a society for non-medical homeopaths, trying to establish non-medical homeopathy; these had all been big issues for Thomas.

When he was alive, everybody had been content to let him be the leader but once he was dead, suddenly there was a kind of motivation to try and make his wishes happen. So Robert Davidson, Martin Miles, Peter Chappell and various people were really motivated to do that. I was on the edge of it at that time because of everything else that was going on my life so I wasn't so involved with the mechanisms of getting it going.

I sat in the classroom the weekend that Sid died, and that was when I decided to become a homeopath. I was guilt driven and one of the issues I had to deal with was that I was doing my homeopathy for Sid for quite a long time. I felt that somehow I had to compensate for his death and that my life now had to be more meaningful. One of the ways of making it meaningful was making the homeopathy work.

Even when I had started at COH, I had never intended to practise. Basically, I was an ex-hippie punk who had used drugs, been a groupie and political activist and was into esoteric pursuits; I wasn't exactly the kind of person who would make a good image for homeopathy.

People like Robert Nichols and Stephen Gordon who were in the class with me when I started at COH, still remember meeting me for the first time. Robert Nichols says he recalls me coming to class with green punky hair, dressed in bin liners and see through fluorescent T-shirts, camouflage trousers and sexshop stilettos. My hair was green one minute, pink another and blonde the next, and I wore heavy punk make-up. When I started actually seeing patients I had to totally change. I had my head almost totally shaved at that point and the little hair that was left I dyed black and I wore a dark red suit in clinic.

ROWENA: So how come you took over COH?

BARBARA: When I was still at COH, I found it old-fashioned. There was no real teaching theory and it was run very much like 'the masters teach the student'; I never cared for that particularly. I had other things going on in my life and I was more aware of student centred learning and critical thinking. College at that time had too much indoctrination going on for my liking.

I was quite active as a student. Robert Davidson and Martin Miles made me the student rep because prior to there being one I would go to the staff meetings and say, "The students need tutors they can speak to, not just the experience of sitting in rows being taught. They need someone who represents them, who has a say in your staff meetings. Students need advocates." Eventually they just said, "Oh well, you do it Barbara. The students need a rep? You do it. They need a counsellor? You do it."

So students would come to me with their problems and I started arranging tutorials, while I was studying. The first time I went to a college clinic, Martin Miles just gave me the keys when I turned up and said, "All the patient notes are on my desk; I am not feeling well and I am going home." He just left me with the whole caseload for the day; wall to wall patients. That was my first experience of really practising like a professional, taking money and doing all that. It threw me straight in at the deep end, in my dark red suit.

By going to college, my homeopathy changed from how I used to practise when Thomas taught me. I had always known a lot of remedies, as Clarke's *Materia Medica*[28] was my bedtime reading for years. I couldn't repertorise before I went to college but I could recognise masses and masses of remedy pictures; the task was fitting them to patients. Often I didn't know the structure of how to find remedies properly except using therapeutics books, like Clarke's *Prescriber*[131], *A Dictionary of the New Therapeutics*[28], or Lilienthal's *Homoeopathic Therapeutics*[132] and I would look up remedies for a condition and then differentiate. But actually doing disciplined, structured repertorisation, taking symptoms and putting them in - I couldn't do that very well before I went to college.

My first day in clinic, this old boy in his eighties came in and I took his case. One thing I always remember about him was asking about his sex life, because I didn't discriminate at that point and I stuck to my format, which had routine questions including sexual activity. The old man burst out laughing, patted my knee, and said something like, "You know, my dear, it takes a lot longer than it used to!" I almost saw a shift in him completely brought on by the fact that this thirty-something woman thought he still had a sex life. He didn't realise I was going through a routine. He thought somehow I had picked up that he was a sexual being and boy did it give him a twinkle!

I started teaching whilst I was still a student in 1980. David Mundy was in my class at the beginning of the course but before the end, he was one of the main teachers and he was suddenly no longer in the class! He had been an acupuncturist before. I started tutoring and organising the more senior students into groups with the first years; that was my role. Robert Davidson also gave me the college clinic to run. A number of us had been practising for years before we had come to college so by the time we were in the fourth year we had added a disciplined study to what we already knew of homeopathy. We became the clinicians. In the fourth year, we had the third year students and others sitting in with us.

Nicholas Carr-Saunders, whom I had stayed with when I first came back to London in 1974, owned and set up Neal's Yard in Covent Garden, London where we ran the clinic. He thought, when it was coming up for sale "What a great place to have an alternative culture." He started with a bakery, therapy rooms and a wholefood warehouse on the ground floor with sacks of rice and things. The next floor up there was a big room that could be used for workshops and the next floor housed small therapy rooms. One of our students, Margot, became the receptionist and on top of all that was Nick's flat. On Thursdays COH ran its clinic from his therapy rooms. Fourth year students saw the patients with the other students sitting in with them. We would have two students in each room in pairs taking the case. I would circulate around the rooms, getting snapshots of what was going on. The students would come out, we would go into a room, talk about the case quickly, give the patient a remedy, off they would go and the next patient would be in.

I remember Gabrielle Pinto sat in a lot with me. Also Tony Hurley, who turned up to sit in with me one day with no shoes on! There is something about Tony, no matter what he does or wears, he always looks neat; maybe it is his yoga teacher background or something about the way he moves. This shock of having a student sitting in with me who didn't have his shoes on left me confused as to what to do with him. I wondered, "Do I tell him he cannot come into the room?" And then I thought, "Oh, just let him!" He came in and sat in the lotus position on the side.

ROWENA: When did you become principal?

BARBARA: I became vice principal in 1984. What happened was that Martin Miles really didn't perceive that COH was his thing as he was a practitioner through and through. Robert Davidson had gone to live in Devon and Robert Nichols, Kathryn Peck and I were concerned that students that were coming through in the years below us should have a more structured course with timetables and so on. So while in our fourth year we started writing timetables and marking student work with feedback. After graduation I continued to do this and other aspects of course management. I was also involved in the Tiverton College of Classical Homeopathy, which Tony Hurley and Anne Bickley had started and I became more and more involved in the organisational aspects of COH.

While in Devon, Robert Davidson became almost as good as a sleeping partner. Though a principal in name, he was never really in London. He came up for college weekends to teach and ran the business side of things including the money but he left organisation of the course and college activities to the college registrar and me. I went down to Devon to stay with Robert in 1984, and he asked me to be vice principal. As soon as the words were out of his mouth, I said, "No!" He said, "Don't answer me so fast! Barbara, go to bed and remember what Thomas said to you about authority, and what you should be learning. This is an ideal opportunity for you to put some of that into practise."

I did two things; I slept on it and I asked Thomas' advice and the next day I came down and sat with Robert Davidson and said, "OK, I'll do it." And that is when I became vice principal and partner. As I said earlier, Martin Miles had dropped his share in the college so Robert gave me a share, which is how I was supposed to get recompensed but I basically ran the college as Robert wanted to focus on business skills. Our relationship was always an interesting one and Robert was much more fixed and classical about his homeopathy until I got hold of him! He once told me that Sheilagh Creasy went all the way to Devon to warn him that I was a bad influence – I never knew if he was joking.

We were both open to many new influences in the 1980s as we were very involved in self-development activities – NLP, Erhard Seminars Training (EST), Exegesis, immortality, prosperity consciousness etc and we were keen on new thinking in areas of science, such as quantum physics and chaos theory. Pursuing these interests in our different ways, Robert Davidson went to live in Arizona in 1988 and I took over as principal.

ROWENA: What a fascinating life you have lead Barbara. You have really given me a feel for the atmosphere surrounding the renaissance of homeopathy here in London and what it was like studying with Thomas in those early years. Many thanks for sharing your story with me.

CHAPTER 31:   SIMON TAFFLER

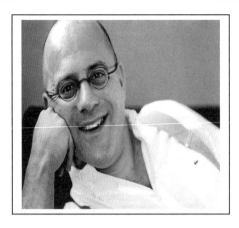

I first met Simon Taffler in Malvern in November 2004 where I met several of the other interviewees as previously mentioned. Simon and I had stayed in touch several times since meeting for joyous conversations about homeopathy and our profession. We set this specific session up for the purpose of the interview and I was very excited about it as Simon is one of the high earners within our profession and he has carved for himself a successful career in homeopathy. It was a cold yet sunny Monday 28 November 2005 that I picked him up from my local train station and took him back to my home for lunch and a long conversation.

"I consider opportunities to teach as gifts because they are usually opportunities to grow and heal."   *Simon Taffler, November 2005*

"I see the need in the UK and in the USA for the vision of homeopathy to change and be clearer, especially about where our profession is going. And I see a lot of common traits that I am not comfortable with. Homeopaths for example, are susceptible to working in their ivory tower alone – forsaken, isolated and separated from the world. With that susceptibility in mind, I think we should be working together and opening centres of excellence that invite research and co-operation in which homeopaths work together to improve and evolve themselves and their profession."   *Simon Taffler, November 2005*

"I think it is easier to be a homeopath now than it was when I started because I think people are taught much better than we were and there is a lot more choice regarding how and where to study."   *Simon Taffler, November 2005*

"I think one needs to practise patient centred homeopathy, rather than remedy centred homeopathy, and that means prioritising the relationship and looking after patients by, for example creating expectations that can be met and helping the patient to be 'process' not 'outcome' oriented."   *Simon Taffler, November 2005*

CHAPTER 31: SIMON TAFFLER

ROWENA: So Simon, tell me how you get into homeopathy in the beginning? Tell me your story.

SIMON: My first experience was over forty years ago! I was eight or nine with a fever that was brought on by an allergic reaction to antibiotics. My grandmother took me to see Margery Blackie and I can remember being feverish in her arms and looking up into her face as she dropped these little white pills into my mouth.

ROWENA: So, this was the early 1960s?

SIMON: Sorry, I know I look younger! Anyway, fifteen years later when I was twenty three or four and living in Israel, I was encouraged to seek homeopathic treatment again. I had suffered from verrucae or plantar warts, as they say in the USA, for ten years and even though I had them gouged and potioned, lotioned and operated on, they kept returning. I went to see a homeopath in a pharmacy and he prescribed for me in about ten minutes. I put my foot up on the counter and he looked at it, gave me two doses of a remedy and ten days later my verrucae were gone and I thought this was absolutely astounding.

I was hooked! Because of my curiosity and enthusiasm he allowed me to sit in his pharmacy all day watching him as well as making him tea and coffee. After that I persuaded him to allow me to be his apprentice – something he had not done before. I was doing other jobs at the time but any spare time I had, I went there to learn from him. I did that for a few years and then I decided I needed to study homeopathy properly and Joseph Reves at this time was working in Israel.

I found his teaching interesting and it appealed to my intellect, but I had come from working in a pharmacy and I didn't have the background philosophy to hold together what he was talking about. I feel I went to him too soon (in terms of my knowledge and experience) and so I studied with him only four or five times and decided that his approach was not for me. I then came back to London to study on the part-time course at Barbara Harwood and Robert Davidson's College of Homeopathy (COH). The year was 1985 and there was an intake of two hundred and fifty students on my course.

Robert Davidson and Barbara Harwood taught us, as did David Mundy. At the time there were only a few UK schools, principally COH in London, the School of Homeopathy in Devon and the North West College of Homoeopathy (NWCH) in Manchester. Also I used to go to two tutorials, alternating every week between tutorials run by the late Kay Samuel and the late Liz Danciger. They were fantastic, inspiring hot houses - brilliant stuff went on there.

ROWENA: Tell me more...

SIMON: There are two types of teachers as there are diamond craftsmen. Liz Danciger was a visionary cutter and Kay Samuel was a nurturing polisher so we had this contrast of learning homeopathy in different ways.

ROWENA: What kind of teacher are you?

SIMON: What am I? I aim to be an appropriate teacher; a healing teacher. There are different ways of facilitating and guiding people, sometimes you need to be a cutter and succuss and sometimes you need to polish, nurture and potentise. I consider opportunities to teach as gifts because they are usually opportunities to grow and heal. After all, the root meaning of the word 'doctor' is derived from the Latin docere, meaning 'teacher'. When I use the word 'doctor' or homeopath I am emphasising the connection between healing and teaching and suggesting that healing is a learning process and learning is a healing process.

So back to my journey - after two years studying at COH I decided to leave, as I did not like the way we were being taught. Some of the teachers would just walk up and down between the desks reading from materia medica. There were also many inconsistencies between the philosophy of the education and the philosophy of the practice. And if homeopathy is about recognising people's individualised health picture, then it should also be acknowledged that everybody learns differently; people have individual ways of taking in material and learn at varying speeds.

I had an argument with Barbara Harwood about this issue as I believed COH should have been about the further education of adults and I didn't want to be treated like a kid having to pass monthly tests and methodological quizzes. It was not a healing experience and reinforced my childhood memories of school as a place that prioritised the art of revision and validated teachers who taught with a hefty dose of fear to submissive passive learners. It was not a confidence building experience for me.

Hence I left and went to the School of Homeopathy, which was totally the right decision for me. I had a fabulous group full of characters - people who, as the years went by, kindly shared their experiences and pathology, which gave us something to work with in class. From epileptic fits to temper tantrums, people shared their lives and personal cases. And I just loved the learning that Misha facilitated. On reflection, his curriculum allocated time for the exploration and integration of content and process, explanation and experience and of consciousness and connections made during the learning process. It felt like I was learning homeopathy in a healing environment in a healing way.

ROWENA: Do you think that students should share their cases? Did everyone share their case?

SIMON: I think that the decision to share a student's case or not should depend on the group and teacher at the time. Not everyone in my group shared their case, but I was quite unwell one time and David Mundy walked into the room and said, as he always did, "What do you want to do today?" pretending that he hadn't prepared anything, when of course he had, and I was feeling rough. He said, "Do you want to do a live case?" and I said, "Yes, do mine because I am really feeling ill." And I think I had got to the point where I couldn't take any more in my life, as there were lots of things going on which were pressuring me. And so I gave my case. David managed to get a lot of experiences that I had not spoken about out of me because he was good at creating a sense of safety.

ROWENA: A constitutional picture?

SIMON: Yes. He gave me *Opium*. To this day, I am a very good teacher of *Opium* because I know it so well. And I hope my fellow learners know *Opium* well from that class experience. But also I know, for example, that *Opium* is a very good fever remedy, and not everyone knows that. I have experienced it a couple of times where I have had high fevers come on quickly. If *Belladonna* doesn't work, then I take *Opium* and it drops the fever, which is really interesting.

ROWENA: And you don't think that is because it has an affinity with you, as opposed to being a good remedy for fever?

SIMON: Good point. Both, I have an affinity for it and it is a good fever remedy. It is just that it is not a remedy I previously associated it with fevers. If I get ill, my fever comes on fast, I get a pounding headache and in the space of seconds my temperature can go from normal to 106° which is a classic *Belladonna* picture and it usually does relieve it. But when it doesn't, then I will just take one *Opium* 1M and it will drop my fever from 106° down to normal in about half an hour to forty five minutes.

ROWENA: That is very impressive.

SIMON: Yes, those kinds of experiences are great, especially as they help increase confidence when treating patients.

My confidence as a practitioner really jumped when after completing at the School of Homeopathy I did Jeremy Sherr's Dynamis course. Misha Norland's teaching was a potentisation and I left certain that I had found a framework of philosophy that worked for me and one that would help me make meaning in the world. Jeremy's was a succussion - a major succussion – I appreciated the Dynamis School and learned huge lessons from him about praxis, about connecting the theory and practice and importantly about provings. He addressed many of my confidence issues around my prescribing process.

By the time I graduated from the Dynamis School I was living entirely as a homeopath, having transformed my naturopathic practice into a homeopathic clinic. My entire studying and upkeep was financed by the clinic, which I had established in 1985.

ROWENA: Were you prescribing homeopathy?

SIMON: Yes, I was. Initially, I was known more as a naturopath and when I prescribed homeopathy it was mainly with acute remedies. As my confidence grew and I learned more, I then prescribed more constitutionally. Over the years of my studies, with tons of supervision, I built up a very good clinic.

ROWENA: Where was it?

SIMON: Around the back of the Royal Free Hospital, it was called Life Works. I started with a shop and I sold loads of remedies, vitamins and minerals and if people needed help, I would close the shop and take them into the back room for an hour. Eventually I had enough people who wanted my help that I could employ someone to work in the shop. And then I took over the flat above the shop and turned that into the clinic and expanded the shop. But over time as the shop and clinic got busier and busier, I couldn't cope with it all, so I closed it and went to Primrose Hill. There I converted three garages into a clinic with a reception room in the middle, a toilet at the back and two clinic rooms. I took one room and an acupuncturist worked from the other. There was a clinic at the end of the mews and another clinic opened upstairs above Life Works and my dream was to make the whole mews into clinic spaces.

But it didn't quite work out as my attention moved away from practising to teaching. I realised that I was teaching homeopathy the same way as I was taught, and I didn't like that. And so I decided to explore homeopathy philosophy and how to teach homeopathy. So I sold my clinic and everything else in 1995 and went to live in San Francisco for five years.

ROWENA: What made you do that?

SIMON: I just knew that I needed to deepen my understanding of homeopathy and move away from the way it was taught. I had some appallingly experiences learning homeopathy and some great ones. I wanted to find a way of teaching, grounded in the homeopathy philosophy that invites learners to be homeopathic and not teach in ways that reinforces allopathic modes of thinking and being. I think that there is a lot of allopathic teaching of homeopathy so practitioners end up prescribing homeopathy allopathically.

ROWENA: So tell me Simon, why San Francisco?

SIMON: I did a search on the net and one of the places that came up was this university in San Francisco called the California Institute of Integral Studies. They emphasise the Integral Philosophy of Sri Aurobindo, and latterly people like Ken Wilber, and offered a course that enabled the integration of philosophy and practise in a person's chosen profession. So I went there, encouraged by a fellow student from the Dynamis School. I flew over and had an interview, told them that they needed me as a student – and I was in. While I studied, I started a teaching clinic in New York because at that time there was nobody teaching homeopaths there in a clinic setting.

ROWENA: How did you manage to do that if you were in San Francisco?

SIMON: I set it up before I left London because I knew I would need income in the USA when I was living there. And I knew I would get a work permit for three years, so I started a teaching clinic in New York encouraged by Jeremy Sherr. Studying in San Francisco was a wonderful experience; it was just stunning. I was in the best place at the right time and was exposed to people that I would never, ever, ever have had the chance to meet over here – phenomenal people.

I sat in a class with sixteen people and when the likes of Deepak Chopra and Fritjof Capra did their stuff we had an opportunity to totally grill them. Phenomenal researchers and thinkers who were writing consciousness changing books at the time were also part of my course - Richard Tarnas who wrote *The Passion of the Western Mind*[133], Brian Swimme and Thomas Berry who wrote *The Universe Story*[134] and various other books and Amit Goswami who wrote *The Quantum Doctor*[135]. I mean, I just sat in the classroom with these people and it was astounding!

It was a really, really brilliant time and I studied a lot of philosophy - Goethe, Hegel, Kant - and I got to understand the philosophical context in which Hahnemann wrote the *Organon*[4]. Incidentally, the Sixth Edition of the *Organon*[4] is available to view in San Francisco. At the same time Wenda O'Reilly, whom I had already met at the Dynamis School, was translating and simplifying the Sixth Edition[136], so I ended up spending a lot of time with her. With Steven Decker's help, I really understand where lots of mistakes had been made in the past with the various translations of the *Organon*[4]. I felt that it was perfect timing for me and ultimately I was teaching all over the USA in other homeopathy schools and running my teaching clinic in New York. Then I came back here, to London in 2000.

I returned and rejoined Life Works with David Mundy. We moved out of Primrose Hill and into Drummond Street, and so for five years we had a clinic there until Camden Council wanted to double the rent and rates in 2005. Unfortunately we had to close it and now I work in Marylebone with friends in an osteopathic clinic.

ROWENA: Do you miss working with David Mundy?

SIMON: I do, yes. I think we worked well together and it confirmed my liking of the whole idea of working with colleagues. I like the idea of co-operation and not competition between practitioners. There is too much of that in our profession and it is something in the future that I want to change.

ROWENA: How?

SIMON: I see the need in the UK and in the USA for the vision of homeopathy to change and be clearer, especially about where our profession is going. And I see a lot of common traits that I am not comfortable with. Homeopaths for example, are susceptible to working in their ivory tower alone – forsaken, isolated and separated from the world. With that susceptibility in mind, I think we should be working together and opening centres of excellence that invite research and co-operation in which homeopaths work together to improve and evolve themselves and their profession.

Perhaps a floor of a building in Harley Street with two-way mirrors in all the treatment rooms so that practitioners and students can observe, learn and give advice. Then, if you have got a problem with a patient, you just walk into the observation room and invite someone who has been observing into the clinic room to help. This is an experience I had in Sri Lanka this summer where I was working. There were ten or eleven of us all practising in one room without any curtains, without barriers and I loved it because people called me down to diagnose something or treat someone and they sent me patients and I did the same. I like that kind of interaction and it has got to be much healthier, in my mind, than working in isolation and competition. This ethos acknowledges our collective susceptibility and offers opportunities for all sorts of learning and healing.

ROWENA: You spoke earlier about going to the USA in order to study further how to teach homeopathy. What were your frustrations with how homeopathy was taught here?

SIMON: It has been changing in the last few years, but there are a number of schools that still have a curriculum that is very allopathic with a disproportionate emphasis on the material aspects of health and not enough importance given to the energetic aspects of life. And homeopathy is a vitalist, energetic medicine. If you take the model in the *Organon*[4] of the mind, body, soul and spirit of homeopathy, then the mind, soul and spirit are the energetic parts of the totality leaving the body as the only physical part. That means three quarters of our being is energetic and one quarter is physical.

In my opinion many curricula are based the other way around – that is three quarters physical and one quarter energetic, if that. And some schools are even more physically inclined, particularly the ones that have gone for university degree status, and that has meant that the way they do anatomy, physiology and pathology is much more allopathic than homeopathic. So, I have a problem with this. The extreme of this occurs at the Royal London Homeopathic Hospital. They were much more homeopathic in their thinking, but not anymore; now they think and prescribe like allopaths. When I went there a few years ago a patient would sit in front of a doctor for say ten or fifteen minutes, the repertory would be opened and they would look at asthma and locate the black type remedies and keep trying them until one of them made a difference. That is not homeopathy.

What I see is that the essence of the curriculum of homeopathy has not changed in the last twenty years and it is very allopathically oriented. What I have found is that many of the people I supervise are allopathic thinkers prescribing homeopathy and I don't get on very well with that concept and I cannot supervise them very easily. So I encourage them to venture forth on a transition process from allopathic to homeopathic thinking. However, everything in our society validates allopathic thinking, so people need to do this journey against the current.

For me, a homeopathic curriculum needs to acknowledge and recognise primarily that the student is there to make this transition, this journey from allopathic to homeopathic thinking. From thinking and considering things from a culturally based model that validates allopathic meaning making, to being prepared to stand behind a philosophy that understands life differently and puts us on the margins of society. When we start thinking differently, we start appreciating different values based on different assumptions and we start having a comprehension of a way of understanding that validates individual experience over notions of collective symptom pictures or syndromes.

In my opinion, one of the biggest problems we have in ensuring the future of homeopathy, is how do we make sure that our curriculum is homeopathic and not allopathic? And this could get worse once we have a single register. The more the Government and conventional Western medicine become involved with homeopathy, the more allopathically thinking and allopathically validating it could become. If homeopaths don't think homeopathically they will not be able to teach their patients nor advocate clearly for their profession.

This is reflected in the media that constantly criticises homeopathy from an allopathic perspective and headlines research that can only invalidate homeopathy given the premises under which the research was undertaken. You cannot double-blind test homeopathy, it just cannot happen and there is no point trying. It just won't work because the essence of homeopathy is about treating everybody as an individual. And that means double-blind testing won't work.

Homeopathy prescribed and researched allopathically is happening all the time. The 2002-3 research into *Arnica* for pain relief after carpal tunnel release surgery is a good example as I don't know a single homeopath who would give *Arnica* for postoperative carpal tunnel pain relief in the first place. But this type of research and the thinking behind it and the media that publishes it, is going on all the time and I think it affects the way homeopaths write their brochures, the way they promote their clinics, the way they think about what they do, the way they address their patients and the way they address the world. And I have problems with that, because to me that is not homeopathy. You can see I feel passionately about this.

ROWENA: Yes, I can see that. So what is the answer Simon; how do we move our profession forward?

SIMON: I think everybody needs to be plopped into a crucible that nurtures and supports them to think homeopathically.

ROWENA: You say that there are certain colleges that are more allopathic than homeopathic. If you were a student now, where would you study?

SIMON: I would go to a college like the Lakeland College of Homeopathy; there is no question about it.

ROWENA: OK, tell me what is it like teaching at the Lakeland College?

SIMON: Well, I like it as the structure of the Lakeland College and curricula emphasises each learner as an individual aiming to develop to their full potential in their own unique way. So I am a facilitator more than a teacher. It feels like a place that I can safely learn and grow as the students learn and grow, because supportive feedback structures exist for the staff and the students. There is a flexible sense about the curriculum, which evolves, and there is plenty of time for exploration of experience and ideas.

ROWENA: What do you teach there?

SIMON: Philosophy around theory and practise, especially case taking and analysis, skills around being in the clinic with the patient and diet and nutrition. I also teach materia medica of remedies that I have experience with.

ROWENA: Are there any particular years you teach?

SIMON: All of them. I teach there because I enjoy it, I like the people who teach there and I like the philosophy of the Lakeland College, and it has more of an emphasis on the energetic. It seems more homeopathic than other schools that I have taught at.

ROWENA: You are a classical homeopath, aren't you?

SIMON: Yes I am.

ROWENA: But it is a nonclassical college; are you the only classical homeopath teaching there?

SIMON: No. It is important that students get exposed to as many different forms of practise as possible. It is not about creating little Simon Tafflers or teaching and making little Rowena Ronsons. It is about everybody becoming the person that they can be and practising in their own way and I think that that is very important. Listen, I started in a class of around two hundred and fifty potential homeopaths of which at the end, I think, fewer than forty graduated. The year I left COH, ten of us transferred to the School of Homeopathy and many more left without completing the course. It was an appalling indictment of the way I was taught and if I think of the people that started with me, I don't know how many of them are still practising.

So learning homeopathy clearly is not just about helping people prescribe; it is about validating the chosen philosophical framework (homeopathic) and then helping them validate their experiences by reviewing their understanding of the world. This is one way of looking at what a remedy does. And that is the starting point because many of the people who graduate don't practise. They need to be exposed to as much personal development, validation and acknowledgment as possible. Then they will know that it is OK that we think differently from everybody else and that we can address medical problems based on the experience of the patient and not on what a test says. They will know that people's health is transitory and that we have assumptions in homeopathy that actually support the way people understand their health.

I think it is good that some people will leave the Lakeland College and just want to work with Flower Remedies and set themselves up as Flower Remedy practitioners, and some people do other things, and that is just fine because homeopathy is one of a number of 'energetic' healing modalities. But nonetheless, they all have an appreciation of totality and they all understand what mind, body, soul and spirit means in homeopathy. My aim is for the students to become aware of the context that Hahnemann found himself in and appreciate a lot more about where homeopathy came from. Provings were a new concept - that was Hahnemann's brilliance. But the most appropriate aspect of the *Organon*[4], which I think is hugely misrepresented, is Hahnemann's case taking. And he was light years ahead of anybody else and still is. There are still issues today, such as the two way impact of the environment that the general population only now is starting to understand is important, which Hahnemann wrote about two hundred years ago.

Case taking in homeopathy is unique and extremely pertinent and relevant to every single practitioner of medicine anywhere in the world. When I teach doctors, I don't start by telling them about remedies. Instead, I tell them how we take a case, because it is an eye opener for them. And when doctors sit in on my practice and I take a case, they ask me where I get the information from. That is because they sit and hear, and I sit and listen. Hearing, for me, is a physical thing you do and listening is an active participation in a conversation without influencing it. I think people need to be trained and it is a skill that they have to have when they leave homeopathy school. And that is much more important than how many remedies they know because you can always look up a remedy.

ROWENA: I agree; that is why I teach practitioner development.

SIMON: Listening is not the first thing I teach. The first thing I teach is how to be present, because you cannot listen if you are not present.

ROWENA: The soul and the spirit; what is the difference within homeopathy?

SIMON: Well, the totality in homeopathy consists of the body, mind, soul and spirit. The mind or to use the German gemüt is the home of emotions, like our fears, anxieties, drives and tempers. It is the place of our participative consciousness, which is the way we participate in the world. The geist or spirit is our transcendent, higher, noetic faculty. It is the way we participate in the universe and it is our connection to the universe. Hahnemann clearly states that if the two are not aligned, if there is a difference between what we know we should be doing and how we are actually doing it; that creates pathology. So he says that everybody has a sense of where they are going and what they are doing and what they should be doing to actualise their potential. He is very clear that all illness starts on an energetic level.

He also says that in between the geist and the gemüt the soul or seele spins. *Aphorism 226*[4] describes how diseases are spun and sustained by the seele so affecting the way ideas, sense and impressions get translated. We are born with subtle influences in our life like astrology, miasmatic tendencies and other obstacles to cure and they affect the way we translate things and manifest health in our bodies. These are the recurring patterns and if you don't see the pattern, it keeps hitting you and it keeps you spinning and so it needs to be addressed. So, for me when I take a case, it is about listening not just to the person's emotions and/or their bodies but also to their soul and spirit.

Homeopathy as I prescribe it, is about addressing the biggest totality possible and the biggest totality has got to be body, mind, soul and spirit. From that place, I find, people get better quite quickly. If I cannot get the kind of case that I need, then I start compromising and I narrow my totality to meet where the patient is, always trying to be appropriate. If someone isn't breathing, I am going the give them a remedy to get them breathing. If they are having a heart attack, I will use the smallest totality to prescribe a remedy that will help them and that is allopathic thinking.

For me, prescribing is about being appropriate and is not a choice between homeopathic thinking and allopathic thinking. Big totality homeopathic thinking is great for chronic cases, small totality allopathic thinking is great for acute cases – allopathy nests very nicely in homeopathy. Homeopathy doesn't nest well in allopathy, because homeopathy has a greater view, it is a larger paradigm, rather like an umbrella with allopathy nesting inside it, so much so that a homeopath and a wise practitioner sometimes needs to think allopathically. It is not one or the other; it is about being appropriate to the patient.

In my opinion, teaching is about how students learn the skills necessary to be appropriate to a patient and I think those skills need to be the core backbone of what one learns, and that is what I teach. And that is why I like working at the Lakeland College, because this philosophy is validated there.

ROWENA: And at the Purton House Homeopathic Centre (Purton House), too. That essence runs through the whole college. So where do you think homeopathy is going? Do you think it will ever become dormant again?

SIMON: I am concerned that homeopathy could die because it could get swallowed into an integrated health care programme where the primary responsibility for a patient is taken by an allopathic doctor who will validate tests and research over personal experience. In other words, I see that conventional Western medical practitioners will validate explanations over experience while homeopaths validate experience over explanation. I cannot envisage an integrated medicine approach working for homeopathy, because as I said before, the homeopathic paradigm has a greater worldview than conventional Western medicine. And therefore, allopathy or Western medicine fits nicely into homeopathy but not the other way around.

I am full of admiration for homeopaths that work in allopathic settings. It is very hard to get heard. I have friends who work in the hospitals in Israel and they don't find it easy because the extra/alternative treatment choices cause a lot of tension. But at least in Israel, there are homeopaths and acupuncturists in the hospitals.

ROWENA: Really?

SIMON: Most hospitals. So here in the UK we are miles behind. I feel that many of my patients' understanding of their health is limited and dogged by fears that they have taken on board from our society and culture. And much of my time is spent dealing with people's fears, not their pathology. We used to have the Iron Curtain, it was the East versus the West and it was a way of keeping an element of fear in our society. Now the Iron Curtain has come down, and the fears are redirected to other dynamics, for example, corporations verses conservation and energetic verses material medicine.

The Canadian UN Climate Conference is going on today, as we speak, and there is so much disagreement about the direction to take, that actually in a way it mirrors the homeopathy verses allopathy discussions. Whose research do you agree with and which way do you view things? Are we going to validate everybody's experience of the change in the weather since we were kids or invalidate those experiences by agreeing with some scientifically based research that says that if you take a graph of climate over the last five hundred years there is no change?

ROWENA: But don't you feel that people who would never have used homeopathy a few years ago are now turning to it?

SIMON: Actually, I am afraid I don't. Well maybe people are consuming more remedies from pharmacies but are there more patients seeing homeopaths? – I am not sure. Because every homeopath I know used to see more patients than they do now.

ROWENA: Really.

SIMON: What I am hearing from my colleagues is that maybe there is still roughly the same number of people using homeopathy. There are more homeopaths now and that is one issue. The other issue is that I feel that yes, there is a change in consciousness coming in our generation but we haven't found a way of breaking through to convert the increased numbers who try remedies purchased over the counter into patients who use homeopathy to treat chronic deep seated ills.

I pick up brochures that say, "I practise homeopathy. What is homeopathy? Homeopathy was started two hundred and fifty years ago by Samuel Hahnemann. He proposed the law of like cures like and minimum dose and we use successed, potentised energetic medicines." But I have never read a brochure from an allopath that says, "I practise allopathy. What is allopathy? Allopathic medicine is the refining of petroleum products into 'nature identical' compounds that are compressed with excipients that are often toxic, into a pill prescribed on the basis of the opposite cures!"

We certainly never hear of the two hundred thousand that died from the side effects of allopathic medicine in the USA alone last year but we do hear of the few people for which homeopathy did not work, even though there were no lasting side effects!

Maybe we need to think about homeopathy differently and not promote like cures like, succussion and potentisation, because these terms don't mean anything to the general public. I suggest that homeopaths need to promote their ability to validate experience of life and disease, their ability to understand different ways of making sense of and the embodiment of chronic illness, in other words all that makes one an individual. Maybe it needs a reorientation away from prioritising the right remedy to prioritising the relationship we create with our patients and our brilliance at understanding uniqueness. Homeopathy is not a quest for the right remedy, it is about the right relationship and I feel very strongly about this.

ROWENA: How easy do you think it is being a homeopath compared with twenty years ago?

SIMON: I think it is easier to be a homeopath now than it was when I started because I think people are taught much better than we were and there is a lot more choice regarding how and where to study. Importantly there is a lot more experience to build on so, for example, there is much more exposure to different prescribing methodologies. On the whole, computers have aided homeopathy enormously. Homeopaths are prescribing a lot better with many more remedies, although when I talk about that, I am talking about people who practise homeopathy in a way that I recognise. I stick with the tenets of Hahnemann's homeopathy, in that I prescribe a minimum dose to the biggest totality and I will only give one remedy at a time.

ROWENA: Are there any circumstances in which you would give more than one remedy?

SIMON: Not in the mouth at the same time, no.

ROWENA: Oh ok, you mean not as combinations.

SIMON: Yes, I won't give combination remedies. If someone turns up in my clinic and they are having a major asthma attack and I don't know what remedy to give them, I will line them up with ten remedies with instructions to take one after another every three to four minutes until they find the one that works. The ten starts with *Arsenicum album* and ends with *Oxygenium*. I have only had to send one person to hospital because they got to *Oxygenium* without any remedy working.

I have patients who might take two different remedies on a day, one in the morning and one at night. Particularly patients who have tumours that are painful and need pain relief. If it stops them sleeping, I might give them something to help them sleep. I try to be as appropriate as I can to the patient. My biggest problem is that as I have gained experience patients get better quicker and I need more new patients to keep the same throughput that I had ten to twelve years ago.

ROWENA: What skills do you think make a good homeopath now?

SIMON: I think one needs to practise patient centred homeopathy, rather than remedy centred homeopathy, and that means prioritising the relationship and looking after patients by, for example creating expectations that can be met and helping the patient to be 'process' not 'outcome' oriented. Patients in my experience arrive at my door or telephone because of recommendation. So I try not to piss people off because it leads to fewer recommendations.

ROWENA: And do you find that sometimes people come to you and it is just not necessarily the right remedy but the relationship that they have with you?

SIMON: Well, often I don't give the right remedy, whatever the right remedy is. What I mean is, often the remedy doesn't produce the kind of dynamic shift that I would like in a patient and I need to change the remedy. It is the quality of my relationship that enables me to say, "Hey, listen, we messed up there, let us try another remedy; I have got another one up my sleeve" or, "You have had one snake remedy, it didn't work; let us try another snake." And that happens often.

ROWENA: And they feel comfortable to open up to you?

SIMON: Yes, I hope so, because I create a climate of safety with the expectation where people know that it may not be about one curative remedy. Changes in health involve a journey that we have to go on together with the patient.

Most people get the remedy before they leave the room, anyway. I do what I call a reality check. I say to my patients, "This is what I am prescribing for. This is what I see. Do you agree with me?" And if they go, "No", then I know I need to think differently, and if they go "Yes", I go, "Great" and then I say, "And that picture matches this picture of this remedy." So patients get involved in the process. I do this little reality check, which I think is very important, otherwise how do I know if I am barking up the wrong tree? I get my students to do it because I think it is one of the most successful things I do.

I encourage students that I supervise and teach to summarise a case in five sentences, as if they were going on a ward round in a homeopathic hospital. And if they cannot summarise the case, then I know they haven't got the case. So there is no point in analysing and giving me remedies if they cannot summarise the case. That discipline gives me the reality check. In my mind, I summarise the case in five or six sentences at the end of a first appointment, and that is what I give to the patient, and the patient goes, "Yes, I agree." And if I cannot do that, then there is no point in going for the remedy; I need more information. And I like to make a difference in two weeks; if they haven't got a change in two weeks, then we review things together.

ROWENA: So have you worked over the years with patients who haven't gone down the chemotherapy route?

SIMON: Yes, many of them.

ROWENA: Do you advise your patients not to have chemotherapy?

SIMON: For me, chemo is the last form of medieval medicine left in the conventional Western medical armoury. It is mostly untargeted, hugely toxic and kills people. So in my experience, the people who survive the best, certainly with the best quality of life, are the people who haven't been on chemotherapy, and that is without question. However, I have treated people on chemotherapy who have come through it and done very well.

ROWENA: Do you advise people against it?

SIMON: I advise people to look at all their options and take the most intrusive last, and chemotherapy is the last option, so hopefully homeopathy has got them better before the time they would have arrived at the last option.

ROWENA: So you wouldn't have chemotherapy yourself?

SIMON: Absolutely not. There is not a chance in hell that you could put chemotherapy in me.

ROWENA: What about an operation?

SIMON: I have had surgery. Thankfully, not for cancer. If it is a definable tumour and you can just take out the lump, then why not, if it is stopping something flowing properly? But I give patients remedies, and their fibroids that they thought were through the wall of the lining of their uterus drop out so they no longer need surgery. And I am sure there are other homeopaths that have had similar experiences.

ROWENA: Do you give constitutional treatment, as opposed to these protocols that people talk about for fibroids?

SIMON: I don't believe in protocols for anything, because how can you be appropriate to a patient if you are limited to a given protocol? The other day I taught methodologies, and I think the class worked out that there were thirty six different methodologies you can use for a case. I cannot be fixed on one way of doing things.

That reflects the way I look at the world. I am in business to find what is unique and different in every patient. It is very easy to suddenly see the world as, "Everybody needs *Carcinosin* "or "Everybody needs *Tuberculinum bovinum*" because everybody is restless (*Carcinosin*) and the grass is greener on the other side of the fence (*Tuberculinum bovinum*). I am in business to appreciate and understand the unique subtleties in people, and their tendencies to behave, think, do, walk and breathe in different ways. We have thousands of remedies. Someone comes to me for asthma and I think there are six hundred and eighty different asthma remedies in the repertory. So I am going to sit there and I am going to work out which five or six of these six hundred and eighty resonate with the person in front of me.

ROWENA: So it is about understanding them as a person?

SIMON: Exactly. And, in my opinion, we should avoid defining remedies as solely acute or chronic. I have a case of cancer cured with *Arnica*.

ROWENA: I took on a fertility case last year. She had had two ectopic pregnancies, and when she came to see me I really prescribed *Natrum muriaticum* and all her headaches went away and she was feeling a whole lot better. But she had some IVF and it wasn't successful. Since then, she has had *Carcinosin, Folliculinum*, as well as *Agnus castus* herbally to lower her Follicle-stimulating hormone levels, with success. She then went to a different specialist who said that she had a massive fibroid. So I don't know why after a year of treatment that fibroid hasn't gone.

SIMON: Because fibroids are very difficult to get rid of. And if the person is very tense in their pelvic girdle, and none of the remedies have released the tension then how are they going to get rid of the fibroids?

ROWENA: What would you have done differently?

SIMON: What would I do differently? I don't know, but because of my training, I look at how my patient walks, how they hold themselves, how they breathe. I do facial, tongue and pulse diagnosis so I build up a picture that reveals an in-depth picture of them. I give them a questionnaire that they fill in before they come to see me so that I don't have to waste time during the consultation on questions like what food do they eat, how regularly do they go to toilet, what are their blood sugar levels and how are their periods.

ROWENA: How do you relate that back to remedies?

SIMON: Their answers give me modalities before I even begin. At the end of the day, if I have got two or three remedies that are in the same family or related, my decision is going to be based on modalities.

ROWENA: Simon, if you wanted to design a college now, what would it be like?

SIMON: Materia medica wouldn't be the core of the school curriculum. I think that after the first year, second, third and fourth years can all study materia medica together. In fact, they can teach each other materia medica. I have never understood why certain remedies are given in the third year. What makes a remedy a second or third year remedy? So I would teach all the materia medica lessons to everybody at the same time.

ROWENA: That would save so much time.

SIMON: Absolutely, because it is not the number of remedies you learn, it is how you learn them which is important. People need to acquire the skills of appreciating and understanding a remedy. For example, *Bellis perennis* isn't just a trauma remedy for spines; it can be a remedy for the totality of trauma in somebody. *Arnica* is good for skin cancer and other cancers too; it is not seen as just a trauma remedy.

The core of a college curriculum for me would be about all the skills, capacities and capabilities that you need to acquire to become a successful practitioner in relationship with the patient, so the relationship becomes the core of the curriculum. As a consequence, by the time a student leaves the school, they are very clear about who they are as well as what they are doing. Taking a case is the most important part of homeopathy and would start from day one in the school.

As far as my understanding goes, from my limited – although ten years of studying it – exposure to the world of quantum physics, homeopathy to me is a prime example of a quantum medicine. And what is lacking in conventional Western medicine is that it hasn't taken the quantum world on board. But it is integral to homeopathy; homeopathy is quantum medicine. So that means that a quantum approach needs to be taught from the start.

ROWENA: Have you seen movie *What The Bleep Do We Know*[137]?

SIMON: I have. I thought it was very good for a layperson; but homeopaths should be way beyond *What the Bleep*[137] ! They should understand about tendency and intention and the subtle forces that are at play, because they explain homeopathy. And it recognises a different language, and that language is based on experience, not on explanation.

ROWENA: How do you feel about homeopathy courses now having degree status? It does seem to be the way that the profession is moving.

SIMON: I think it is the way that some people in the profession are moving. Personally, I don't think it is necessary to have a degree to be a homeopath; it is adult education. I have a problem that some of the homeopaths that I am now being asked to supervise are nineteen or twenty years old. How do you explain to someone of that age about the subtleties of life that need to be observed in order to prescribe, when they haven't been taught that for the three years in their school already? It has to go in from the beginning with a seventeen year old; they have to start understanding what the differences are between hearing and listening, and what it means to be present. As you know, Hahnemann discusses freedom from bias, healthy senses, attention while observing and fidelity in recording. That is a high standard to attain. It is all about participating in something without influencing what goes on; transference and countertransference. That means they have got to be immersed in that for three years. And I don't see that happening.

ROWENA: Do you think people are capable of being homeopaths at any age?

SIMON: I think so, yes, but you cannot suddenly introduce practitioner and personal development in the fourth year and expect them to pick it up when they are meant to be taking cases already.

ROWENA: Do you think that you can with somebody who is older?

SIMON: With someone who is older, maybe, but I still think it should be introduced earlier on anyway. Homeopathy for me is a perfect profession for adult learners and you have got to treat them as adults. You have got to support them in learning as adults. They need to have some immersion time; they need to be immersed in homeopathy for five days in a row, maybe twice a year. If you are going to do sea remedies, take them to the sea or at least an aquarium. You know what I mean? It helps to take people to different environments and have them immersed in homeopathy. It works well with for the Open University, for the Dynamis School.

ROWENA: And some of the other colleges do it too; the Welsh School of Homoeopathy for instance.

SIMON: That is good to hear. I also think that the final year of a course should include a solid grounding in how to set up a practice, how to run a small business and how to refine your prescribing process so you can actually make money.

We need a profession for people to go in, where they can earn a decent living. It is ridiculous that homeopaths down the road are charging half of what I charge. How are they surviving?

ROWENA: Do you think you should charge more, the more experience you have?

SIMON: Well, not necessarily. I think we should charge a valid, decent rate that affords a good standard of living as expected in other professions. There is a poverty mentality that has shadowed the development of homeopathy, hopefully it will go.

ROWENA: Who inspires you now Simon?

SIMON: I am hugely inspired by the students I facilitate, and by Jeremy Sherr and Jan Scholten. But the people who inspire me the most are my patients.

ROWENA: One cannot argue with that! Thank you so much for our chat today Simon; I have found it inspiring.

CHAPTER 32:   JEREMY SHERR

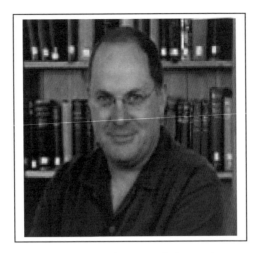

On Monday 5 December 2005 I ventured up to Malvern. It was a year and a week since I had attended the teachers' seminar there, when I had met several of the teachers on my list with whom I then went on to interview. Jeremy Sherr was the most challenging of all to organise because of his busy schedule. But I managed to tie him down for a few hours, the evening after one of his clinics and at the start of a Dynamis School teaching week. He was extremely welcoming and open to talking endlessly with me on a subject we both feel so passionately about – homoeopathy - which he insisted I spell in the old way for his interview!

"I am concerned about AIDS and twenty five million people dying in Africa. Whole populations are being wiped out and billions of US dollars are being poured into allopathic nonsense. People are going through untold suffering, not only the dying but also those that are left behind. If homoeopathy can help, then it has to; that is the one thing that we need to achieve."   *Jeremy Sherr, December 2005*

"Nearly every patient to whom you give a good remedy will come back with a lesson for you. They will come back and say one little sentence that will resonate with you; they will come and give you their gift back."   *Jeremy Sherr, December 2005*

"The second prescription is in my mind the highest art of homoeopathy. That first prescription is like moving your first pawn forward but it is not checkmate. Checkmate comes after a lot of moves and a lot of careful following through with long-term case management."   *Jeremy Sherr, December 2005*

"I know that as long as I am capable of practising, I will practise. As long as I can move or even think, I will practise homoeopathy."   *Jeremy Sherr, December 2005*

CHAPTER 32: JEREMY SHERR

ROWENA: I have already done some research on you, Jeremy, so I know you first heard about homoeopathy in a bar in London. Could you tell me more about that?

JEREMY: That is right. You know what they say about the 60s; if you can remember it, you weren't there! But I was there, because I cannot remember it. All I remember is that I was very drunk or stoned. I had this conversation with somebody and I said, "What are you doing?" and he said "Homoeopathy." And I asked, "What is it?" and he replied, "Like cures like." You know, whoever is meant to be a homoeopath has susceptibility and all they need is a single dose. And that is the way it was, even though it took two or three years until I actually started to study because there were no colleges then. But I knew that is what I was going to do. I was living in a squat in Huntley Road at the time and then I went back to Israel and had a motorcycle accident followed by a few months in hospital and that sealed the deal.

ROWENA: You were quite a wild boy then?

JEREMY: Yes, I was a wild boy and still am but in different ways. When it comes to 'wild' experiences, I have done it all and I have dropped a lot of stuff by the wayside; from whiskey to coffee to dope. I am very clean living now but I replaced the old journeys with provings, so I am still dropping stuff but in homoeopathic form. I am doing a proving right now.

ROWENA: Do you know what it is?

JEREMY: I know what it is because I choose the remedy for my class, but they don't know. They have been on it for a few weeks but I only took it last week. My wife took it as well, so we are doing the proving together.

ROWENA: Do you get any cures during a proving?

JEREMY: There is a difference between a cure and a proving. The proving is hopefully an inaccurate prescription, whereas a cure is hopefully an accurate prescription. But it might end up that your prescribed remedy is inaccurate and therefore a proving, or that your proving remedy is unintentionally accurate and therefore a curing. You never know.

I observed that in every class that does a proving, there are twenty to thirty percent who feel better. And it is often people who have been looking for their constitutional remedy for years; they take the proving and loads of symptoms vanish. I can recall at least one case of cure in every proving.

ROWENA: So do you think spiritually they were just there because they were meant to be?

JEREMY: That might be the case. Or it might just be a random event, but the statistics are higher than you would expect. A lot of people benefit from provings. Another strange thing is that in many classes there will be a few who are petrified of doing the proving. Some of them will do it anyway and some will run away. The strange thing is that the people who are most petrified often have curative responses. This is not a law, just an observation – I have seen it four or five times in different provings.

I remember a lady who was absolutely terrified of doing a proving; she cried during the whole first year. In the second year we did the proving of *Jade* and she did fantastically on it - a perfect cure. I remember similar cures during the provings of *Germanium*, *Sapphire* and *Salmon* (*Onchorynchus tschawytscha*). They were all terrified of the proving but courageously went ahead and did it and enjoyed excellent cures. I am talking about cures of persistent physical, mental and emotional symptoms. It differs from remedy to remedy. Some provings 'accidentally' help a lot of people and some, just one or two, but I have never seen a proving that hasn't cured someone.

ROWENA: That is fascinating.

JEREMY: Another strange phenomena is that, in a couple of cases, the people who left the classes because they didn't want to do a proving, came back to see me in clinic three or four years later and the remedy they escaped from was the remedy that they needed and helped them. If they had done the proving earlier, it might have saved them some three years of suffering. Again, this is not a law; it is just anecdotal.

I believe very much that the correct sequence in homoeopathy must be provings first, followed by cases and finally, materia medica. The provings should suggest a basic materia medica and the picture should be developed through clinical cases. I publish provings without my opinion unless I have used the remedy for a few years. I avoid premature essences, and sometimes I get criticism for that as people are looking for the cherry on the cake. If somebody just gives an 'essence, you will lose the totality of the proving, its tempo, language and deeper secrets. The essence is only five percent of the totality and you might as well not have done a proving for that.

ROWENA: So how does one get one's head around a proving when it is just a long list of symptoms? I struggle with that.

JEREMY: It is difficult and this is a problem in homoeopathy. If you have a proving that is not divided into themes it is very difficult. It takes two to three days to study a proving full-time to get an idea of what is going on but it is hard work. You have to know what you

431

are doing and it is not easy. If somebody has divided it into themes for you – anger, irritability, delusions – then it is a bit easier because they have chewed on it for you, but you are going to have to swallow it and digest it and that is hard.

As there are approximately ten new provings a month, people cannot get to grips with all this information. I am partly responsible as I helped create the proving boom in the first place. Looking back, it is twenty three years since I did the *Scorpion (Androctonos amurreuxi hebraeus)* proving. At the time it was the only new proving. When there is only one new proving a month, learning it is manageable. But now, there are so many provings that nobody can swallow them all. I have many of the new published proving books and I am not keeping up. So on the one hand, I don't want to succumb to the essence idea but on the other hand we need to devise a way where it is easier to get to grips with so much information.

Yet there is no doubt that we need these provings. A famous homoeopath came to me and said, "Look, there are enough remedies, we don't need any more provings." The next month I had a case of a patient with MS who had been seen by this homoeopath for many years and had been given many remedies. I gave her *Germanium* and she did really well on it, which proved to me yet again that each new remedy is needed. I have successfully prescribed many of the new remedies; *Lac leoninum, Butterfly, Plastic (Polystyrenum), Raven (Corvus corax), Ozonum* and *Neptunium* and of course all my own provings. I am devising a computer programme, which is going to chew up all the information, digest it and make it easier to study without losing sight of the totality and all the symptoms. That is my big project for the next few years and I am very excited about it.

ROWENA: How do you have the energy?

JEREMY: It is easy because I love what I do. My passion is my driving force and it gives me energy.

ROWENA: So you are Hahnemann's zodiac sign.

JEREMY: Actually I am proud to say that I was born exactly two hundred years after him. He was born in April 1755 and I was born in April 1955. It is not a big thing but I like to brag about it!

ROWENA: I am an Aries too.

JEREMY: You can always tell an Aries by how smug they are about being an Aries!

ROWENA: I know exactly what you mean!

432

JEREMY: Aries like to start new ventures and have plenty of new challenges, but we need Virgos and Capricorns around to perfect and finish the job or we create a lot of unfinished projects. I am very fortunate to have many friends and students that help me. Tina Quirk in the USA is marvellously meticulous. We have spent the last five years working on planning an AIDS project in Africa. I believe AIDS in Africa is one of the most important diseases for us to treat because really that is the big issue.

ROWENA: Absolutely. What about the other current epidemics? What about bird flu?

JEREMY: There are many other diseases and epidemics around the world that need treating, malaria, cholera, tuberculosis (TB) etc. However, I think that the bird flu scare is an irrelevant. They are just feeding it to us in order to generate more money for vaccinations and pharmaceutical companies. When and if it comes, it will be relevant but it is not here now. What has been created around it is just spin.

ROWENA: Do you think bird flu will come? What should our approach to it be?

JEREMY: Eventually, yes, it will, but Hahnemann specifically says of epidemics, "Don't worry or speculate about it until it comes." He states the reason very clearly in *Aphorism 100*[4], which says, "Always treat the epidemic that is here. Don't look at last year, or the year before." The reason for this is that viruses mutate quicker than we can develop solutions. If you get stuck in the past and lag behind them, you have lost the battle because they will have mutated fast forward into the future.

Allopaths always prescribe last year's vaccine because it takes them so long to develop it, but we can do it homoeopathically in one or two weeks. The only way to help is to be absolutely 'here and now' when an epidemic happens. Yesterday I read about a doctor who gave a vaccine to sixty patients with bird flu in Thailand. It didn't work and it made them worse because it is not related to the current epidemic. So as homoeopaths there is no use speculating what remedy will be needed, as it limits our freedom from prejudice. We need to wait for the real symptoms to appear, and you cannot get those from allopathic reports. As a result, I don't care about bird flu; when it comes, it comes.

But I am concerned about AIDS and twenty five million people dying in Africa. Whole populations are being wiped out and billions of US dollars are being poured into allopathic nonsense. People are going through untold suffering, not only the dying, but those that are left behind. If homoeopathy can help, then it has to be our mission; that is the one thing that we need to achieve. There are a lot of very great and noble homoeopaths that have gone out to Kenya or Swaziland, and sit in clinics and treat one person after another and that is fantastic; I really admire them. In some ways I would really like to do that but I don't see that as necessarily being my role. My aspiration is to help in a formal, academic way.

I believe we have got to go out there and say, "Look, this is what homoeopathy can do in AIDS cases; here are the figures, here is the research, it is all watertight." Billions of US dollars go to AIDS in Africa every year; if a small fraction went to homoeopathy, can you imagine what we could do? But nobody is going to give money or resources to anything anecdotal. I can show fantastic AIDS cases on video, where you clearly see people getting better and coming off their drugs. We can go and show these and a lot of other evidence to Bill Gates and Elton John charities or any other AIDS charity, but that is not going to impress them. They won't give us money on anecdotal evidence. They want to see academic figures; that is the way.

I personally am too impatient for academics, research and statistics but I feel that it has got to be done. Therefore I have been working to set up a proper research study of homoeopathy treating HIV and AIDS patients. And because I have contacts and a bit of a name, maybe I can get it off the ground, with a little luck and help from my friends. But it has been very frustrating, because the academic wheels grind far too slowly for me. You have to find willing partners and get a protocol through an ethics committee, and you need to talk their language. I hope it will work but if not, I will just go and do it on a small scale myself - I am determined to do that.

ROWENA: So what would your project involve?

JEREMY: Ideally it would involve treating three to five hundred AIDS patients over a couple of years. The aim is twofold; one, to treat individually and show the efficacy of homoeopathy for these patients and two, to look for a genus epidemicus for AIDS, providing it is an epidemic. Epidemics have certain characteristics and AIDS is one foot in and one foot out. I do not want to hear what this or that homoeopath gave an AIDS patient; I just want to collect the symptoms for myself, as Hahnemann said we should do with epidemics, and see.

I went to Tanzania as I have a friend there, Sigsbert Rwegasira; a homoeopath and a lovely guy. He also has a hundred percent success in treating malaria, which is still the biggest killer the world has ever known. The allopaths are poisoning people with pharmaceuticals such as Lariam, which is causing absolute devastation. He has treated five thousand AIDS patients. I went for a week and treated twenty AIDS cases and collected all the symptoms, and we are getting really good results.

ROWENA: Did you take malaria prophylaxis yourself?

JEREMY: No, because I just went to Dar es Salaam, which is a city and not a malarial region. If I went to a malarial region, I would. You know, there is nothing against prophylaxis in homoeopathy; it is perfectly classical. Practitioners have used it from Hahnemann onwards and it is only some neopseudoclassical delusion that says that homoeopathic prophylaxis isn't homoeopathy, because if you can prevent suffering we should prevent it!

ROWENA: And do you prescribe *Malaria officinalis*, or do you go for the *Natrum muriaticum* and *China* option?

JEREMY: Malaria officinalis, which is made from decomposed vegetable matter, can be useful. However, I prefer *Natrum muriaticum* or *China sulphuricum*. They have worked very well in my experience. There is a certain sequence in prophylaxis prescribing; the best remedy is the main one of the genus epidemicus of the epidemic that is happening at the time, because you want to hit the mutation that is happening now. If it has not been worked out yet, then you can work with the known remedies for the specific epidemic. If you don't have that, then you prescribe the nosode or something similar. But when you are talking about malaria, it is not really an epidemic; it is endemic, so there are fixed remedies that are known to treat malaria.

ROWENA: What are your thoughts about there being a hospital here in the UK where professional homoeopaths can practise?

JEREMY: A homoeopathic hospital anywhere would be wonderful. Every homoeopath plays with that idea and, of course, I have done so too. My dream would be a university hospital; it just needs somebody to come along with fifty million bucks. For some people that is small cash and I can see exactly how it would work.

ROWENA: I remember I read an interview where you talked about this before, but it was written before the universities such as the University of Westminster and Lancashire validated a degree in homoeopathy. So do you think that now that we have those within our profession we are getting closer to your dream?

JEREMY: No, I don't think the degree is even tickling it. There is a long way from a BA or MA to a medical university hospital. All respect to them but, in my opinion, the universities don't yet offer a better homoeopathic course than the other colleges. In some ways it is a step forward and in other ways it isn't, because they have had to compromise in order to fit into the system. We need a full-time course with all the facilities that stands on its own and isn't designed to fit into the allopathic paradigm.

In the USA, you can study a five year naturopathy course leading to a kind of Doctor's degree (ND), with homoeopathy as part of the syllabus. I have taught in all these establishments but I cannot say that the homoeopathy is any better compared to how we teach it here in the UK because it is viewed through naturopaths' eyes. Homoeopathy has always been the black sheep even within alternative medicine. If you ask any homoeopathy class how many were the black sheep of the family many will raise their hands. It is like

435

that with homoeopathy too; people don't want it because it doesn't conform. They would much rather play with safe stuff like herbs, needles, vitamins and water therapy. Even the naturopaths regard homoeopathy with a bit of caution. We need a course that leads to doctor status in the field of homoeopathy, not naturopathy. There are other countries that are closer, for instance in South Africa and India they have five year homoeopathy medical courses.

ROWENA: Can you see that happening?

JEREMY: Maybe the reason it has not happened so far is because we are not really ready. We are only in the toddler stage of our development as a profession but we are moving forward. Twenty five years ago we were still embryonic. Martin Miles would give a brilliant evening talk once a month and we would all go; it was the only talk there was. Today there are so many teachers and projects. My wife was involved in Homoeopathy For A Change; she went to Honduras for three months and taught and prescribed there. Schools are opening in Africa. I have taught in China. Homoeopathy has just taken off in Japan and the Far East.

ROWENA: You must know homoeopaths that would be keen.

JEREMY: There are many keen people, but keen is one thing, and able and willing to commit to a project and come up with the goods is another. When I did the *Jade* proving, the thought that went around in my head all day was, "There are three kinds of people - doers, thinkers and wankers." That is part of the *Jade* picture. Doers are top of the hierarchy, then people who just think about it and lastly those who don't do anything.

ROWENA: Talk to me about how this is a symptom?

JEREMY: I wasn't the only one that had these thoughts, other people had this symptom in different guises as well. It is about people who don't do anything in their lives, they just think about it. *Jade* is a remedy that really puts you in your power spot. It did for me, and was curative. It kind of gives you the power of an emperor; the wizard's hat. Of course it can take it away as well, leaving you powerless!

ROWENA: Do you feel that the UK is saturated with homoeopaths and there are not enough patients?

JEREMY: Yes, that is the case, which is evident because not everybody can make a living. I think those who really want to make a living from it, will, because there are plenty of sick people around, but it is not easy. It takes a long time to build a homoeopathic practice. There are two things that bring people to a homoeopath - the carrot and the stick. I have seen four new patients today and at least three of them have come because of the stick –

arthritis and MS - they didn't know anything about homoeopathy but somebody mentioned to them that it might help. Those that come from the carrot of awareness, of course, make the best patients.

ROWENA: How long, would you say, does it take to build a practice?

JEREMY: At least two years. A lot of people want to study homoeopathy because it is fascinating. At least thirty percent of them are not practitioner material. They like to study and write excellent essays but when it comes to sitting all day with patients, they decide it is not for them. I still think they should study homoeopathy, but there should be a differentiation and filtering process to help students find out if they do actually want to actually practise, so that if they don't, the guilt at not succeeding is taken away. They could become a homoeopathic historian, develop computer programs, organise charities or treat friends and family.

ROWENA: Or do administration in a hospital?

JEREMY: Exactly that. There are all kinds of support roles our profession needs. We could do with more people writing articles for the press. But those students who do not practise can end up feeling guilty; they try to build a practice but it only half works. Many want to be practitioners but have all kinds of restraints – financial constraints, kids, divorce - so it is difficult to hold on until a practice gets going. Then you have got the forty percent who get through the initial hurdles and succeed.

Part of the problem financially for us is the fact that we see patients once every four to six weeks. In comparison, an acupuncturist or an osteopath sees a patient one or two times a week. Patients book in for six treatments and they hear their neck cracking and are happy with what they see as an immediate result. With homoeopaths there is a four to six week wait so there is a high drop out rate. Patients think, "He gave me one little white pill but I didn't hear a crack and there were no fireworks. I am not going back just to talk."

ROWENA: Prescribing LMs helps.

JEREMY: Yes, daily repetitions, phone contact and booking patients for a follow up at the end of the first appointment all help as they make the process conscious. This is basic business management but it is still going to be a very slow, logarithmic build up. Eventually there will be a build up of patients, especially after you find the golden patients who recommend you to another thirty. But you have to get past those first two years and not everybody makes it. Working part time can also stop practitioners from building their practice, as subconsciously they might want to keep it part time before giving up their day job. The market is saturated to a degree, but it doesn't have to be. If some of those people who write beautiful essays but do not want to practise did some research, wrote articles or gave talks it would raise public awareness.

ROWENA: So tell me why graduates come to study with you at the Dynamis School. What is it all about?

JEREMY: Homoeopathic colleges are just a first step. There is much more to be taught in homoeopathy than what is learnt in undergraduate college. People who come to the Dynamis School want to go deeper into the philosophy and practical aspects. Some Dynamis students study alongside their undergraduate course while others may have up to twenty five years of practise. I have never had a problem with the diversity of levels because I am not teaching horizontally; I am going deeper. You can always go deeper, it doesn't matter what stage you are at. And the deeper you go, the better the results and the more pleasure you get from practise. We build strong philosophical roots so people know exactly where they are coming from and where they are going to, and that makes all the difference. A lot of people want to get continued support and share knowledge, and a lot of people just love studying homoeopathy.

ROWENA: Are you going to keep the Dynamis School going? If I delay studying with you for, say, a couple of years, will I have missed my opportunity?

JEREMY: Since I started the Dynamis School eighteen years ago, there have always been rumours that it is going to stop and I don't make those rumours up myself! I should, but I don't! I love Dynamis; that is where I have fun. It gives me great satisfaction to teach the same group for two years and see their progress. The truth is two years isn't enough but I do two years because people wouldn't come if I did four! But at the end of the course most students say they would love to continue.

Part of the course is long-term live cases; that way students can learn much more than the first prescription, like case management, remedy reaction and second prescription. When one takes cases in front of students you really have to have faith and drop the ego. But the group energy helps. I do my best but if I fail then everybody can share the failure and we try to learn from it. And if I succeed, then everybody can share the success too. There is always learning to be had, whatever the outcome. You have to come to a place in yourself where you believe that you will be able to solve the case in that hour in front of all those students. It is a good challenge!

ROWENA: How many remedies have you proved Jeremy?

JEREMY: I don't know exactly, but I think it is somewhere between twenty seven and thirty.

ROWENA: How do you choose them?

JEREMY: I have two methods of choosing; intellect and omens. An intellect choice is like when I decided to prove all the noble gases because I know that they can increase our knowledge of the whole periodic table.

ROWENA: Are they for very spiritual people?

JEREMY: Yes, there is something spiritual about the noble gases, because at their full potential they can really touch heaven.

ROWENA: So they feel very connected to the source; to God?

JEREMY: They can be very connected to the source, if they are in the right place. But their problem is that they don't know how to disconnect from it. They feel they are in such a perfect position and everything is so right that they cannot step into life and get dirty, and if you don't get dirty, you are not living. You have to suffer if you want to sing the blues.

So proving the noble gases was an intellectual decision but other remedies I chose through omens or synchronicities. *Swan (Cygnus cygnus)* was an omen choice. I was sitting by the sea with a very sore neck, and this swan sailed by. I had previously asked for an omen and you have to ask for one otherwise you don't get it.

ROWENA: Like in Paulo Coelho's *The Alchemist*[138]?

JEREMY: Yes, absolutely. To get omens, you have to believe in them, ask for them, and not miss them when they are revealed to you. When I asked for an omen before choosing fallow deer, in one day five people mentioned deer to me or showed me pictures of deer and then I saw a TV documentary and that sealed the deal.

ROWENA: Do you think sometimes that your patients move you spiritually on your own journey?

JEREMY: Definitely. Patients come who are in a high place spiritually and they will impart something to you, but nearly every patient to whom you give a good remedy will come back with a lesson for you. They will come back and say one little sentence that will resonate with you; they will come and give you their gift back.

ROWENA: A lesson about the remedy, or a lesson for yourself?

JEREMY: Both a lesson for me and a lesson about the remedy, and that is a gift in itself. It will often be just what I need to hear for that day and will pick me up and make me feel better about life.

ROWENA: Do you think that you get those patients that need your remedies or do you think we are all getting them but we just don't recognise the remedy picture?

JEREMY: A bit of both. Maybe some get attracted to me because they need those remedies, maybe because I know those remedies I recognise them in patients and maybe other people miss them because they don't know them. There was an interesting experiment in India that some homoeopaths did ten or so years ago. They did sixty provings and then created a homoeopathic network in a few centres across India, and for two years, they worked exclusively with those remedies, and they got great results.

I could probably survive only prescribing my thirty remedies and just about get by, but it would not be great homoeopathy. Hahnemann only used twenty remedies for many years until he proved a hundred. You can work with a small number of remedies that you know very well and get reasonable results, because similars work, not just simillimums. If only simillimums worked, we would all be out of business! Hahnemann says there is no such thing as a simillimum.

ROWENA: Really?

JEREMY: He says it is just a theoretical concept and I agree with him. It does give us a beacon to work towards but it is a delusion that gets planted into people at college until they start practising and hopefully realise there is no such thing. If there is a simillimum for each person, and we have only proved three thousand remedies, then how are we finding the simillimum for millions of patients around the world? We cannot be.

There are a hundred thousand minerals and plants and a hundred million animals and insects. Curing like with like is about metaphor and analogy, not sameness, so there cannot be one simillimum and we don't want there to be a simillimum either, just like there can never be only one perfect poem for each person.

Homoeopathy is poetry or music because it is analogy. You don't say to somebody, "Your eyes are beautiful, like eyes!" You say, "Your eyes are like the lake in the spring and your hair is like the wind blowing through the soft leaves as they fall to the ground in the autumn." If it is the right music, rhythm and words, it will touch. So many poems touch you and they will do so in different ways. Some poems will be better than other poems, and they will touch deeper and longer and carry you further. And some will be crap and not touch much at all!

We want to work 'in the image of' and it is better that way because it means that every level of practitioner can get results. It allows practitioners the possibility of not being perfect. If you take a case in any class, if you have got twenty homoeopaths, it is likely that you will get fifteen different remedy suggestions.

ROWENA: And do you think all fifteen remedies will work?

JEREMY: Probably three or four would act beneficially; some more, some less. It is a matter of how close you get by percentage. Those within ten percent of the target would get a good result, those within twenty percent would get a medium result and with those out of range, nothing much would happen or they would suppress the case. It is a grey area between the unattainable Holy Grail of the theoretical simillimum and suppression. It is not black and white 'suppressed' or 'cured'. The problem with the simillimum concept is that it messes people's heads up. All these cases that are published as a definite case of a particular remedy encourage practitioners to have fixed ideas of how that remedy looks. Students see a video and think that this is how the face of that remedy looks, and your little essence is formed and it gets neatly stuck instead of remaining fluid and dynamic.

ROWENA: What about what practical homoeopaths call 'part-patient' homoeopathy?

JEREMY: Obviously practical homoeopathy is not my way and I have a lot of fear for the damage it can do to homoeopathy. These practices use potentised remedies and homoeopathic principles in a very crude manner. But I am not knocking the individuals who study there, because I get a lot of wonderful students that have been to colleges that teach in a practical way and sometimes get results in cases where classical homoeopathy won't, especially where there is a lot of heavy pathology. This is not because classical homoeopathy cannot deal with these cases, but because it is much more sophisticated and therefore more difficult to apply. Hence people opt for 'easypathy'. But when you start from the easy short cuts it is very difficult to work up. I prefer to start from the highest ideal, and then know when to compromise, but if we start from the bottom of compromise, we will forever compromise.

ROWENA: OK, I am following you.

JEREMY: Some do manage to move to a higher level of homoeopathy, because they are climbers and have a bigger vision, but it is very difficult to change once you have that mind set. An old homoeopath who had been an engineer once told me, "You can bend a pipe into any shape you want, but you can never straighten it again." In my opinion, if you cure the person behind the drug picture, you will get the cure on all the levels from the inside out, including heavy pathology and obstacles. It isn't always easy to see the case but prescribing for isolated parts of the case or trying to clean out exciting causes and allopathic drugs is not the best that homoeopathy can offer. It is just symptom ping pong.

441

ROWENA: Sheilagh Creasy says that homoeopaths still get cancer because of homoeopathic suppression. What do you think?

JEREMY: I remember there was a debate in homoeopathy at one time on the subject of why patients who have been treated homoeopathically still get cancer. One of our delusions as homoeopaths is thinking that if we take our so-called constitutional remedy on a regular basis, we are immune to every disease forever but this is rubbish. Cancer is a statistical possibility in all of us at all times; it is a process that is potentially happening in our body at every moment, as cells duplicate. If we lower our resistance with drugs, alcohol, cigarettes, vaccinations, radiation and stress, it will start to perpetuate. And if we strengthen ourselves and are healthier, there is less of a chance.

Let us say, somebody has a thirty seven percent chance of getting cancer, because their parents had it, or they were exposed to cadmium in childhood, or because they cooked in a microwave; you treat them homoeopathically for five years, and now they only have an eighteen percent chance of having cancer. But it is still eighteen percent, and that eighteen percent can happen. If you don't treat them well and you give them drugs that cause suppression, toxic food and bad thoughts, then that thirty seven percent could increase to fifty two percent chance of getting cancer. If they are poisoned by a radioactive substance it will increase to ninety five percent, and so on.

Remedies change throughout treatment. In eighty to ninety percent of cases, a person needs one remedy for life. Let us say, they were born *Aurum metallicum*, and they had their first grief, *Aurum*, their second grief, *Aurum*, their first love disappointment, followed by a job loss, still *Aurum*. They always develop situations and react as *Aurum*. Now, if they get *Aurum* over two or three years, you are really saying, "Come on, and learn the *Aurum* lesson so you can stop being *Aurum*!" If they are not going to learn the lesson and move on, we are wasting our time. When they have finally learned the lesson of *Aurum* and they don't need to be *Aurum* anymore, they need to graduate to the next lesson and need another remedy. So when I say eighty to ninety percent of the cases need one remedy for life, I mean until they have actually received the remedy in sufficient amounts to eradicate their constitutional pathology. Hence, one of the laws I formulated is: The remedy will truly change only when its susceptibility has been fully satisfied.

That is called the second prescription, which is in my mind the highest art of homoeopathy. That first prescription is like moving your first pawn forward but it is not checkmate. Checkmate comes after a lot of moves and a lot of careful following through with long-term case management. That is the problem with the simillimum concept, because it makes you imagine that if you give a person one remedy that is the end of their case.

The remedy needed will truly change once its susceptibility has been satisfied. If the person needed *Aurum metallicum* all their life and you gave ten different remedies, except

Aurum, things will change but they won't truly change. But when you give the *Aurum* and repeat it, that susceptibility is fulfilled. Then you will see the next susceptibility and you will move on. So what do we mean when we say 'one remedy for life?' Are we referring to the entire patient's life, from now until they die, from conception until death? Or do you mean that they need it from their birth until they get the remedy? It is like when somebody sells you a light bulb and they say that it is guaranteed for life. I always wonder, do they mean guaranteed for the life of the bulb, or for my life? Which is it? Once a person has had their simillimum, their life should change dramatically and they, for example, can stop playing *Aurum* and play another game.

Go and look in anybody's practice and show me how many five year and ten year cases on the same remedy they have. If they have got a busy practice it will be about a few percent. I love to see the first remedy change after a couple of years and when it changes, I know homoeopathy has eradicated that level and now they can move onto the next thing. You wait and watch carefully until the next remedy is clear and use all the laws of the second prescription to move further down into the case, deeper and deeper. You can thrash around with part-patient methods and you might get some results, but in the long run the case didn't go anywhere except round the hill, hence these methods are not curative. People say, "Yes, but it works." Sure! Steroids work, Chemotherapy works, raspberry jam therapy works. Whether something 'works' is not a criteria for me. We need to ask ourselves what really needs to be cured and did it get cured?

ROWENA: I tell my patients that they are going to go through a process.

JEREMY: A long process. Homoeopathy is really all about chronic long-term case management. Five years, ten years, if you can get them to continue with homoeopathy that long. That is the game, and it involves obstacles to cure, case management, follow up prescriptions, understanding miasms and the way diseases move and change, how remedies influence a case, unintentional provings, stronger dissimilar disease, acutes and epidemics.

ROWENA: I understand what you mean. So tell me Jeremy, who has inspired you?

JEREMY: Robert Davidson was the first homoeopath who inspired me. In my first lesson in homoeopathy, what he did in two hours, that single dose, was enough to get me going. And even by the second year when I didn't agree with a lot of what he said, it didn't matter because he had given me that gift. He inspired me.

ROWENA: So how did you get to a place of disagreeing with him? What clicked for you?

JEREMY: In homoeopathy you can always tell a person's approach by the first book they read. The first book I read was Kent's *Lectures*[61] and I developed my approach from there. You can agree or disagree with particular things Kent says, but you cannot doubt that he always follows the highest ideal. Robert Davidson took a different path, always searching for something new. He is the perpetual revolutionary. What was the first book you read?

ROWENA: I knew you were going to ask me that, because of the research I have done on your website today! We were told to read George Vithoulkas' *The Science of Homoeopathy*[31], which had a massive impact on me.

JEREMY: That is great, a lot of people started with that book. George Vithoulkas' first book was Boericke[39] it was the only book he had for many years, and hence he has a great knowledge of small remedies. After Kent I read the *Organon*[4] and I started to develop my belief. After that I was inspired by Vassilis Ghegas and Joseph Reves. Since then I am constantly inspired by my students, by proving remedies and by my patients.

ROWENA: Do you think homoeopathy will become dormant again?

JEREMY: It is strong now and I think its time has come, so I think it will prevail. In the USA, as far as I remember, at the start of the twentieth century, there were a hundred thousand homoeopaths, so they say. A lot of them were taught in a practical way, the 'eclectics', as they were called. In Europe I guess there were twenty thousand at that time. In comparison now, just in Brazil alone there are thirty thousand homoeopaths, Mexico probably has forty thousand, Argentina probably has thirty, and India, a hundred thousand. There are now a thousand students in Japan. So do I think it will become dormant again in our time? No.

I think the biggest blow we have received in twenty five years was *The Lancet Article*[109]. We will recover from it, but it will take two to three years. Students of mine in Ireland and in Israel have certainly felt its impact in their practices. The people who paid for this research got what they wanted and there is not much doubt that the drug companies were behind it. The biggest gun the allopaths have is *The Lancet*[110] so it is a blow but not a terminal one. Homoeopathy is very strong at grass roots level. But homoeopathy is weak in the propaganda department. There should have been a huge response and there was no response.

ROWENA: The Society of Homeopaths did try.

JEREMY: The Society is pretty good as societies go but you can shout much louder than that.

ROWENA: The newspapers didn't want to know.

JEREMY: Of course. They had already had their pound of flesh. But then you have to keep on writing articles, making movies and writing books. You have to organise a lot of serious research and show that it works. The Society of Homeopaths is good relative to a lot of others, but it needs to do a lot more. Israel's reaction to *The Lancet Article*[109] was a total flop. I sat eating ice cream with the ten people who were supposed to respond and everybody threw out ideas but at the end of the day, inertia blocked it.

ROWENA: What about the movie idea?

JEREMY: Let me give you an example of one little project that can make an impact. My wife Camilla Sherr and Kate Gathercole, a Dynamis School graduate who practises here in the UK, set up a free treatment scheme for a halfway house of people who have been in and out of mental asylums. They were not capable of caring for themselves, were on a load of psychiatric drugs and totally dependent. During the last year ten patients were treated and they have had fantastic results. A lot of them are now off their drugs, and they are starting to work and be independent again. All that is on video. So if marketed correctly it could have a big impact. If it is shown to all halfway houses, they are going to be impressed.

There are many excellent projects like this happening, as well as some good research, it just needs to be published and displayed. We need more watertight research, which they cannot shoot holes in it. Somebody needs to put it all together and I have confidence it will happen.

ROWENA: I just hope it is going to happen in our lifetime.

JEREMY: I hope so too but even if homoeopathy becomes semi-dormant again, we will carry on bearing the torch. I know that as long as I am capable of practising, I will practise. I don't care if they outlaw me. As long as I can move or even think, I will practise homoeopathy.

ROWENA: So what happens if they outlaw it?

JEREMY: It is outlawed in many states in the USA but people still find a way to practise. In the USA one day, they just singled out a homoeopath in Connecticut and charged her with illegally practising medicine. Two homoeopaths were recently arrested in Florida. The government walked into their practices and confiscated all their books and remedies and took them to court. It is the biggest delusion that it is the world of the free over there. That can happen to anybody in the USA, yet people are still practising and teaching. However, the good news is that six states have now legalised professional homoeopaths and more are on the way.

ROWENA: They are not allowed to practise unless they are doctors in the USA?

JEREMY: Sometimes even less so if they are doctors.

ROWENA: There was a book of fiction, *The Law of Similars*[139], written about that.

JEREMY: I didn't read it but you can take the true story of George Guess, a homoeopathic doctor practising in North Carolina. He treated somebody with asthma. Nothing bad happened but he didn't comply with the accepted standards of allopathic medical practise. He was disqualified by the allopathic medical society because he was a doctor who used homoeopathic remedies. In order to practise homoeopathy he had to move out of that state. If he hadn't been a doctor he would have been safer.

ROWENA: Did his Society support him?

JEREMY: A lot of people supported him and the other homoeopaths who have been in trouble; people contributed from all over the world. The people who get into those situations in the USA are not looking at less than one hundred thousand US dollars before they start moving again. The question is can we and will we support all those who get arrested.

ROWENA: I read that you started your journey with homoeopathy when you were twenty four. Do you feel it helps if you are older and/or when you have more life experience? Or does it depend on the person?

JEREMY: It is better to start younger because you get your life experience prescribing; you get triple life experience with people. Of course it also helps if you have been around the block a couple of times. If you are young, for the first few years you don't have a lot of experience but you will do ten years later! My wife started when she was nineteen straight out of school. I have students that were sitting in my class when they were fourteen and they are now practising. They went straight from school into homoeopathy and they are doing great work. I think you can start at any age. Many students start at sixty five or seventy, and they are doing great too. Everybody's cruising on their path.

ROWENA: A few little things. If you are not fed up with me!

JEREMY: Rowena, I love homoeopathy. I could talk about it all day!

ROWENA: Do you think different remedies sometimes suit different countries? For example, do you think you get more Scorpions in Israel than in the UK because scorpions live there?

JEREMY: I teach homoeopaths and practise all over the world and the same pictures emerge in the USA, Finland, Germany, Israel and Japan or the UK. In my opinion, there is no difference in terms of race.

ROWENA: Some homoeopaths say that because the UK is an island surrounded by salty seas, *Natrum muriaticum* is often indicated. Do you find that you prescribe it a lot in Israel?

JEREMY: Actually, it is not a remedy I use that much. Not in the UK either.

ROWENA: Why do you think that is?

JEREMY: It is because I have learned to work with a bigger range of remedies and the more you do that, the less you focus on a few polycrests and essences.

ROWENA: Massimo Mangialavori gets patients that respond to remedies made from parasites in his clinic. You don't think it is because there are more parasites in Italy, then?

JEREMY: The fact that he gets them doesn't mean that this was the person's remedy. More likely it is the way he is thinking and it was a good remedy for that person. The mistake would be to say that because Massimo Mangialavori gave a person a parasite it is exclusively a case of a parasite and cannot have been a case of anything else. Possibly if you gave *Natrum muriaticum*, they would have done fairly well too; there are many levels of similarities.

ROWENA: How do you see homoeopathy progressing from here?

JEREMY: As a profession we need deep roots into the past; into the philosophy, and we need to grow new branches into the future. If we are running forward all the time, there is not enough time to develop a solid base. Everybody is looking for a new technique, a gimmick, to find the remedy. That is why they are running; that is why they go to seminars. Homoeopathic treatment is not about finding the remedy; usually it is a series of remedies carefully managed. It is just as important to focus on the second prescription, how to manage a case or what to do when nothing happens. Homoeopathy is like a game of chess; it is not a one shot.

ROWENA: That is how Mike Bridger practises; he sees it in zigzags.

JEREMY: You have to zigzag a lot of the time, unless you happen to get it bang on the first prescription, which happens once in twenty cases and can take you a long, long way down the line. It is like sailing a boat - you need to stay close to the wind so that your remedy will continue to benefit for as long as possible.

ROWENA: I have a cancer patient who is taking *Natrum muriaticum LM* but I think her cancer is probably ticking away. What you have just said has made me think. If she is doing well in herself, and that seems to be the remedy that is indicated then maybe all I can do is palliate and maybe she is not meant to overcome her cancer. What is your take on that?

JEREMY: You have got to be careful with the concept of the 'meant to'. Destiny can be changed by circumstance and remedies, otherwise we are doing nothing. There should be room for miracles but there is a certain border where you pass with cancer, where it is difficult to pull the patient back.

ROWENA: She has had ovarian cancer for five years.

JEREMY: It is different with every cancer and with every patient; the stage and type of the cancer, the person, the treatment that they have had, their spirit and their support systems all make a difference. It is like someone standing on the edge of a cliff and just about falling over. There is a point where you can catch them and pull them back, and there is a point where they are going to fall. It is different in every case. When you see that they are too far gone, you have to move into palliation; palliation is a very important and proper part of homoeopathy.

ROWENA: Do you sometimes not know if you are palliating? Sometimes I am not sure whether I am palliating or working towards cure. I am just going with the picture of where they are at when they sit in front of me.

JEREMY: If it is on the cusp it can be confusing in which case you have got to do that. You might get a situation where the cancer is too advanced in which case you are not going to pull them back and you have got to start palliating. In that case you prescribe in a different way and you change techniques. Everybody said that, from Kent to Grimmer. There is a certain point where you let go of the big war and you go for the little battles.

ROWENA: Using organ support?

JEREMY: I don't use organ support in a routine way. But I do choose remedies that fit the organ and pathology as well as the totality I choose to work with. When patients go into heavy, incurable pathology, you have to constrict your totality and prescribe more palliative remedies. These would be local and dealing with recent issues. First you prescribe for the whole person, the soul and the body together, but there comes a time where the body is too wrecked and the soul is half detached. You then have to try to patch up the body and make it easier and less painful. But during the last few hours before death, the soul begins to leave the body and then you can see the whole picture again and prescribe for that. At that point you don't worry about the body and you go for the big picture and it will show clearly if they are not drugged. Then you can help their passage before they die. Kent says that there is nothing more beautiful to see than homoeopathic euthanasia and that is exactly what it is; you go back to the soul.

ROWENA: I have just taken on another cancer case and as you have written a book on the syphilitic miasm, I thought I might ask you this question. The patient has had so many terrible things happen to her; one accident or tragedy after another. I was taught at college that when this is apparent in a case one should look for a syphilitic remedy but none have come through the repertorisation as far as I can see.

JEREMY: It is a generalisation to say the syphilitic miasm is destructive. It is true that some syphilitic cases are like that. It is not that black and white. Is it true syphilitics have a lot of accidents all of the time? Definitely not. Is it true that all people who have accidents all the time are syphilitic? Definitely not. Is it true that it happens some of the time? Yes. Is it true that maybe it happens in sycotic or psoric cases as well? For sure. It could be that psorics, sycotics and syphiltics have different kinds of accidents. Saying that people who have such a history are only syphilitic is simplistic. The concept is much more delicate and sophisticated.

When I do a case in class and ask, "What miasm do you think this is?", half the students shout syphilis, half sycosis and half psora! Nobody ever knows. That is why I wrote my book *Dynamic Materia Medica – Syphilis*[140]. It is a philosophy book, disguised as a materia medica. In it I try to reach the essence of syphilis through studying purely syphilitic remedies. Each of the eleven remedies I have chosen is written in a different style to demonstrate how you can study remedies in many diverse ways.

ROWENA: On a different subject, what do you think about the single register?

JEREMY: I gave up on homoeopathic politics about fifteen years ago so I am not that knowledgeable about what is going on with the single register. I want to have a register of classical homoeopaths who think in a similar way. I don't want to be in the same register as people who throw six different high potencies remedies in a day at anything that moves. Politically our profession needs a single register to show a united front to the outside world. But how we practise on an individual basis is another matter. This can be equated to epidemics.

A genus epidemicus is like a unified register, you go by the common denominator. What is common to all practitioners of homoeopathy across the board? They use potentised remedies and that is the big picture of the epidemic. Then you have to individualise; different patients within the epidemic get different remedies within the genus. Each one has a different point of view. That one gets that remedy and that one gets another. In a similar way we need a unified register for the outside and individualised registers for the inside. All politics can be understood using homoeopathy philosophy. That is the way I decide on everything; who I vote for and what I believe in.

ROWENA: I think that is an excellent place to finish. Thank you so much, Jeremy.

The Process

My two and a half year year journey is coming to its end and I find myself in a very different place from where I started. When I had the inspiration for this project it was over a typical Grecian lunch after the interview with George Vithoulkas in August 2004. Nigel Summerley and I were passing time while waiting for our ferry to make the short trip back from Alonissos to Skopelos. We had enjoyed our time with George; he had welcomed us into his Academy and generously shared his home-grown figs and stories and spoke with passion and enthusiasm of his experiences in our profession. We were both left with that warm feeling you get when you meet someone who has done so much for something that is dear to you. He has had such a huge influence on homeopathy for the last forty years.

I knew this project was an ambitious idea but that has never stopped me before! However, looking back from where I am now, I can see I was very naïve about the amount of work the project would actually involve but I was determined and just as much as homeopathy is described as a 'calling', I too felt a calling to have these conversations.

In some ways everything slotted so easily into place. I scheduled an achievable timetable for the interviews to fit in alongside my practice and with the graciousness of good timing, I attended a seminar organised specifically for teachers of homeopathy held in Malvern by the Homeopathic Symposium[3] in November 2004. By then I had compiled a list of possible interviewees and a synopsis of what I wanted to achieve. During those couple of days I met many of the homeopaths that I then went on to interview in 2005, and had a thoroughly enjoyable time in the process. The first chapter was with Linda Gwillim and Bill Rumble of the Welsh School of Homeopathy and it took place in the bar of the hotel in which the seminar was being held.

It took me a few weeks to make contact with the homeopaths that I had met at that seminar and by mid-January the interviews became a regular part of my life. 2005 soon revealed itself to be one of the most enjoyable challenges I had ever experienced. There is a common belief within our profession that you can never know it all in homeopathy – the subject is so vast and multifaceted. Even if we were to be familiar with all three thousand plus remedies, new ones are being created every day. Even if we were to know anatomy, physiology and pathophysiology as well as all the allopathic specialists combined, we would still need to learn about the many new drugs that are regularly being trialed. Even if we perpetually reflected on our own issues and prioritised our interpersonal relationships with our patients, we would still find those that would challenge us to keep us moving forward. Learning homeopathy is an endless process.

What I learnt – thoughts, reflections and questions for the future

Having been inspired by my final interviewee, Jeremy Sherr, to think in analogy, I wanted to create a summary for the book that wasn't just a linear list of highlights from each chapter and as I sat and meditated on it, my mind started wandering to the sea. After all it was at the ferry port on Alonissos that the idea for the book first came to me and since then my laptop has accompanied me to several beaches for the writing and editing process. During each retreat I spent several hours staring out to sea as well as looking at the pebbles surrounding me in the shallow waters. I studied the pebbles as the waves breathed in and out and stirred them around. Some stayed firm, while others tossed and turned creating ripples of their own before journeying back out to sea. I began to observe some similarities with what I had learned on my travels.

Hahnemann's homeopathy could be compared to the firm and stable rocks on the beach where the sea meets the land. Ever present and strong and more than capable of weathering a storm, influential on its surroundings but at the same time able to evolve with the flow over time. As each wave arrives it brings with it graduating homeopaths, newly proven remedies and innovative methodologies, ways of practising, prescribing and taking cases. These can all be observed in the myriad of colours and shapes that are created by the numerous shells, pebbles and stones. Some waves bring positive press and, as a result, new patients to our doors; a rise in awareness of our healing art. Other waves have a more detrimental effect and the negativity they create can wash away the looser stones as well as dislodge some of the larger ones. As they retreat they can take with them the less established homeopaths that might then travel to distant shores for other adventures.

The tides too assert their influence. A high tide in the sixties and seventies brought a whole new cove supported by some very strong and sturdy rocks, the building blocks for our renaissance. A whole community of animal, mineral and plant life has gathered here since. The cove continually changes in appearance. There is a vast matrix of colours, shapes and textures to be found if you look closely and the overall picture is breathtaking. Endlessly complex and perpetually developing and maturing, the beach invites, and increasingly attracts, visitors of all ages to come and explore. Some feel the experience changes their perception of their health, their life and their world around them. Others say the more often they visit, the more beneficial the experience.

On a cloudy day though, when the waters are a little muddied with disturbed sand, some of the shapes are difficult to decipher by the untrained eye. Sometimes the weather and the darkened water can put off the more cautious beachcomber. They might ask themselves if it is safe or whether they should just venture on the dry land that is familiar to them. Are they taking too much of a risk for themselves and their family and if they were to hedge their bets, which stone should they choose?

451

Perhaps we can ask ourselves how we can make our beach more appealing to people who have not visited us before or those who have only passed through without stopping long enough to take a closer look? How can we stop litter deposits from unwelcome guests whose aim is, intentionally or otherwise, to destroy our seascape? How can we create a safe haven for a variety of stones and pebbles without loosing sight of the rocks that have held the beach in place since its infancy? Food for thought.

Rowena J Ronson
March 2007

Appreciations

One aspect that I didn't consider, in terms of my workload, was the transcribing of the interviews. I knew that the organisation of the interviews and the interviews themselves would be a very large time commitment but that is as far as I had projected. However, the right people stepped in to assist just at the opportune moments. I had a whole team of students and practitioners transcribing for me and I owe a lot to them for their support and feedback. Throughout 2005 tapes were flying in and out of Rivendell, my home, on a regular basis.

Many, many thanks to my team of transcribers: Sue Gee-Pemberton, Kate O'Connor, Petra Wood, Mary Krizka, Fee Jones, Jane Perry, Georgi Gill, Jemima Kallas, Gill Upham, Monica Hayward, Diane Goodwin, Lea Horvatic, Linda Cooke, Prue Fox, Alison Larkworthy, Caroline Heatlie, Rachel Mcdonald, Caroline Mcneill, Jean Watt and Rebecca Knorr.

Once the scripts returned the writing, rewriting and editing began and that part of the project took eighteen months. For the last six months I had two assistants to speed up the process. Rebecca Knorr had originally volunteered to transcribe a couple of the interviews in the early part of 2006; she had found out about the project through the homeopathy grapevine. She then went on to do some proof reading for me and in the summer I asked her to take on a fuller role and work as an editor. I will be forever in her debt as she came in and saved me when I was swamped and drowning.

My second editor was Adam Samuels, my amazing partner in life. From a completely sceptical place at the start – after all, he is an accountant(!) – he has been working on this project with me since last August. We have lived and breathed it together as he was responsible for the complex index system which we hope you will utilise to find your way around the book. His analytical mind and attention to detail enabled us to eradicate inconsitencies as well. The book is a much more polished piece as a restult of his hard work. Thank you my dear Adam.

Of course my endless appreciation goes to the interviewees who kindly spared the time for not only their conversation with me but checking through their chapter afterwards. Some were very meticulous and took several days out of their busy schedules, so thank you, thank you, thank you.

My appreciation also goes to Nigel Summerley for igniting my passion for writing back in 2004 and giving me the chance to scribe Double Take with him for the Society of Homeopaths' Journal[46] and of course to former editor Jo Evans for agreeing to publish the column.

I would also like to thank Michelle Shine. Michelle gave me the opportunity to work for her soon after I graduated. I learned a great deal during that year and we have been good friends ever since. She introduced me to the world of book writing when she wrote and published *What About Potency*[141]? She also encouraged and supported me to self-publish under her publishing company banner Food For Thought. Thank you Michelle.

In the final weeks before going to print Francis Treuherz came on board to preview the book. However, in addition he couldn't quite resist going through each chapter with a fine toothcomb correcting errors that only he would have ever spotted. Francis also helped me compile the lengthy bibliography and checked over some of the index – after all he is not called the Homeopathy FT Index for nothing! Thank you so much Francis; what would the profession do without you!

At the same time Jill Leuw, an editor, and Robin Cowan, a homeopath, also rambled through the manuscript and came up with some useful feedback and previews for the back cover. Thank you to you both.

Some words from Rebecca Knorr

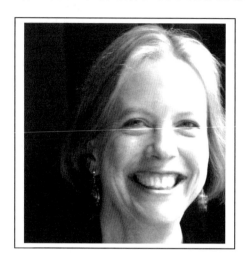

I am a graduate of the School of Homeopathy, a fledgling homeopath in my second year of solo practice, and a newly registered member of the Society of Homeopaths. There is a real synchronicity around my involvement in this project. My stated aim for my first Continuous Professional Development cycle includes developing a deeper understanding of homeopathy philosophy and principles and this book has given me the opportunity to listen to many different points of view and to weigh up different methods of practising and teaching. It has helped me to appreciate more deeply the education that I have received so far and to make an important decision about my postgraduate study. It has inspired me greatly. And the wonderful thing about editing is that because you must read, and reread, and reread, the golden nuggets have a tendency to stay with you.

This book challenged my own ideas; at times, I felt distinctly uncomfortable with arguments that seemed watertight yet contradicted my own training. I found myself wondering, what is the purpose of doing this? Will we be exposing to the public the lack of congruity among homeopaths in methods of prescribing and taking the case? Is this appropriate reading for the first year student, or someone who is trying to decide where they want to study? Will they come away more confused, rather than less? And yet as I read on, my uneasiness lessened. How else can you make an informed decision other than by being exposed to different points of view that often contradict one another? Being made uncomfortable is something I needed to stay with and explore, rather than run away from. And in the end, I found I had greater clarity, not less. I also have a much better grasp of the history of homeopathy, the esoteric philosophical ideas that have influenced various practitioners in their methods of practise, and the development of these ideas over time.

I had never met or even spoken to Rowena when I agreed to help edit this book, but through reading and listening to so many interviews I felt honoured when she chose to include me in her project. She has boundless enthusiasm, a wonderful sense of humour, an endlessly enquiring mind and she infuses everything with her love of homeopathy. This is a very personal journey made by Rowena. It is her story, but like all the best stories, it is relevant to us all.

Rebecca Knorr
December 2006

Contacts

Linda Gwillim: Welsh School of Homoeopathy 22 Bridge Street Carmarthen SA31 3JS 01792 366540 www.welshschoolofhomoeopathy.org.uk www.welshschoolofhomoeopathy.org.uk Linda's practice: Covent House Maengwyn Street Machynlleth Powys SY20 8EB 01970 832 039 linda.gwillim@talk21.com	Bill Rumble: Borva Cottage Port Eynon Swansea SA3 1NN 01792 391539
Brian Kaplan: 140 Harley Street London W1G 7LB www.drkaplan.co.uk	Myriam Shivadikar: 4 Ingleway Finchley London N12 0QJ myriam@doctor.com
Ellen Kramer: The College of Practical Homeopathy 760 High Road, Finchley, London N12 9QH Tel: 020 8445 6123 www.college-of-practical-homeopathy.com	Peter Chappell: Peter chappellhom@yahoo.co.uk www.vitalremedies.com www.healingdownloads.com
Robert Davidson: 5 Linton Close Milton Keynes MK13 7NR 01908 315387 07973 133230 robert.homeopath@gmail.com	Misha Norland: The School of Homeopathy Yondercott House Uffculme Devon EX15 3DR 0800 0439 349 UK Free phone -☐0845 257 8887☐ Fax: 0845 257 8885 info@homeopathyschool.com www.homeopathyschool.com

Annette Gamblin: Surbiton Natural Health Centre 14 Claremount Road Surbiton Surrey KT6 4QU 020 8399 2772 annette.gamblin@ukonline.co.uk For the University of Westminster's contact details see Sue Sternberg below.	Francis Treuherz: 2 Exeter Road (side entrance) London NW2 4SP 0208 450 6564 07795 845 9446 fran@gn.apc.org The *Homeopathic Helpline*[18] is open 9am to midnight 365 days a year, all calls cost the BT Premium Line rate, currently £1.50 per minute. Regulated by ICSTIS. 09065 343404 www.homeopathyhelpline.com
Charles Wansbrough: Centre for Bioliminal Homeopathy 25a Amerland Road SW18 1PX 020 8870 1808 charles_wansbrough2002@yahoo.co.uk www.biolumanetics.net/tantalus	Jerome Whitney: Flat 5 64 Auckland Road London SE19 2DJ jerome@jwhitney.demon.co.uk www.jwhitney.demon.co.uk
Mike Bridger: For information about homeopathic training at the Contemporary College of Homoeopathy in Exeter, Devon or Mike Bridger and Dion Tabrett's Orion advanced training postgraduate course in London (and their CDs of the course) visit www.conhom.com 0845 6032878 Mike practises at Ainsworths in London.	Dion Tabrett: The Fairbourne Clinic 17 Wendan Road Newbury Berkshire RG14 7AG 01635 44200
Ernest Roberts: 3 The Lane Sunderland Point Morecambe LA3 3HS 01524 850 490 and North West College of Homoeopathy 23 Wilbraham Road Fallowfield Manchester M14 6FG	Gordon Sambidge: BSc(Hons) Homeopathy part-time and full-time courses at:- The Centre for Homeopathic Education 020 7359 7424 www.homeopathycollege.org www.homeopathycollege.org

0161 225 1028 and 0161 257 2445 info@nwch.co.uk www.nwch.co.uk	
Sheilagh Creasy: 10 The Gables Leighton Buzzard Bedfordshire LU7 2PQ 01525 382964 For her postgraduate workshops held bi-monthly in London, contact Angelika Metzger 17 Blackstone Road London NW2 6DA 020 8830 6020 metzang@aol.com	Kate Chatfield: University of Central Lancashire Corporation Street Preston PR1 2HE kchatfield@uclan.ac.uk 01772 893697 www.uclan.ac.uk Galway College of Homeopathy admin@galwayhomeopathy 00353 91776886 www.galwayhomeopathy.com
Roger Savage: 01799 524442 07889 989398 roger.jo@virgin.net www.RSHom.com	Subrata Kumar Banerjea: Allen College Of Homoeopathy "Sapiens" 382 Baddow Road Great Baddow Chelmsford, Essex CM2 9RA 01245 505859 allencollege@btinternet.com www.homoeopathy-course.com
Yubraj Sharma: School of Shamanic Homoeopathy Unit 1c, Delta Centre Mount Pleasant Wembley Middlesex HA0 1UX 020 8795 2695 yubraj@world-of-light.com www.shamanic-homoeopathy.com	Kaaren Whitney: kaaren.whitney@talk21.com

Anne Waters: The Lakeland College of Homeopathy Postal Building Ash Street Bowness on Windermere Cumbria LA23 3EB 015394 47666 mail@thelakelandcollege.co.uk www.thelakelandcollege.co.uk anne.waters@mac.com	Rebecca Preston: beccaprestonhom@aol.com www.scothomeopathy.com
Martin Miles: 136 North Cray Road Bexley London DA5 3NB 01322 558334	Carol Wise: 24 Rose Bank Burley in Wharfedale Ilkley West Yorkshire LS29 7PQ
Linda Razzell: 82 Point Hill London SE10 8QW 020 8694 4958 practice@linda-razzell.co.uk	Nicky Pool: 01753 644541 nickypool@btinternet.com and The Purton House Homeopathic Centre Room D18 Thames Valley University Wellington Street Slough SL1 1YG 01753 697781 enquiries@purtonhouse.com www.purtonhouse.com
Lesley Gregerson: 57 Wise Lane Mill Hill London NW7 2RN 020 8959 1893 and The London School of Classical Homoeopathy 159 Ladysmith Road Enfield	Sue Sternberg: 3rd Floor Copeland Building University of Westminster 115 New Cavendish Street London W1M 8JS sternbs@wmin.ac.uk

London EN1 3AH 020 8360 8757 info@homeopathy-lsch.co.uk	
Lionel Milgrom: 17 Skardu Road London NW2 3ES l.milgrom@ic.ac.uk drillsma-milgrom@lineone.net 020 8450 8760 07970 852156	Barbara Harwood: bjmharwood@hotmail.com
Simon Taffler: 1 Oldbury Place Off Nottingham Street London W1U 5PA 07967 645960 www.simontaffler.com	Jeremy Sherr: Dynamis School for Advanced Homoeopathic Studies - a 2-3 year postgraduate course. www.dynamis.edu
Rebecca Knorr: Abercromby Place Homeopathic Practice 13a Abercromby Place Edinburgh EH3 6LB www.edinburghhomeopaths.com www.edinburghhomeopaths.com rebecca.knorr@btinternet.com	George Vithoulkas Alonissos 37005, Greece 0030 24240 65142/65190 Fax: 0030 24240 65147 george@vithoulkas.com www.vithoulkas.com

INDEX

A

ALLOPATHIC MEDICINE

Amitriptyline, 54
antibiotics, 24, 31, 36, 40, 119, 130, 131, 165, 282, 342, 353, 380, 410
Antimalarials
    antimalarial, 48
    antimalarials, 47
blood thinners, 53
Chemotherapy, 443
    chemo, 40, 314, 424
    chemotherapies, 217
    chemotherapy, 42, 217, 252, 266, 423, 424
conventional allopathic painkiller, 259
conventional medication, 258, 259
conventional medicine, 35, 146, 148, 152, 153, 251, 252, 259, 308, 379, 383, 387
conventional Western medicine, 420
cortisone, 40
Drugs
    allopathic drug, 34, 41, 52, 53, 217
    allopathic drugs, 183, 441
    Allopathic drugs, 217
    allopathic medication, 32
    allopathic medicine, 35
    Allopathic medicine, 169
Hormone Replacement Therapy, 52, 53
Lariam, 434
Lithium, 358
Methylphenidate, 292
opium, 124
paracetamol, 33
penicillin, 152, 241
Pharmaceutical
    Big Pharma, 89
    drug companies, 124, 444
    drug companies' lobby, 346
    multinational drug companies, 251
    pharmaceutical companies, 383, 433
    pharmaceutical company, 89, 224
    pharmaceutical industry, 164
    pharmaceutical procedure, 214
    pharmaceuticals, 302, 388, 434
Prednisolone, 368
radiotherapies, 40
radiotherapy, 252, 266, 314

Ritalin, 292
Steroids, 368, 443
    steroid, 259
    steroid/inhaler, 259
    steroids, 40, 56, 258, 368
Tamoxifen, 53, 173, 217
the Pill, 53, 152, 216, 323, 347, 349
    contraceptive pill, 323
therapeutic medicines, 70
Ventolin, 291
western allopathic medicine, 269
Western medicine, 420

ALLOPATHY

Allopathic, 421
    allopath, 40, 421
    allopathic, 154, 323, 415, 416, 417, 429, 433, 446, 450
    allopathic approach, 296
    allopathic doctor, 420
    allopathic interference, 34, 41
    allopathic intervention, 198
    allopathic medicine, 421
    allopathic modes of thinking, 413
    allopathic paradigm, 435
    allopathic perspective, 268, 271, 416
    allopathic pollution, 198
    allopathic reports, 433
    allopathic settings, 420
    allopathic terms, 168
    allopathic thinkers, 416
    allopathic thinking, 416, 419, 420
    allopathically, 215, 413, 416, 420
    allopathically oriented, 416
    allopaths, 70, 134, 382, 416, 434, 444
    allopathy, 1, 85, 86, 92, 122, 168, 177, 269, 420, 421
allopathically thinking, 416
atrophy, 247, 255
bacteria, 24, 31, 71, 72, 101
biomedical, 385
blood sugar levels, 425
blood test, 30, 31, 37
bronchodilator
    conventional allopathic bronchodilator, 259
cloning, 276
CT scans, 263

dentist, 120, 137
DNA, 276, 382
Doctors
  allopathic doctors, 210
  conventional doctor, 263, 390
  doctor, 25, 30, 31, 35, 36, 37, 95, 124, 130,
    131, 132, 149, 166, 177, 201, 203, 209,
    212, 224, 242, 269, 278, 291, 308, 312,
    342, 353, 370, 371, 380, 411, 416, 433,
    436
  doctor of biochemistry, 316
  doctor using homeopathic medicines, 181
  doctor's surgery, 95
  doctors, 26, 27, 29, 30, 31, 32, 36, 39, 40, 57,
    73, 82, 95, 102, 108, 118, 129, 147, 155,
    177, 185, 186, 202, 203, 207, 224, 252,
    257, 292, 302, 309, 319, 329, 331, 341,
    355, 369, 391, 418, 445
  Doctors, 26, 77, 108, 118, 330, 337
  doctors' practices, 329
  GP, 25, 35, 48, 57, 128, 129, 130, 158, 209,
    253, 261, 368, 372, 380
  medical doctor, 35, 132, 224
  medical doctors, 269
  orthodox doctor, 25
  orthodox doctors, 401
general nursing, 353
Genetics
  gene therapy, 276
  genes, 276
  genetic, 43
  genetic code, 275, 276
  genetic sequence, 276
  genetic sequences, 276
  geneticists, 400
  genetics, 268, 275, 276, 400
  genetics class, 275
  spiritual genetics, 276
immune system, 31
jaundiced, 273
lumber puncture (spinal tap), 24, 31
Macmillan nurse, 313
mastectomy, 218, 266
obstetrics, 347
ontological, 385
  ontologically, 385
pharmacist, 129, 221, 291, 354
protozoa, 71
Psychiatry
  psychiatric, 356
  psychiatric drugs, 445
  psychiatric nursing, 353
  psychiatric ward in hospital, 292

psychiatrist, 292, 353
psychiatry, 25
Radiation
  radiation, 272, 314
  radiation treatment, 53
  radiography, 256
rheumatologist, 38
saline suspension, 39
sterilisation, 347
Vaccination
  conventional vaccines, 47
  surgeries, 40
  vaccinate, 47, 331
  vaccinated, 47, 328
  vaccination, 55
  vaccinations, 55, 131, 329, 331, 433, 442
  vaccine, 56, 433
  vaccine induced illness, 152
  vaccines, 40
  Vaccines, 56
  whooping cough vaccine, 331
viruses, 71
X-ray
  x-ray, 37
  X-ray, 96, 263

ANATOMY AND PHYSIOLOGY

anatomy, 14, 35, 111, 149, 252, 271, 416, 450
  spiritual anatomy, 268
antibodies, 382
blood cell, 382
bowel, 58, 348
  bowel movement, 56
  bowels, 44, 56, 58, 129, 255
  bowels not to move, 56
  stool, 56
brain, 25, 318, 322, 323
cytokines, 382
dry mouth, 358
endocrine glands, 311, 324, 326
endocrine system, 323, 348
endocrinology, 324
epigastric area, 261
heart, 317, 328
hormones, 40
immune system, 31, 47, 72
in-depth anatomy, 293
insulin, 70, 73
insulin levels, 73

intestine, 41
kidneys, 42, 52, 290, 298, 324, 368
large intestines, 56
liver, 42, 52, 53, 56, 58, 128, 208, 266, 290, 298,
   324
lung, 130
lungs, 290, 298
lymph, 42
nerve cell, 382
nervous system, 318
ovaries, 323
phagocytes, 382
physiology, 14, 35, 111, 149, 252, 271, 293, 416,
   450
pituitary gland, 323
pregnancies, 401
renal, 31
skin, 37, 44, 56, 165, 242, 280, 291, 426
skin cell, 382
stomachs, 178
testicles, 69
thymus gland, 323, 328
thyroid gland, 44, 323
tonsils, 48
uterus, 424
vocal chords, 247

B

BOOKS, FILMS, JOURNALS, WEBSITES, GUIDELINES, REPORTS AND SONGS

A Guide to the Methodologies of Homoeopathy,
   71, 181, 296
A Study on Materia Medica with Repertory, 253
Allen's Key Notes, 305
Alternative England and Wales, 402
Alternative London, 402
American Journal of Homeopathic Medicine, 123
Bhagavad Gita, 392
BNF, 60
Boericke, 120, 126, 152, 202, 241, 242, 331, 444
Bridge Across Forever, 326
British Homeopathic Journal, 127
Caduceus, 275
Chronic Diseases, 200, 214, 349
Chronic Diseases, A Working Hypothesis, 101

Clarke's Materia Medica, 94, 120, 202, 206, 331,
   406
Clarke's Prescriber A Dictionary of the New
   Therapeutics, 406
Clarke's Repertory, 206
Code of Ethics, 126, 241, 247
Comparative Materia Medica, 219
Concordance, 204
CORH booklet, 209
Cyclopedia of Drug Pathogenesy, 153
Dimensions of Homeopathic Medicine, 181
Divided Legacy, 123, 124, 152, 210, 220
Dogmatism in Homeopathy, 187
Drug Pictures, 265
Dynamic Materia Medica – Syphilis, 449
Emotional Healing with Homeopathy, 72, 75
essay by Pierre Schmidt, 134
Essence of Materia Medica, 102, 208
Everyday Homeopathy, 48, 49, 52
Far from the Madding Crowd, 396
Films
   Dead Poets Society, 229
   Modesty Blaise, 396
   The Great Rock 'n Roll Swindle, 404
   What The Bleep Do We Know, 426
   Wizard of Oz, 168
First Aid Homoeopathy in Accidents and
   Ailments, 331
First Class Mail, 379, 393
Grimm's Fairy Stories, 18
Hamlet, 356
Health Science Press, 206
Homeopathic Education Services in California web
   site, 127
Homeopathic Helpline, 52, 129, 130, 131
Homeopathic Medical Repertory, 35
Homeopathic Psychology, 181
Homeopathy an Introductory Guide, 25
Homoeopathic Acute Prescribing, 295
Homoeopathic Therapeutics, 406
Homoeopathy
   Principles and Practice, 181
Homoeopathy and Human Evolution, 198, 311, 312
House of Lords report, 374
   Big Five, 375
How Not to Do It, 181
HPTG web site, 26
I Ching, 275
Journal of the Faculty, 150
Kabbalah, 202
Kent's Lectures, 166, 198, 202, 443
Kent's Lectures on Homeopathic Materia Medica,
   238

Kent's Repertory, 47, 65, 132
The Book of Knowledge, 275
Killed by Homeopathy, 346
Leaders in Homoeopathic Therapeutics, 265
Lesser Writings, 121, 127
Links, 102, 103
Materia Medica of New Homoeopathic Remedies, 276
Materia Medica Viva, 183
Matters of Life and Death, 125
Miasmatic Prescribing, Its Philosophy, Diagnostic Classification, Clinical Tips, Miasmatic Repertory and Miasmatic Weightage of Medicines, 255, 261
National Occupational Standard guidelines, 271, 272, 374, 375
Oeconomia Regnum Animalis – The Economy of the Animal Kingdom, 133
Organon, 5, 8, 17, 44, 54, 65, 70, 72, 91, 103, 109, 110, 114, 154, 163, 180, 198, 200, 202, 203, 210, 214, 254, 256, 264, 267, 298, 349, 356, 369, 414, 415, 418, 444
    Aphorism, 5, 6, 214, 215, 254, 256, 267, 356, 419, 433
    Aphorisms, 70, 254, 259
Positive Health, 275
Prisma, 106, 160
Prometheus, 161, 327, 341
Pura, 200, 214
Ramakrishnan method, 72, 172
Robin Murphy's cancer tapes, 32, 84
Robin Murphy's tapes, 84, 164
Secret Doctrine of Madam Blavatsky, 269
Secret Lanthanides, 307
Sensation in Homeopathy, 180
Smallwood Report, 374
Spiritual Bioenergetics of Homoeopathic Materia Medica, 268
Supervision in the Helping Professions, 27
Synthesis, 1, 106
Talmud, 384
Tapes by George Vithoulkas, 84
Techniques For 24-Hour Lucid Dreaming, 18
The Alchemist, 439
The Best of Burnett, 164
the Bible, 86, 131, 235, 400
The Big Issue, 19
The Chronicles of Narnia - The Lion, the Witch and the Wardrobe, 387
The Classical Homeopathic Lectures of Vassilis Ghegas, 187
The Complete Homeopathy Handbook, 103
The Dancing Wu Li Masters, 354

The Drunkards, 197
The Dynamics and Methodology of Homoeopathic Provings, 308
The Ethics of the Fathers, 125
The Faces of Homeopathy, 124, 209
The Family Guide to Homoeopathy, 103
The Field, 386
The Genius of Homoeopathy, 18
The Guiding Symptoms, 153
The Harbinger, 132
The Healer, 284
The Homeopath, 125, 127, 302, 453
The Homeopathic Conversation, 29, 302
The Integrity of Homeopathy, 221
The Lancet, 337, 444
The Lancet Article, 337, 384, 444, 445
The Law of Similars, 446
The Medicine of Experience, 123
The Nature of Influence, 103
The Passion of the Western Mind, 414
The Prince's Foundation for Integrated Health Response, 374
The Quantum Doctor, 414
The Rheumatic Remedies and Repertory to the Rheumatic Remedies, 187
The Science of Homeopathy, 102, 122, 163, 208, 225, 444
The Second Similimum, 72
The Secret Life of Plants, 104
The Soul of the White Ant, 353
The Tanya, 202
The Tempest, 387
The Universe Story, 414
Therapeutic Pocket Book, 219
Thomas Maughan's Materia Medica, 65
Twelve Levels of Health, 183, 186, 187, 188
Vitalistic Medicine from Ancient Egypt to the 21st Century, 148
Whale Nation, 402
What About Potency, 454
Within you without you, from the album Sgt Pepper's Lonely Hearts Club Band, 392
work of Bert Hellinger, 76
Working With The Dreaming Body, 18
www.biolumanetics.net/tantalus, 139
www.vithoulkas.com/EN/interview_vithoulkas_philosophy.html., 1

c

COMPLEMENTARY AND ALTERNATIVE MEDICINE AND TERMINOLOGY

Age of Aquarius, 314
   New Age concepts, 276
alchemy, 44, 311, 316
Alexander Technique, 26
ancestral mutations, 276
Anthroposophical
   anthroposophical doctor, 353
   anthroposophical medicine, 269
   anthroposophical textbooks or articles or
      journals, 277
   anthroposophy, 121, 150
aromatherapy, 374
   aromatheraphy oils, 391
   massage, 35
Astral
   astral level, 105
   astral plane, 104
   astral realms, 104
   the astral body, 269
Astrology
   astrologer, 109, 277
   astrological chart, 105
   astrological charts, 94
   astrological data of asteroids and some
      esoteric planets, 277
   astrological profile, 277
   astrology, 35, 109, 277, 288, 311, 326, 419
   natal chart, 105
barefoot medicine, 40
   barefoot doctors, 237, 248
Bioacoustics, 138, 142
bodywork, 371
chakra, 71
   chakra diagnosis, 228
   chakras, 288, 290, 298, 311, 321, 324, 326,
      348
   heart, 71, 328
   heart chakra, 244
   lowest chakra, 242
   solar plexus, 328
   solar plexus, 328
   throat chakra, 290, 298
Channelling
   channel, 171, 277
   channel nformation, 322

channel universal information, 322
   channelled, 269, 273, 277, 278
   channelling, 269, 277
   channelling courses, 273
   channels, 41
   channels of energy, 41
chelates, 139, 140, 142
   chelate remedies, 142
Chiropatric
   chiropractic, 375, 376
   chiropractor, 376
   chiropractors, 376
clairaudient, 151
colonics, 26
Complementary medicine
   Complementary and Alternative Medicine, 384,
      388
   complementary medicine, 38, 372, 374
   complementary medicines, 36, 37
   complementary therapies,, 371
cosmosgenesis, 269
counselling
   co-counselling, 64
   co-counsellors, 64
   counselling, 185
   counsellor, 76, 246, 406
Cranial
   cranial sacral, 277
   cranial sacral practitioner, 277
   cranial sacral profile, 277
   cranial sacral system, 277
   cranial work, 271
crystals, 136, 138, 271, 274
   amethyst, 139
detox, 42, 65
   detox therapeutic, 53
   pollution, 323
   toxic, 52, 58, 421, 424
   toxic food, 442
   toxic state, 43
   toxicity, 42, 56, 65, 245
   toxicology, 277
   toxins, 66
dowse, 107, 273
   dowsing, 268, 272
Druidism, 67
   Ancient Order of Druids, 400
   Asterix Druid, 66
   chief Druid, 146
   Chief Druid of England, 66
   Druid Order, 67, 147, 280, 281, 282
      spiritual self-development organisation, 67
   Druid teaching, 146

Druid teachings, 146
druidic practices, 100
Druids, 67, 100, 137, 281, 282, 400
Golden Dawn Tradition, 67
old druid symbol, 193
role of Druids, 146
Stone Circle, 300
ego, 168, 170, 197
ego based decisions, 196
the ego, 174, 197, 269
electromagnetic field, 400
Erhard Seminars Training (EST), 408
esoterics
esoteric, 229, 338
esoteric classes, 145
esoteric medicine, 270
esoteric models of herbalism, 271
esoteric perspective, 268, 271
esoteric philosophical ideas, 455
esoteric philosophy, 269
esoteric pursuits, 394, 405
esoteric teachings, 100
esotericism, 400
Eurythmy, 380
eurythmy, 380
Flower Essences
Alaskan essences, 296
Bush flower remedy, 373
flower essence practitioner, 272, 296
flower essences, 35, 271, 274
Flower Remedies, 418
flower remedy, 27, 373
Flower Remedy practitioners, 418
Rescue Remedy, 78
healer, 9, 14, 17, 22, 107, 158, 270, 272
healer guide, 359
healers, 94, 311, 326
Herbalism
combination of herbal tinctures, 42
dried herbs, 274
herbal book, 163
herbal dispenser, 361
herbal formula, 274
herbal level, 44
herbal medicine, 111
herbal modules, 378
herbal remedies, 361
herbal tinctures, 42, 274, 300
herbalism, 190, 212, 272, 362, 376, 378
herbalist, 53, 163, 190, 272, 361, 363
herbally, 425
herbs, 35, 38, 361, 366, 370, 436
hippies, 152, 155, 308, 317, 394, 398, 402

Holistic
holism, 242
holistic approach, 108, 118
holistic medicine, 353
holistic perspective, 226
holistic sense, 337
holistic therapies, 356
non holistic approach, 113
not holistic, 336
Inergetix Diagnostic and Treatment Technology, 87
Integral Philosophy of Sri Aurobindo, 414
Iridology
iridologist, 272
iridology, 271
isotonic, 39
Karma
bad karma, 178
karma, 40, 172, 174, 197
karmic issues, 272
latent karma, 276
patient's karma, 83
laser therapy, 38
laws of vibration, 278
Learning patterns
auditory, 340
kinaesthetic, 273, 340
visual, 273, 340, 341
visual image, 273
materialistic biochemical paradigm, 148
Meditation
meditate, 321, 322, 399
meditating, 67, 325
meditation, 277, 300, 325, 343
meditation classes, 399
meditation groups, 273, 398
meditation instruction, 399
meditation work, 273
meditative proving. See Homeopathic term Proving
Transcendental Meditation, 398
mysticism, 397, 398, 400
mythology, 18
Naturopathy
Doctor's degree (ND), 435
naturopath, 148, 244, 296, 413
naturopathic, 413
naturopaths, 435
naturopathy, 58, 111, 182, 210, 435
NLP, 317, 408
NLP (Neuro-Linguistic Programming), 317
Nutrition
additive free, 295

additives, 291
bad diets, 323
diet, 35, 44, 54, 56, 58, 353, 417
dietary changes, 55
E numbers, 291
food allergies, 323
Gerson diet, 32
high roughage diet, 56
nutrition, 35, 54, 91, 111, 228, 291, 295, 353, 355, 371, 417
nutritional support, 53
nutritionist, 53
supplements, 56, 89
vitamin, 353
vitamin supplements, 353
vitamins, 89
Occultism
occultism, 397, 400
the occult, 398
Osteopathy
osteopath, 38, 190, 342, 376, 437
osteopaths, 247
osteopathy, 355, 375, 376
pendulums, 268, 272
Photodynamic Therapy, 382
Provocative Therapy, 24, 30, 175
psychic powers, 137, 151
Psychology
psychojargon, 36
psychological, 25, 32, 95, 174, 340
psychological disorders, 25
psychologist, 132, 292
psychology, 24, 32, 95, 400
psychosis, 90, 97
Psycotherapy
psychotherapeutic, 7, 144
psychotherapeutic models, 7
psychotherapist, 175
psychotherapy, 27, 30, 76, 162, 172, 176
Radiation from mobile phones, 323
reflexology, 26, 339, 342, 374
remedial exercises, 35
Shamanism
Power Animal, 301
shaman, 278
Shaman, 107
shamanic, 278
shamanic journey, 301
shamanic training, 273
shamanic work, 301
shamanism, 9, 12, 353
social workers, 292
Spiritualism

a spirit, 104
a spirits, 104
manifestation of spirituality, 33
philosophy of a spiritual science, 269
soul and spirit, 419
spirit, 76, 149, 178, 282, 296, 318, 419, 448
spirit of life, 352, 356
spiritual, 13, 90, 149, 177, 194, 199, 204, 269, 270, 277, 278, 318, 392, 439
spiritual agenda, 28
spiritual anatomy, 271
spiritual awakening, 269
spiritual awareness, 275
spiritual books, 275
spiritual characteristics, 83
spiritual concept, 148, 275, 276
spiritual concepts, 268, 271
spiritual experience, 65
spiritual force, 321
spiritual foundation, 67
spiritual genetics, 276
spiritual healing, 177
spiritual impressions, 273
spiritual knowledge, 269
spiritual level, 99, 105
spiritual mathematics, 74
spiritual philosophies, 151
spiritual philosophy, 150, 269, 311, 316, 326
spiritual realm, 76, 275
spiritual teacher, 66, 109
spiritual teachers, 328
spiritual teaching, 312
spiritual teachings, 148
spiritual way, 376
spiritual worker, 270
spirituality, 76, 189, 192, 272
spiritually, 313, 431, 439
Terminology
geist, 419
gemüt, 419
gestalt, 25, 29
seele, 419
subtle bodies, 269
taxonomy, 144
taxonomy in plants, 143
the dreaming, 12
therapeutic effect, 25
therapists, 26
therapy, 37, 76, 142, 159, 356, 374, 382, 407
Traditional Chinese Medicine, 35
Acupuncture

acupuncture, 26, 35, 36, 37, 38, 111, 153,
    159, 242, 246, 282, 353, 355, 370, 375,
    376
  acupuncture colleges, 398
  acupuncture needle, 38
  acupuncture points, 41
  acupuncturist, 66, 159, 190, 354, 407, 413,
    437
  acupuncturists, 36, 39, 159, 247, 420
  needled, 159
  needles, 436
chi deficiency, 277
Chinese diagnosis, 277
Chinese herbs, 38
Chinese Medicine, 44, 269, 277, 290, 298
concepts of damp and spleen, 277
facial, tongue and pulse diagnosis, 425
oriental medicine, 277
TCM, 38
Transpersonal
  transpersonal, 13, 358
  transpersonal psychology, 357
  transpersonal therapist, 356
UFOs, 398
water therapy, 436
witch doctors, 212, 353
yoga, 25, 159, 184, 342, 407
yogic, 35

H

HOMEOPATHIC TERMS

acute, 49, 58, 113, 114, 159, 239, 323, 328, 425
  acute, 131
  acute cases, 420
  acute clinic, 47
  acute condition, 186
  acute crisis, 243
  acute helpline, 52
  acute illnesses, 48
  acute prescribing, 355
  acute prescription, 127
  acute remedies, 48, 355, 413
  acute situation, 155
  acute symptoms, 49
  acutes, 34, 40, 49, 113, 131, 183, 281, 299,
    443
  acutes clinic, 18
aetiology, 34, 40, 42, 54, 194
  aetiologies, 85
Affinity

affinities, 69
affinity, 323, 412
  organ affinities, 182
Aggravation
  aggravate, 171
  aggravating, 216
  aggravation, 51, 54, 163, 194, 216, 242
  aggravations, 37, 55, 57, 80, 169, 324
  an aggravated, 58
  an aggravation, 37, 56
becoming dormant, 30, 58, 103, 134, 144, 164,
    188, 210, 308, 391
  become dormant, 152, 220, 235, 265, 301,
    329, 420, 444
  dormant, 88, 197, 249, 284, 374
  dormant state, 20, 249
  semi-dormant, 445
blue note, 3, 11, 12, 13
  blue notes, 12
Cases
  case histories, 161
  case history, 38, 333, 401
  case management, 366, 438, 443
  case taken, 309
  case taking, 5, 9, 12, 26, 37, 117, 165, 176,
    195, 244, 272, 273, 309, 354, 417, 418
    case history, 25
    case-taker, 246
    giving me her case, 155
    seeing the case, 174
    take a case, 117, 140, 176, 337, 418, 419,
      441
    take cases, 116, 273
    take friend's cases, 299
    take his case, 291, 332
    take the case, 27, 68, 155, 262, 297, 324
    take the cases, 11
    taken cases, 106
    taken their case, 44
    takes cases, 438
    taking a case, 32, 139, 182, 247, 306
    Taking a case, 426
    taking cases, 283, 427, 451
    taking the case, 12, 117, 183, 203, 217, 272,
      407, 455
    taking the cases, 273, 372
    took a case, 186
    took her case, 332
    took his case, 368, 406
  casework, 11, 26, 188, 306, 389
  centre of the case, 159
  clear the case, 217
  constitutional prescription, 259

first prescription, 41, 65, 66, 101, 129, 429, 438, 442, 447
follow up prescriptions, 443
hold the case, 265
linear cases, 141
long-term case management, 429, 442, 443
nonlinear cases, 141
remedy reaction, 438
second prescription, 429, 438, 443, 447
start most cases, 101
start the case, 53
cell salts, 54, 151
tissue salts, 42
chronic, 113, 114, 239, 328, 425
artificial chronic disease, 258, 259
chronic cases, 114, 420
chronic complaint, 112, 113, 131
chronic disease, 252, 274
chronic diseases, 71, 73
chronic illness, 421
chronic picture, 113, 114
chronic susceptibility, 114
Classical
classical, 29, 81, 106, 116, 141, 144, 154, 162, 176, 181, 191, 226, 230, 267, 277, 327, 335, 349, 369, 373, 376, 381, 408, 434
Classical, 82, 154, 162, 176, 267
classical approach, 27, 31
classical background, 227, 242
classical case, 56
classical college, 154, 335, 364
classical colleges, 154, 350, 376
Classical colleges, 227
classical constitutional prescriber, 155
classical course, 29
classical fanaticism, 84
classical foundation, 226
classical foundations, 46, 226
classical homeopath, 48, 109, 181, 185, 191, 238, 367, 368, 373, 381, 417, 418
classical homeopaths, 54, 154, 180, 194, 381
classical homeopathy, 31, 112, 116, 136, 140, 159, 180, 181, 182, 188, 193, 194, 243, 266, 365, 368, 369
unicism, 243
Classical homeopathy, 85, 150, 154
classical homeopathy training, 188
classical homoeopaths, 449
classical homoeopathy, 441
classical only homeopaths, 242
classical prescriber, 194
classical prescribers, 369
classical principles of homeopathy, 349

classical remedy, 85
classical thinking, 242
classical totality remedy, 194
classical training, 25, 105, 154, 173, 250, 267
Classical training, 156
classical training in homeopathy, 48
classical type of homeopathy, 27
classical way, 220, 229, 267, 375, 381
classicalists, 154
classically, 142, 266, 308, 364
classically trained homeopath, 1, 34, 40
classicists, 218
neoclassical homeopathy, 142
neopseudoclassical delusion, 434
nonclassical college, 418
nonclassical ethos, 1
practise classically, 360
practise very classically, 229
prescribe classically, 327
prescribing classically, 369
taught classically, 266
Clinical
clinical cases, 431
clinical decisions, 38
clinical development, 195
clinical experience, 161, 187, 232
clinical experiences, 140
clinical hour, 374
clinical hours, 374
clinical practise, 111, 140
clinical results, 161
clinical signs, 273
clinical skills, 195
clinical supervisor, 11
clinical training, 22, 23, 63, 76, 77, 232
clinical work, 248
Combination
combination formulae, 243
combinations, 109, 265
combinations of epidemic diseases, 71
Constitutional, 346
constitution, 32, 43, 160
constitutional remedy, 26, 65, 115, 183, 324, 368, 369, 430, 442
constitutionally, 32, 36, 39, 44, 101, 323, 324, 413
remedies constitutionally, 43
consultation, 8, 43, 117, 235, 299, 302, 306, 312, 358, 389, 425
consultations, 273, 377
Cost of consultation
consultation, 164, 182, 235, 377

first consultation, 34, 40, 108, 118, 160, 174,
182, 279, 286, 287, 377
Continuous Professional Development, 18, 103,
134, 376, 455
Continuous Professional Development
programme, 181, 246
degrees, 203, 204, 215
inner degree, 204
outer degree, 204
dis-ease, 41, 194, 358
disease state, 5, 12
disease states, 358
Doctors
doctor homeopath, 31
doctor homeopaths, 150, 151, 369
doctors, 181
homeopathic doctor, 206
homeopathic doctors, 150
homoeopathic doctor, 446
medical doctor homeopaths, 182
medical homeopath, 368, 376
medical homeopaths, 181, 369, 391
non-doctors, 148
Doctrine of Signatures, 103, 161, 277
archetypal energies, 98
archetypal level of signature, 99
signature, 99, 101, 104, 161
signatures, 98, 151, 277
dose, 72, 101, 125, 216, 220, 238, 240, 242, 244,
245, 274, 286, 328, 331, 348, 421, 422, 430,
443
doses, 219, 369, 410
dosing, 274
low dose, 266
overdose, 346
repeated doses, 183
double-blind, 302, 387
double-blind test, 416
Dreams
bad dreams in childhood, 287
dream, 244, 287, 288
dream analysis, 279, 286, 287
dream proving. See Proving
dream section, 287
dream work, 288
dream workshop, 287
dreams, 145, 165, 279, 286, 287
dreams from childhood, 287
dreams mean, 287
dreamt, 287
lucid dreaming state, 148
nightmares, 145, 279, 287
recurring dream, 287

recurring dreams, 279, 287
repeated nightmares, 145
significant dreams, 287
emotional aetiology, 194
energetic entities, 12
Epidemics
epidemics, 433, 434, 443, 449
genus epidemicus, 434, 435, 449
Essence
essence, 81, 256, 420, 431, 432, 441
Essence, 254, 255, 257
essence concept, 81
essence of homeopathy, 416
essence of syphilis, 449
essences, 209, 431, 447
internal essence, 257
psychic essence, 255
psychic essences, 257
spiritual essence, 74
Totality Essence Keynote, 254
Hahnemannian, 5, 91, 162, 163, 176, 285, 298
Hahnemannian disciple, 251
Hahnemannian homeopathy, 180
Hahnemannian path, 1
Hahnemannian technique, 266
Hering's three legged stool principle, 37
homeopuncture, 37
intercurrents, 71, 154
isopathy, 375
Kentian
Kentian, 5, 27, 34, 40, 42, 59, 85, 162, 176
Kentian approach, 28, 266
Kentian homeopathy, 162, 176
Kentian ideology, 257
Kentian prescribing, 149
Keynotes
keynote prescribing, 29
keynotes, 29
Keynotes, 254, 255, 257
keynotes of a remedy, 37
Kingdom
an animal, 27
animal, mineral or vegetable kingdom, 75
kingdom domains, 141
kingdoms, 27, 165, 340
mineral, 27, 246
mineral table, 246
plant, 27
plant based remedies, 128
plant kingdom, 246
snake, 27
the kingdom approach, 140
vegetable kingdom, 325

Law of Similars
    Law of Similars, 203, 235
    levels of similarities, 447
    remedy similarity, 245
    similar, 367, 368, 369
    similar remedies, 304, 307
    similar simplex, 265
    similarity, 85, 244, 386
    similars, 440
    symptomatic similarity, 259
    The homeopathic principles of similarity, 140
Like cures like, 43
    like cures like, 94, 368, 421
    Like cures like, 430
Machine
    Abrams machine, 207
    bioresonance, 244, 245
    Bioresonance machine, 36
    cybernetic circuit, 42
    De La Warr machine, 207
    energetic medicine, 244
    machine, 36, 39, 40, 41, 42, 43, 44, 112, 136, 139, 140, 141, 322, 373
    machine's energy, 139
    machines, 28, 31, 39, 78, 139, 207, 268, 272
    meridian based technology, 41
    meridians, 41
    radionic instrument, 244
    radionic practitioner, 94
    radionic session, 244
    radionics, 207, 242, 243, 244, 245
    radionics machines, 207
    Rae machine, 207
    Rae machines, 336
    The frequency generator, 138
materia medica, 11, 23, 27, 28, 33, 47, 52, 53, 60, 65, 69, 80, 86, 98, 102, 106, 111, 140, 142, 158, 169, 262, 263, 264, 268, 277, 290, 298, 305, 306, 311, 326, 340, 341, 394, 411, 417, 425, 431, 449
    materia medicas, 185, 265, 314
Methodology
    active layers, 272
    cancer layer, 32
    classical method, 54
    classical methodology, 85
    Eizayaga's layers, 34, 40
    Eizayaga's layers methodology, 85
    emotional layer, 115
    Kentian method, 169
    layer, 40, 165, 169, 188, 274, 328
    layer clearance, 245
    layer model, 106

layer of susceptibility, 115
layers, 40, 41, 85, 105, 169, 183, 188, 215, 237, 238, 260, 274, 315, 323
layers approach, 68
multilayered, 274
multilayered cases, 183
Murphy method, 171
outer layer, 256
part patient, 54, 58
part patient homeopathy, 441
Rajan Sankaran's new system, 69, 180
Scholten method, 181
second layer, 256
Tautopathy, 52, 53
    drugs back in potency, 52
    tautopathy, 52, 53, 54, 115, 217, 375
top layer, 42, 183
traumatic pattern, 75
whole patient method, 54
Miasm
    antimiasmatic remedy, 256
    antipsoric, 101
    antisycotic medicine, 257
    antisyphilitic remedy, 256
    cancer miasm, 71
    CEEDS - chronic effective epidemic diseases, 71
    change of miasm, 260
    chronic miasms, 72
    combinations of miasms, 72
    conceptual domain of miasms, 142
    constitutional miasms, 40
    dominant miasm, 324
    fourth miasm, 253
    genetically, 44
    miasm, 72, 255, 256, 259, 261, 262, 266, 272, 360, 364, 449
    miasm changes, 260
    miasm theory, 116
    miasm work, 229
    miasmatic, 254
    miasmatic consideration, 256
    miasmatic diagnosis, 255, 256
    miasmatic diagnostic technique, 261
    miasmatic dyscrasia, 256
    miasmatic ideas, 309
    miasmatic influences, 257
    miasmatic nature, 256
    miasmatic observation, 256
    miasmatic remedy, 43, 389
    miasmatic technique, 253
    miasmatic tendencies, 419
    miasmatic theory, 142

Miasmatic Totality, 254
miasmatic unfolding, 215
miasms, 34, 71, 72, 125, 166, 211, 219, 250,
    254, 259, 262, 276, 311, 316, 324, 337,
    443
MTEK, 254, 259, 262
multimiasmatic, 260
nosode, 43, 324, 435
nosodes, 152, 324
other miasms, 214
psora, 114, 214, 255, 261, 449
Psora, 71
psoric, 255, 256, 449
psoric miasm, 348
psorics, 449
remedies for miasms, 72
surface miasm, 255, 256
sycotic, 255, 256, 257, 261, 449
syphilis, 70, 210, 255, 449
syphilitic, 255, 256, 261, 262
syphilitic miasm, 260, 449
syphilitic remedies, 449
syphilitic remedy, 260, 449
syphilitic syphilitic miasm, 328
syphilitics, 449
the syphilitic state, 358
trauma miasm, 75, 76
tubercular, 44, 255, 256, 261, 293
tubercular miasm, 253, 261
mixopathy, 28
non-medical homeopaths, 405
Organopathy
    drainage, 160
    organ drainage, 53, 54, 58
    organ support, 42, 128, 171, 182, 186, 228,
        324, 389, 448
    organ support system, 229
    organ therapy, 160
    organopathic medicines, 258
    organopathy, 148, 152, 154
Palliation
    not palliated, 35
    palliate, 239, 266, 324
    palliated, 240
    palliating, 182, 239, 302, 448
    palliation, 182, 218, 219, 239, 240, 243, 245,
        448
    Palliation, 217
    palliative, 70
    palliatively, 309
    serial palliation, 240
payment scheme, 50, 51
periodic table, 165

peripatetic homeopath, 290, 297
personal development, 13, 92, 165, 176, 275, 294,
    356, 418, 427
    personal development workshops, 352
    self-disclosure, 21, 22
Philosophy
    homeopathy philosophy, 38, 108, 123, 148, 217,
        218, 228, 298, 355, 361, 413, 455
    homoeopathy philosophy, 449
    overreaching philosophy, 103
    perrenial philosophy, 100
    underlying philosophy, 20
physical generals, 85, 169
placebo, 141, 143, 291, 335, 346
plussing, 43
polypharmacy, 28, 31, 43, 44, 54, 142, 265, 266
    Polypharmacy, 266
Potency
    different potencies, 44
    differential analysis, 100
    high potencies, 138, 181, 244, 449
    high potency, 27, 180, 216, 239, 274
    higher potency, 285
    in potency, 53, 173, 217
    LM potency, 32, 44, 113
    LM system, 163
    LMs, 43, 44, 216, 219, 228, 329, 389, 437
    low potencies, 58, 244, 285
    low potency, 42, 43, 171, 245, 274
    lower potencies, 286
    particular potency, 348
    potencies, 43, 44, 128, 133, 203, 204, 214,
        216, 220, 245
    potency, 41, 58, 66, 99, 106, 117, 128, 129,
        219, 240, 241, 244, 377
    potentisation, 421
    potentise, 411
    potentise electromagnetic frequencies, 138
    potentise sound, 137
    potentised, 52, 296, 449
    potentised remedies, 441
    potentised remedy, 99
    potentised sound, 138, 142
    potentised the crystals, 138
    potentising, 241
    remedy potencies, 94
Practical Homeopathy
    classical/practical issue, 80
    divide between practical and classical, 266
    practical approach, 101
    practical homeopath, 53, 58, 60
    practical homeopaths, 60

practical homeopathy, 54, 58, 59, 162, 176,
193, 267
Practical homeopathy, 46
practical homoeopaths, 441
practical homoeopathy, 441
practical versus classical, 267
practical way, 148, 441, 444
practitioner development, 6, 33, 46, 61, 111, 165,
195, 198, 272, 298, 352, 356, 419
Prescription
accurate prescription, 430
change my prescription, 260
classical prescriber, 194, 369
classical prescribers, 369
correct prescription, 33, 254, 255
first prescription, 41, 65, 66, 101, 129, 429,
438, 442, 447
follow up prescriptions, 443
homeopathic prescription, 154
inaccurate prescription, 430
inappropriately prescribed, 55
Kentian totality prescription, 54
mental and emotional prescribers, 165
not prescribe straight away, 8
over-prescribed remedy, 389
pathology prescriber, 166
prescribe a different remedy, 159
prescribe again, 130
prescribe classically, 327
prescribing classically, 369
prescribe constitutionally, 323, 324
prescribe for the whole person, 448
prescribe immediately, 117
prescribe in many different ways, 10
prescribe inappropriately, 188
prescribe like allopaths, 416
prescribe non-judgementally, 158
prescribe on physicals, 162, 176
prescribe on states, 142
prescribe on that level of chakras and
endocrinology, 324
prescribe on the greatest totality, 238
prescribe on the spot, 117, 389
prescribe on the symptoms, 5
prescribe one remedy, 322, 323
prescribe single remedies, 128
prescribe that one remedy, 323
prescribe the right remedy, 26
prescribe the 'right remedy', 81
prescribe the simillimum, 149
prescribe therapeutically, 191
prescribed combinations, 109
prescribed in the correct sequence, 183

prescribed more constitutionally, 413
prescribed on mentals, 169
prescribed on the basis of few available
symptoms, 259
prescribed on the basis of symptomatic
similarity, 259
prescribed on the symptoms, 169
prescribed palliatively, 309
prescribes on old symptoms, 164
prescription of a homeopathic remedy, 155
second prescription, 429, 438, 442, 443, 447
single remedy prescriber, 128
the prescription, 25, 113, 155, 182, 260, 264,
337
a prescription, 117, 130, 256, 261, 262, 273
totality prescriptions, 52
process, 6, 7, 15, 26, 112, 194, 198, 240, 297,
300, 387, 391, 409, 411, 422, 450
a process, 8, 112, 216, 306, 324, 329, 443
case process, 298
creation is a process, 392
creative process, 392, 393
disease process, 233
filtering process, 437
group process, 14
healing process, 299, 357, 411
homeopathic process, 6
individual's process within homeopathy, 10
inner process work, 191
inner processes of life, 151
internal process, 9
journey work, 294
learning process, 354, 411
my process, 295
personal growth, 298
prescribing process, 413, 427
process of deep cure, 183
process through it, 9
process way of teaching, 8
process work, 6, 7, 14, 18
process works well, 25
processes, 17, 321
psychological process, 27
scientific process, 180
the process, 8, 18, 25, 218, 250, 267, 288,
330, 335, 357, 423
the process conscious, 437
the process stuff, 11
to process, 26
transition process from allopathic to
homeopathic thinking, 416
whole process, 23
Proving

art of proving, 246
classical Hahnemannian proving, 335
conventional proving, 325
conventional provings, 322
double-blind meditation, 325
dream provings, 187
Hahnemann's proving, 187
Hahnemannian proving, 265, 322
Meditation
    body consciousness, 322
    circle to meditate, 320
    meditate, 322, 325
    meditating, 137, 321
    meditation, 321, 325, 326
    meditation circles, 326
    meditation groups, 318
    meditations, 326
    meditative, 322
    meditative proving, 266, 325
    meditative provings, 137, 160, 175, 228,
        321, 325, 330, 335
    meditatively, 321
    meditators, 324
modern provings, 187, 266
new proving, 335
new provings, 271, 305, 308, 309, 432
newly proven remedies, 451
old proving symptoms, 258
prove, 274, 325, 439
proved, 107, 161, 266, 321, 335, 432, 438, 440
proven, 216, 263
prover, 310
provers, 304, 310
proving, 6, 124, 144, 304, 310, 314, 321, 326,
    335, 351, 430, 431, 432, 436, 439, 444
proving symptoms, 265
provings, 7, 11, 44, 102, 106, 144, 161, 175, 191,
    276, 304, 308, 309, 314, 320, 327, 330,
    335, 351, 413, 430, 431, 432, 440
Provings, 7, 418
reprove, 175
unintentional provings, 443
well proved, 216
quantum homeopathy, 336
Remedy
    acute remedies, 48, 355, 413
    acute remedy, 43
    ampoules, 39
    archetypal remedies, 75
    bowel nosode, 101
    bowel nosode programme, 339, 347, 348
    bowel nosodes, 66, 348
    chronic remedy, 114

classical totality remedy, 194
combination of remedies, 71
combination remedies, 66, 350, 422
Combination remedies, 350
combination remedy, 127
combinations, 323, 422
constitutional remedy, 26, 65, 115, 183, 324,
    368, 369, 430, 442
constitutionally, 43, 113, 323
degree of remedy, 245
energy of homeopathic dilutions, 153
energy of the remedy, 140
field of the remedy, 12
Holy Grail, 307, 328, 441
Holy Grail of homeopathy, 106
Holy Grail remedy, 328
homeopathic bronchodilators, 258
how remedies work, 5
immunity boosting, 368
keynotes of a remedy, 37
little white pills, 410
    little white pill, 437
LM remedies, 128
macerated solution, 274
mixed remedies, 127
mother tincture, 128, 274
mother tinctures, 128, 272
new remedies, 33, 63, 77, 117, 160, 175, 187,
    271, 274, 276, 277, 311, 314, 318, 322,
    326, 351, 432
new remedy, 274, 432
newer remedies, 266, 322
nosode, 43, 324, 435
nosodes, 152, 324
one basic remedy, 105
one curative remedy, 423
one remedy, 105, 113, 119, 131, 227, 238, 273,
    286, 298, 307, 322, 323, 329, 350, 442
one single remedy, 327
partial remedies, 106
polycrest, 66, 183
    polycrests, 447
potentised remedy, 128
Prophylaxis
    malaria prophylaxis, 434
    prophylactic dose, 305
    prophylaxis, 434, 435
relationship of remedies, 43, 169, 215, 218,
    219
remedies for belief structures, 76
remedies in combination, 316, 328
remedy minerals, 246
remedy pattern, 104

Remedy Pictures
  Arsenicum albums, 80
  Aurums, 70
  drug picture, 441
  Drug Pictures, 257
  Miss Phosphorus, 257
  Mr Lycopodiums, 257
  Mr Nux Vomicas, 257
  Mr Psora, 256
  Mr Tubercular, 256
  Mrs Pulsatillas, 257
  picture of this remedy, 423
  remedy picture, 238, 328, 369, 389, 440
  remedy pictures, 406
  Sepias, 70
  small pictures, 175
  the picture of the remedy, 187
remedy potencies, 94
remedy profile, 277
remedy relationships, 168
remedy similarity, 245
right remedy, 165
sarcodes, 152
several remedies, 367, 369
similar remedies, 304, 307
single remedies, 128
single remedy, 127, 312, 329, 350
single remedy classic prescribing, 125
single remedy practice, 106
single remedy prescriber, 128
single remedy treatment, 243
Theme
  antimiasmatic remedy, 256
  antisyphilitic remedy, 256
  asthma remedies, 425
  bird theme, 341
  detox remedies, 66
  disease remedy, 72
  drainage remedies, 154
  drainage remedy, 53
  electromagnetic remedies, 138
  epidemic remedy, 134
  fever remedy, 412
  genetic remedies, 276
  liver remedies, 183
  liver remedy, 56
  meditative remedies, 316
  Mercury remedies, 43
  miasmatic remedy, 43, 389
  Milk remedies, 244
  Natrum theme, 341
  noble gases, 439
  not divided into themes, 431

  organ remedies, 11, 182, 183
  organ remedy, 182
  palliative remedies, 448
  plant based remedies, 128
  remedies for diseases, 72
  remedies for miasms, 72
  remedy epidemicus, 134
  sea remedies, 427
  snake remedy, 423
  syphilitic remedies, 449
  syphilitic remedy, 260, 449
  themes, 142, 340, 432
  trauma remedy, 50, 426
  tubercular remedies, 44
totality of symptoms of the remedy, 182
totality remedy, 59, 80
triads, 101
triturate, 274
vaccines in potency, 55
vaccinosis, 164
Repertory, 47, 126, 132
  a repertory curriculum, 306
  Cara, 305
  Homeonet, 126
  Isis, 305
  MacRepertory, 126, 132, 305
  Radar, 305
  repertories, 110
  repertorisation, 100, 110, 128, 354, 406, 449
  repertorise, 110, 406
  repertory, 17, 29, 41, 52, 53, 60, 65, 69, 102,
    110, 126, 132, 158, 191, 263, 264, 287,
    301, 305, 306, 311, 325, 326, 354, 416,
    425
  repertory books, 258
  repertory of personality characters, 258
rubrics, 68, 100, 110, 132, 158, 354
sequential, 54, 182
  sequentials, 85
shift, 24, 112, 139, 172, 304, 310, 407
  dynamic shift, 423
  shifted, 8, 66, 82
  shifting, 136, 144, 337
Simillimum
  disease simillimum, 69
  first simillimum, 69, 73
  individual archetypal simillimum, 75
  individual simillimum, 75
  second simillimum, 69, 73
  simillima, 106
  simillimum, 28, 114, 140, 141, 142, 145, 149,
    154, 237, 239, 304, 307, 350, 352, 357,
    358, 375, 440, 443

simillimum concept, 441, 442
simillimum prescribing, 155, 237, 240
simillimum principle, 101
simillimums, 440
theoretical simillimum, 441
spheres, 203, 215
succussion
succuss, 411
succussed potentised energetic medicines, 421
succussion, 412, 421
succussions, 214
supervision, 32, 77, 106, 188, 365, 366, 413
Suppression, 176
suppressed, 176
suppression, 54, 71, 176, 215, 218, 243, 266,
269, 347, 441, 442
Swedenborgian, 133, 150, 151
Swedenborgianism, 150
Symptom
acute symptoms, 49
assessement of symptoms, 255
available symptoms, 259
characteristic symptoms, 169
CLARITY OF SYMPTOMS, 254
clinical symptoms, 265
collective symptom, 416
complete symptoms, 244
early symptom, 239
emotional symptoms, 149, 181, 182, 431
individualising symptoms, 28
language of symptoms, 356
main symptoms, 53
mental symptom, 155
mental symptoms, 149, 181, 182
no symptoms, 72
old proving symptoms, 258
old symptoms, 164, 180, 218, 245
outer symptoms, 149
partial symptom pictures, 243
pathological symptoms, 153
physical symptoms, 149, 171, 186, 286
picture of symptoms, 416
power of symptoms, 351
presenting symptoms, 265
proving symptoms, 265
psychological symptoms, 168
real symptoms, 433
return of symptoms, 164
scarcity of symptoms, 256
SRP symptoms (strange, rare and peculiar
symptoms), 254
PQRS symptoms, 254, 255, 257
suppressed symptoms, 256, 259

symptom, 5, 29, 115, 116, 165, 169, 217, 242,
436, 441
symptom maker, 5
symptom picture, 130, 151
symptomatic prescribing, 29
symptomatically, 31
symptoms, 5, 8, 28, 37, 49, 52, 54, 55, 57, 60,
85, 112, 115, 149, 153, 163, 165, 169, 171,
172, 180, 187, 239, 242, 254, 257, 259,
260, 261, 262, 266, 303, 331, 335, 358,
369, 430, 431, 432, 434
SYMPTOMS, 258
symptoms around an organ, 169
symptoms improve, 49
symptoms of the acute, 328
taking symptoms, 406
totality of symptoms, 101, 256
Totality of symptoms, 254, 255, 257
totality of symptoms of the remedy, 182
uncontaminated symptoms, 258
whole symptom picture, 152
totality
Big totality, 420
biggest totality, 419, 422
classical totality remedy, 194
greater totality, 357
greatest totality, 238
Kentian totality prescription, 54
Miasmatic Totality, 254
new surface totality, 257
presenting totality, 257
proper totality, 256
qualitative totality, 257
quantitative totality, 264
small totality, 420
smallest totality, 419
the totality, 239
totality, 5, 59, 80, 215, 218, 219, 220, 244,
261, 266, 415, 418, 419, 431, 432, 448
Totality Essence Keynote, 254
totality in homeopathy, 419
totality of a disease, 72
totality of experience, 357
totality of symptoms, 101, 256
Totality of symptoms, 254, 255, 257
totality of symptoms of the remedy, 182
totality of that disease, 70
totality of trauma, 426
totality prescribing, 5, 52
totality prescriptions, 52
totality remedy, 59, 80
Transference
countertransference, 24, 32, 427

transference, 24, 27, 32, 427
vibrational library of memories, 272
Vital force
  a vital force, 115, 217
  disturbed vital force, 113, 116
  divided vital force, 382
  energy centre, 328
  energy disturbed, 176
  energy field, 140, 268, 272, 400
  energy flowing, 290, 298
  energy levels, 73
  energy medicine, 56, 301
  energy of compassion, 71
  energy will flow, 75
  energy work, 268, 272
  fields of energy, 7
  homeopathic vitalism, 148
  levels of energy, 133
  looking at energy, 168
  psychic vital energy, 401
  shifting energy field, 337
  subtle energy, 136, 139, 144
  the vital force, 5, 7, 12, 41, 53, 57, 72, 99,
    113, 148, 151, 178, 216, 217, 219, 285, 286,
    328, 382
  vibrational library of memories, 268
  vital energy, 57, 69, 104, 218, 268, 272, 276
  vital field, 400
  vital force, 12, 149, 215, 216, 217, 400
  vitalism, 148, 153
zigzagging
  zigzag, 447
  zigzagging, 115, 168, 172
  zigzags, 447

HOMEOPATHY ORGANISATIONS, HOSPITALS, PHARMACIES, COLLEGES, CLINICS AND INSTITUTIONS

Clinic
  Homeopathic Physicians' Teaching Group
    (HPTG), 26
    HPTG, 27
    HPTG web site, 26
  Life Works, 413, 414
  Manchester Homeopathic Clinic, 120

Colleges
  Allen College Of Homoeopathy
    Allen College, 250, 252, 262, 263, 267
  Bengal Allen Homeopathic College, 253, 333
  Bombay School, 309
  Braintree Forest School, 331
  British School of Homeopathy, 126, 369, 372
  Burren School, 306
  Centre for Homeopathic Education (CHE), 59,
    163, 189, 290
    CHE, 191, 193, 194, 195
    Regent's College, 189
  City Lit, 343
  College of Homeopathy (COH), 4, 39, 47, 67,
    80, 110, 121, 137, 147, 163, 184, 190, 283,
    320, 343, 353, 362, 381, 394, 410
    COH, 39, 80, 83, 84, 87, 110, 122, 126, 143,
    147, 156, 157, 164, 167, 184, 185, 186,
    188, 193, 320, 343, 344, 354, 355, 381,
    404, 405, 406, 407, 410, 411, 418
    Imperial College, 123, 213
    YWCA in Great Russell Street, 123, 362,
    404
  College of Practical Homeopathy (CPH), 46,
    66, 157, 192, 375
    CPH, 46, 50, 53, 54, 57, 59, 60, 61, 87, 192,
    375
  College of Practical Homeopathy in the
    Midlands (CPH Midlands), 45, 49, 88, 157,
    192, 271, 293
    CPH Midlands, 60, 88
    the Homeopathy College, 157, 271, 293
  Combined Colleges of Homeopathy (CCH), 157,
    193, 394
    CCH, 394
  Contemporary College of Homeopathy
    (Contemporary College), 163
    Contemporary College, 164, 177
  Darlington postgraduate collective, 305
  Dynamis School for Advanced Homoeopathic
    Studies
    Dynamis course, 412
    Dynamis School, 305, 337, 356, 412, 413,
    414, 427, 429, 438, 445
  Greek Seminars, 123
  International Academy of Classical
    Homeopathy (I.A.C.H.)
    Alonissos, 1, 102, 119, 131, 155, 180, 185,
    188, 208, 333, 450, 451
  Lakeland College of Homeopathy, 45, 271, 290,
    417
    Lakeland College, 45, 290, 293, 294, 298,
    299, 301, 303, 417, 418, 420

Lakes, 290, 294
London College of Classical Homeopathy
    (LCCH), 19, 48, 49, 106, 108, 110, 126, 154,
    173, 193, 200, 214, 229, 250, 279, 306,
    344, 356, 364, 367, 372, 381, 394
    LCCH, 49, 110, 155, 156, 157, 204, 214, 229,
    230, 306, 381
    Morley College, 48
    Russian Embassy, 344
London School of Classical Homeopathy
    (LSCH), 214, 360, 372
    LSCH, 363, 364, 365, 366
Medical School at the University of Athens,
    122
National Extension College in Cambridge, 372
New College of Homeopathy (New College),
    136, 193, 311, 339
    New College, 136, 142, 143, 144, 340, 344,
    345, 349
North London Group, 150, 319
North West College of Homoeopathy (NWCH),
    127, 179, 214, 224, 290, 410
    NWCH, 180, 182, 185, 186, 188, 225
Northern College, 127, 332
Orion, 162, 163, 170, 171, 177
    Orion class, 162
    Orion Postgraduate Course, 163
Practical College in Iceland, 45, 60
Practical Colleges, 116
Rajan Sankaran's school, 245
School of Homeopathy, 4, 98, 99, 106, 410,
    411, 412, 418, 455
School of Shamanic Homoeopathy, 45, 157,
    268, 278, 301
Scottish College, 295
South Downs School of Homeopathy, 127, 157
South London Group, 150, 151
Thames Valley University
    Slough campus, 352
    The Purton House Homeopathic Centre
    (Purton House)
    Purton House, 352, 354, 355, 356, 357,
    359, 420
Tiverton College of Classical Homeopathy, 213,
    408
University of Calcutta, 254
University of Central Lancashire, 223, 226,
    228, 230, 232
University of Greenwich, 339, 351
University of Westminster, 108, 111, 116, 156,
    157, 367, 369, 370, 376, 383, 435
    Department of Complementary Therapies,
    370

Pathways for Complementary Therapies
    programme, 157
Polyclinic, 111, 116, 117, 374, 377
School of Integrated Health, 111
Welsh School of Homoeopathy, 3, 427
    Welsh School, 3, 7, 13, 14, 15, 17, 18, 19,
    427, 450
Yorkshire School of Homeopathy, 126, 305,
    330, 334
    Yorkshire School, 305, 306, 335
Guidelines
    European Guidelines for Homeopathic
    Education, 339, 345
Hospitals
    Glasgow Homeopathic Hospital, 302, 376
    Royal London Homeopathic Hospital, 29, 31,
    113, 181, 269, 270, 316, 368, 416
Institutions
    Alliance of Registered Homeopaths (ARH)
    ARH, 270
    conference, 34
    Spring Conference, 237, 339
    American Institute of Homeopathy, 150
    British Homeopathic Association (BHA)
    library, 121
    Cooper Club, 148
    Council for Homeopathic Colleges (CHC), 157,
    270, 294
    CHC, 271
    Registration and Continuous Professional
    Development working groups, 270
    Council of Organisations Registering
    Homeopaths (CORH), 157, 253, 294, 375
    Accreditation
    accreditation, 373, 376
    accredited, 376
    accredited course, 376
    accrediting body, 270, 271
    new accreditation process, 271
    single register Accreditation Working
    Group, 157
    CORH, 253, 301
    CORH booklet, 209
    regulations, 30
    regulatory bodies, 30
    single register, 119, 127, 145, 160, 161, 302,
    373, 374, 416, 449
    statutory, 91
    statutory regulation, 392
    voluntary regulation, 392
Faculty, 27, 29, 31, 127, 129, 147, 150, 181,
    269, 369
    Faculty homeopath, 241

Fellowship of Homeopaths, 190
Guild of Homeopaths (Guild), 137, 160
  Guild, 138, 160
Homeopathic Education Services in California,
  127
Homeopathic Medical Association (HMA), 270
  conference, 91
  HMA, 91
Homeopathic Symposium, 2, 450
  teachers' seminar in Malvern, 2, 3, 24, 108,
    162, 223, 304, 409, 429, 450
Homoeopathy For A Change, 436
Institute for Homeopathy, 157
Not Just Classical Club, 82
Society of Homeopaths, 1, 3, 33, 46, 63, 67,
    91, 119, 121, 122, 125, 126, 129, 147, 189,
    213, 219, 233, 237, 246, 250, 270, 271,
    283, 311, 320, 330, 334, 339, 363, 373,
    374, 375, 379, 384, 391, 444, 445, 455
  Code of Ethics, 126, 241, 247
  First Class Mail, 379, 393
  Society Cases Conference, 129
  Society of Homeopaths' Conference, 173
  Society of Homeopaths' Continuous
    Professional Development group, 339
  Society of Homeopaths' register, 343
The Northern California Institute of Classical
  Homeopathy, 214
Pharmacies
  Ainsworths, 47, 50, 162
  Galen's pharmacy, 66
  Helios pharmacy, 320
  Neal's Yard, 407
    Neal's Yard Remedies, 130
  Nelsons Homeopathic Pharmacy, 162, 242, 379
    Nelsons, 162, 163

O

OTHER ORGANISATIONS, HOSPITALS, COLLEGES, CLINICS AND INSTITUTIONS

Clinic
  Clissold Park Natural Therapy Centre in Stoke
    Newington, 47
    Clissold Park, 47
  Fitzrovia Medical Centre, 128
  Islington Green Centre of Complementary
    Medicine, 51
  Marylebone Health Centre, 128
  NHS clinic, 108, 118
  osteopath's clinic in Hampton, 355
    osteopath's clinic, 353
Colleges
  Aberystwyth University, 96
  American International Schools, 147
  British School of Osteopathy and
    Naturopathy, 365
  BCOM, 365
  Cambridge University, 74
  Imperial College, 382
  LAMDA, 96
  London College of Traditional Acupuncture, 45
  London University, 120, 121
  New York University, 146
  Open University, 120, 121, 427
  School of Oriental Studies, 137
  Steiner school, 193
  Westminster College, 96
Hospitals
  Great Ormond Street Hospital, 67
  Hammersmith Hospital, 96
  Kensington General Hospital in Johannesburg,
    211
  Royal Free Hospital, 413
  University College Hospital, 354
Institutions
  Association of Natural Medicine, 270
  California Institute of Integral Studies, 414
  Eclectic Institute of Cincinnati, Ohio, 148
  Institute of Complementary Medicine, 221
  Medical Research Council, 96
  National Health Service, 128
    NHS, 16, 35, 108, 128, 129, 301, 302, 374
  National Institute of Health in America, 276
  New Church of Jerusalem of Emmanuel
    Swedenborg, 132
  Online Mendelian Inheritance in Man (OMIN),
    276
  South Bank University, 156
    South Bank, 156
  Transpersonal Psychology Centre, 356
Other organisations
  British Medical Association, 391
  CAT – Child Aid Trust, 402
  Hyperactive Children Society, 291
  Roof, 402
  Shelter, 402
  Terrence Higgins Trust, 171
  the ANC, 211

P

PATHOLOGY, DISEASE AND THE COMMON COLD

acne, 56
ageing degenerative sequences, 276
AIDS, 38, 70, 71, 72, 73, 74, 115, 171, 429, 433, 434
allergic, 256
allergies, 255
alopecia, 255
anxiety, 131
appendectomy, 24, 31
appendicitis, 24, 31
Arthritis
    arthritis, 31, 99, 131, 437
    chronic rheumatism, 194
    chronic rheumatoid arthritis, 274
    rheumatic-gouty, 256
    rheumatism, 38, 184, 187
    rheumatoid arthritis, 43, 113
asthma, 12, 38, 163, 291, 331, 416, 424, 446
    an asthmatic, 291
    asthma attack, 422
autoimmune disease, 307
baldness, 255
Blood Pressure
    drug dependent hypertensive, 259
    high blood pressure, 53, 276
    hypertension, 255, 276
    hypotension, 255
bone pains, 255
bradycardia, 255
bronchitis, 380
bruising, 99
Cancer
    breast cancer, 53, 125, 173, 217, 224, 346
    breast malignancy, 266
    buboes, 218
    cancer, 31, 32, 35, 38, 41, 42, 58, 59, 66, 69,
        71, 72, 73, 115, 171, 172, 173, 182, 199,
        224, 252, 266, 268, 272, 274, 311, 313,
        314, 317, 329, 357, 382, 424, 425, 426,
        442, 447, 448
    Cancer, 172, 442
    cancer care centre, 199, 218
    cancer case, 218, 449
    cancer cases, 172
    cancer of the prostate, 72

cancer of the testicles, 72
cancer patient, 382
cancer patients, 58, 244, 377
cancer research, 96
cancerous, 96
cancers, 32, 58, 149, 181, 314, 426
carcinogenic, 383
carcinogenic substances, 382
carcinogenicity, 383
carcinogens, 96
Hodgkinson, 205
hyperplasia, 255
incipient cancer, 72
leukaemia, 314
liver cancer, 351
lump, 219, 224, 424
    lumps, 218
lung cancer, 66, 317
malignant melanoma, 31
ovarian cancer, 448
prostate cancer, 72, 240
tumour, 58, 382, 424
tumours, 314, 382
Candida, 244, 245
carpal tunnel pain relief, 417
carpal tunnel release surgery, 416
chest infections, 48, 380
chicken pox, 331
cholera, 433
    cholera epidemic, 120
    cholera epidemics, 120
chronic degenerative disease, 323
colds, 44, 48
colic, 396
    colicky, 256
constipation, 255
coughs, 44, 332, 342
Crohn's, 43
Daithesis
    eruptive diathesis, 256
dandruff, 255
degenerative diseases, 317
dermatitis, 48
diabetes, 73
    diabetic, 70, 73
diarrhoea, 115, 255
    diarrhoeic, 256
diplopia, 132
drug dependent asthma cases, 258
dyscrasia, 256
dysenteric, 256
dysentery, 255
dyses, 255

dyslexic, 50
dysplasia, 255
dystrophy, 255
earache, 241
eczema, 44, 49, 50, 55, 56, 196, 221, 331
epilepsy, 35
   epileptic, 35
   epileptic fits, 411
Female health issues
   cystitis, 183
   ectopic pregnancies, 425
   fertility, 323, 346, 347, 348, 425
   fibroid, 425
   fibroids, 69, 424, 425
   Follicle-stimulating hormone levels, 425
   hot flushes, 52
   infertile, 323
   infertility, 347
   IVF, 347, 425
   IVF hormones, 347
   menopause, 52, 64
   polycystic ovaries, 163
fever, 410, 412
   feverish, 410
   fevers, 353, 412
   high fevers, 412
Flu
   bird flu, 433
   flu, 130, 396
   flu epidemics, 134
gallstone, 396
gastric ulcer, 256, 261
gastroenteritis, 342
haemoptysis, 128
haemorrhage, 218
   haemorrhages, 255
   haemorrhagic, 256
   haemorrhagic diathesis, 256
   haemorrhagic secretions/discharges, 256
hay fever, 168, 172, 245, 255, 302
headaches, 42, 183, 425
heart attack, 99, 100, 147, 360, 364, 419
hepatitis, 120
HIV, 115, 138, 434
hyperactive, 256
hypertrophy, 255
indurations, 219
infections, 342
joint pains, 43, 255
kidney infection, 48
lithic-uric acid, 256
malaena, 255
Malaria

malaria, 47, 71, 433, 434, 435
   malarial region, 434
measles, 47, 70, 131
Meniere's Disease, 302
meningitis, 24, 31, 155
menorrhagia, 255
Methicillin resistant Staphylococcus aureus
   (MRSA), 134
migraine, 183
multiple sclerosis, 38, 132
   MS, 132, 244, 432, 437
mumps, 47, 131
myalgic encephalomyelitis (ME), 142, 297
nephrotic syndrome, 368
neuralgic pains, 255
neurodegenerative disorder, 137
pain, 218
painkiller dependent migraine cases, 259
pains with exhaustion, 255
pancreatitis, 364
Pathology
   constitutional pathology, 442
   mental pathology, 111
   pathological, 71, 169
   pathologies, 58
   pathology, 14, 34, 41, 42, 43, 54, 69, 70, 95,
      111, 122, 125, 126, 129, 132, 149, 153, 166,
      170, 182, 183, 187, 194, 223, 228, 232,
      233, 239, 240, 411, 416, 419, 420, 441,
      448
   Pathology, 71
peptic ulcer, 186
plantar warts, 410
pneumonia, 130, 380
polio, 47
proliferative diathesis, 256
pulmonary embolism, 396
pus, 36, 218, 255
schizophrenia, 172
sepsis, 131
septicaemia, 131, 283
sexually transmitted diseases, 70
   AIDS, 38, 70, 71, 72, 73, 74, 115, 171, 429,
      433, 434
   chlamydia, 70
   gonorrhoea, 70
   hepatitis, 120
   herpes, 70
   HIV, 115, 138, 434
   syphilis, 70, 210, 255, 449
smallpox, 70
sore throat, 48, 353
steroid dependent arthritic cases, 258

stroke, 40, 52, 124, 177, 273
suppurative-ulcerative, 256
tachycardia, 255
tinnitus, 29
tonsillitis, 172, 241, 342
tuberculosis (TB), 71, 331, 433
ulceration, 219, 256, 262
ulcerative colitis, 328
verrucae, 410
vitiligo, 37
wheezing, 291
whooping cough, 305, 331
worms, 210
yaws, 210

PEOPLE

CELEBRITIES, FAMOUS PEOPLE, FILM STARS, ARTISTS, WRITERS, MUSICIANS AND BANDS

Albery, Nick, 402
Bailey, Alice, 269
Baker, Douglas, 269
Blake, William, 400
Bolan, Mark, 403
Bowie, David, 403
Brown, James, 397
Carr-Saunders, Nicholas, 401, 402, 07
Caruso, Enrico, 107
Chaplin, Charlie, 98
Christie, Julie, 396
Collins, Jackie, 397
Collins, Joan, 397
Emerson, Ralph Waldo, 132
Fitzgerald, Ella, 23
Gates, Bill, 434
Goethe, Johann, 414
Hardy, Oliver, 17
Hawkins, Coleman, 397
Hendrix, Jimi, 397
Icke, David, 90
James, Henry, 132
Jefferson Airplane, 398
John, Elton, 434
Keaton, Buster, 98
Keeler, Christine, 396
Laurel, Stan, 17

Lawrence, DH, 400
Lerman, Oscar, 397
Marley, Bob, 397
McLaren, Malcolm, 403, 404
Mozart, Wolfgand Amadeus, 107
New Romantics, 404
Oliver, Jamie, 296
Picasso, Pablo, 10
Prince Charles, 302
Quant, Mary, 396, 398
Raft, George, 397
Reid, Jamie, 404
Roosevelt, Teddy, 179, 181
Savalas, Telly, 397
Serelis, Vytas, 397
Shakespeare, William, 86, 143, 356, 387
Shrimpton, Jean, 396
Sinatra, Frank, 396
Slim, Eddie, 397
Spungen, Nancy, 404, 405
Stamp, Terence 396
Strange, Steve, 404
Tarnas, Richard, 414
The Doors, 398
The Heartbreakers 403
The Krays, 397
The New York Dolls, 403
The Rolling Stones, 399
The Sex Pistols, 403 404
The Slits, 403
Twiggy, 396
Vicious, Sid, 403, 404, 405
Westwood, Vivienne, 403
Williams, Heathcote, 402
Yeats, William Butler, 400

HOMEOPATHS OF THE DISTANT PAST

Allen, John Henry, 251, 253, 263, 264
Beauharnais, Nash Eugene, 265
Boericke, William, 120, 126, 152, 202, 241, 331, 444
Burnett, James Compton, 123, 131, 148, 149, 150, 152, 163, 164, 169, 171, 171, 228
Clarke, John, 94, 120, 123, 131, 148, 164, 202, 206, 331, 406
Close, Stuart, 18
Cooper, Thomas, 148, 164
Farrington, Ernest, 219

Hahnemann, Samuel, 5, 6, 8, 12, 21, 33, 34, 41, 43, 44, 54, 58, 69, 70, 72, 73, 85, 101, 112, 103, 114, 116, 121, 123, 127, 131, 132, 143, 149, 150, 151, 154, 161, 162, 163, 164, 166, 168, 180, 169, 182, 187, 198, 202, 203, 204, 215, 218, 219, 220, 228, 235, 240, 241, 251, 254, 256, 268,298, 272, 299, 312, 330, 335, 348, 350, 352, 356, 414, 418, 419, 421, 422, 426, 432, 433, 434, 440,451

Hering, Constantine, 37, 148, 149, 150, 153, 161

Honigberger, John Martin, 251

Hughes, Richard, 153

Kent, James Tyler, 28, 47, 54, 65, 85, 101, 106, 112, 121, 121, 123, 126, 131, 132, 133, 148, 149, 150, 151, 154, 162, 164, 166, 168, 169, 176, 179, 180, 181, 182, 183, 198, 202, 204, 206, 219, 220, 238, 239, 244, 253, 263, 264, 265, 389, 443, 444, 448

Künzli, Jost, 109

Lilienthal, Samuel, 406

Quin, Frederick, 202

Skinner, Thomas, 202

von Boenninghausen, Clemens, 153, 219

NON-HOMEOPATHS, HOMEOPATH'S FAMILY AND FRIENDS, HISTORIANS, PRINCIPALS, LEADERS AND OTHERS WHO WORK IN THE FIELD OF HOMEOPATHY

Berry, Thomas, 414

Clarke, Mary, 126

Coulter, Harris, 123, 124, 152, 210

Creer, Daphne, 356, 357

Hocking, John, 147, 156

Hood, Mary, 193, 230, 394

Maughan, Jennifer, 147, 316, 398

Sokolov, Joan, 401

Wallace, Maggie, 301

Winston, Julian, 124, 209

NON-UK BASED HOMEOPATHS – PAST AND PRESENT

Assilem, Melissa, 190, 191

Bailey, Philip, 181, 295

Bose, BK, 263

Boyce, Carol, 262

Braunger, Jane, 109

Candegabe, Eugenio, 68, 333

Castro, Miranda, 103, 128

Choudhuri, NM, 253

Coulter, Catherine, 123

Davis, Dr, 281

Decker, Steven, 414

Dey, SP, 125

Eizayaga, Francisco, 34, 39, 68, 85, 132, 163, 333

Feldman, Murray, 4, 184, 191, 213, 225, 357

Ghegas, Vassilis, 4, 5, 26, 28, 68, 121, 122, 123, 155, 208, 332, 333, 338, 444

Gray, Bill, 102

Grimmer, Arthur, 448

Guess, George, 446

Haggiag, Michael, 181

Herscu, Paul, 295, 296

Logan, Robin, 121, 122, 167

Lozdan, Jack, 120

Mangialavori, Massimo, 27, 113, 114, 142, 143, 447

Morrison, Roger, 68, 122, 208, 265, 332

Murphy, Robin, 32, 35, 57, 84, 164, 171, 172, 191, 195, 274, 295, 296, 333

O'Reilly, Wenda, 414

Payrhuber, Dietmar, 181

Peck, Kathryn, 407

Quirk, Tina, 433

Ramakrishnan, A.U, 58, 72, 182

Reves, Joseph, 354, 355, 356, 410, 444

Robert, Herbert, 187

Rwegasira, Sigsbert, 434

Sankaran, Rajan, 35, 39, 68, 71, 83, 102, 125, 143, 144, 180, 183, 185, 198, 226, 239,246, 247, 265, 296, 304, 309, 355

Scholten, Jan, 35, 69, 102, 142, 151, 181, 238, 246, 265, 304, 307, 308, 309, 310, 428

Schroyens, Frederik, 1, 106

Shah, Jayesh, 185

Sherr, Camilla, 445
Ullman, Dana, 127
Vermeulen, Frans, 106, 160, 265
Vithoulkas, George, 1, 4, 26, 27, 28, 29, 31,
   33, 39, 68, 81, 82, 83, 84, 101, 102, 103, 106,
   107, 119, 121, 122, 123, 131, 149, 150, 155,
   163, 175, 180, 181, 183, 185, 186, 188, 206,
   207, 208, 209, 225, 226, 238, 263, 264,
   308, 309, 333, 354, 390, 391, 400, 444, 450
Warkentin, David, 126

SCIENTISTS, PHILOSOPHERS, THERAPISTS, CAM TEACHERS, PRACTIONERS AND OTHERS – PAST AND PRESENT

Aristotle, 86, 385
Bach, Edward, 101, 121
Benveniste, Jacques, 137
Capra, Fritjof, 414
Chopra, Deepak, 414
Cronquist, Arthur, 143
Crookes, William, 240
Democritus, 385
Descartes, René, 385
Döbereiner, Johann Wolfgang, 109
Firebrace, Peter, 147, 398
Freud, Sigmund, 95
Fuller, Buckmaster, 74
Garth Wilkinson, JJ, 132
Gordon-Brown, Ian, 356
Goswami, Amit, 414
Hegel, Georg, 414
Hellinger, Bert, 76
Heraclitus, 385
Holford, Patrick, 295
Holligan, Sally, 291, 292, 293
James Snr, Henry, 132
James, William, 132
Jayasuriya, Anton, 36, 37, 38, 40

Johnson, Steve, 296
Jung, Carl, 352, 356
Kant, Immanuel, 414
Krishnamurti, Jiddu, 146, 208
Ledermann, Eric, 29
Leucippus, 385
MacGregor Reid Robert, 400, 404
Newton, Isaac, 385
Paracelsus, 44, 148, 149, 150
Paterson, John, 101
Plato, 242, 385
Rademacher, Johann, 131, 148, 149
Rae, Malcolm, 94
Richards, Patrick, 139
Russell, Rosemary, 94
Sangarachita, 146
Shohet, Robin, 27
Steiner, Rudolph, 121, 150, 194, 269
Swedenborg, Emanuel, 123, 132, 133, 148, 149,
   150, 151, 202, 203, 204, 220
Swimme, Brian, 414
Temple, Jack, 284
White, Ian, 296
Wilber, Ken, 414

UK HOMEOPATHS – PAST AND PRESENT

Abbott, Ros, 381
Adams, Peter, 121
Ball, John, 122
Banerjea Kumar, Subrata, 250, 333
Barker, Ellis, 164
Barker, Rob, 354
Berg, Stella, 121, 354
Bickley, Anthony, 213, 343, 354, 363, 364,
   369
Blackie, Margery, 120, 410
Bridger, Mike, 6, 162, 190, 196, 339, 343, 381,
   447
Burger, June, 127
Chappell, Peter, 4, 63, 91, 100, 147, 282, 316,
   317, 319, 401, 403, 405
Chatfield, Kate, 162, 223
Creasy, Sheilagh, 4, 106, 108, 122, 185, 200,
   235, 239, 240, 243, 246, 248, 262, 343,
   349, 354, 355, 356, 360, 362, 363, 389,
   408, 442
Crump, Sue, 372
Curtin, David, 122, 127, 167, 181, 185, 402
Curtis, Susan, 121, 354

Damonte, John, 65, 94, 99, 100, 101, 106, 107, 120, 123, 147, 155, 213, 319, 320, 399, 401
Danciger, Liz, 156, 332, 410, 411
Davidson, Robert, 4, 6, 21, 49, 50, 51, 57, 59, 61, 65, 67, 78, 100, 121, 122, 137, 147, 160, 164, 167, 191, 192, 193, 213, 214, 243, 244, 282, 283, 295, 317, 319, 320, 343, 349, 355, 362, 364, 401, 403, 404, 405, 406, 407, 408, 410, 443, 444
Dorrian, Hilery, 190, 196, 262, 343
Douch, Geoffrey, 380
Duckworth, Jean, 162, 223, 228, 229, 230
Dyson, Roger, 191
Eising, Nuala, 107, 288, 296, 306
Evans, Dave, 179, 182, 290, 293, 294
Evans, Madeline, 296, 334
Fernandez, Marcus, 193
Fordham, Bob, 363
Foubister, Donald, 29, 72, 101, 125
Francis, Paul, 299, 301
Gamblin, Annette, 108, 367
Gathercole, Kate, 445
Gemmell, David, 48, 49
Gordon, Stephen, 121, 372, 394, 406
Gregerson, Lesley, 121, 214, 343, 354, 360, 372
Griffith, Colin, 137, 190, 191, 324, 326, 327, 328
Gwillim, Linda, 3
Hammond, Christopher, 271
Hannon, Dorothy, 331, 332, 334, 336, 337
Harling, Marianne, 29
Hart, Lorraine, 301, 343
Harwood, Barbara, 4, 6, 110, 121, 137, 190, 193, 213, 230, 320, 343, 362, 394, 410, 411
Hebbourn, Kay, 290
Howard, Terry, 324
Howell, David, 50, 82, 88, 192, 295
Hurley, Tony, 6, 121, 164, 167, 190, 191, 193, 196, 225, 342, 343, 355, 407, 408
Jackson, Anjie, 293
Jaffey, Joel, 343
Josling, Sue, 137, 193
Kaplan, Brian, 24, 46, 48, 175, 186, 212, 302
Kennedy, Charles Oliver, 241
Kramer, Ellen, 173, 375
Larkin, Anne, 154, 156, 157, 214, 364
Lewith, George, 127
Lockie, Andrew, 27, 103
Lovell, Lynn, 282
Maclaughlin, Dee, 306, 402
Martanda, Adam, 18

Maughan, Thomas, 63, 64, 65, 79, 84, 100, 101, 120, 123, 145, 146, 147, 151, 152, 154, 155, 160, 184, 193, 213, 280, 281, 282, 312, 318, 320, 328, 350, 394, 398, 399, 404
Meldrum, Janet, 356, 357
Micallef, Janice, 137, 324, 326, 327, 328
Miles, Martin, 65, 67, 100, 137, 147, 152, 184, 187, 190, 193, 198, 213, 283, 311, 331, 339, 351, 355, 362, 401, 405, 406, 407, 408, 436
Milgrom, Lionel, 379
Millum, Christine, 334
Mitchell, Jillian, 298
Moon, Deirdre, 293
Morgan, John, 121, 333, 343, 354
Mundy, David, 4, 6, 122, 167, 184, 185, 186, 187, 191, 362, 407, 410, 412, 414, 415
Needleman, David, 129, 131
Nichols, Robert, 121, 333, 394, 406, 407
Norland, Misha, 4, 6, 9, 21, 65, 120, 122, 167, 181, 184, 185, 189, 193, 213, 245, 246, 355, 362, 399, 412
Peters, Sonyo (Julia), 343
Pinto, Gabrielle, 407
Pitman, Diane, 324
Pool, Nicky, 343, 352
Preston, Rebecca, 304, 334
Probert, Valerie, 143, 341
Puddephatt, Noel, 206, 207, 208
Razzell, Linda, 143, 339
Reiley, David, 302
Relton, Clare, 225
Riley, David, 376
Roberts, Ernest, 179, 214, 224, 354
Roy, Margaret, 295, 343, 344
Rumble, Bill, 3, 162
Sambidge, Gordon, 137, 143, 189
Samuel, Kay, 356, 357, 410, 411
Saunders, Anne, 213, 225, 408
Savage, Roger, 237
Shannon, Linda, 262, 333, 343
Sharma, Yubraj, 268, 301
Shemmer, Yair, 110
Sherr, Jeremy, 4, 69, 74, 102, 117, 121, 156, 184, 193, 213, 237, 238, 240, 246, 304, 305, 306, 308, 309, 335, 337, 352, 354, 355, 356, 412, 414, 428, 429, 451
Shine, Michelle, 345, 454
Shivadikar, Myriam, 34, 290
Singer, Wendy, 213
Smart, Jackie, 109
Smeaton, Keith, 343
Smith, Julie, 367, 369, 372

Snowdon, Janet, 4, 121, 181, 184, 245
Southam, Tony, 295
Speight, Phyllis, 155, 206
Sternberg, Sue, 367, 383
Tabrett, Dion, 162
Taffler, Simon, 409, 418
Thompson, Michael, 65
Tibbs, Stan, 121
Titchmarsh, Mary, 65, 282, 317, 319
Townsend, Ian, 223, 228, 229, 230, 363
Treacher, Sylvia, 121, 324, 344
Treuherz, Francis, 119, 158, 262, 333, 343, 354, 362, 454
Twentyman, Ralph, 29
Tyers, Beth, 293
Tyler, Margaret, 27, 181, 265
Wansbrough, Charles, 136, 193, 340, 341
Waters, Anne, 271, 290
Watson, Ian, 6, 57, 71, 137, 164, 181, 193, 225, 291, 292, 293, 294, 295
Whitney, Jerome, 65, 145, 271, 279, 280, 282, 317, 319, 398, 400, 401
Whitney, Kaaren, 65, 100, 146, 147, 184, 279, 317, 319, 398
Winton, Barbara, 362
Wise, Carol, 262, 330
Wright, Jill, 324

Buddha, 136, 268
Buddhist, 38, 385
the Friends of the Western Order, 146
Christianity, 64, 385, 395
Christian, 132, 150, 276
Christian religious teaching, 151
esoteric Christian, 150
fundamentalist Christians, 150
Jesus Christ, 268
The Christians, 385
traditional Christian philosophy, 151
Hindu, 385
Judaism
Hebrew, 400
Jew, 95
Jewish, 95, 125, 130, 131, 202, 203, 397
Jewish background, 204
Jewish books, 202
Jewish leader, 204
Jews, 95, 97
Judaism, 202, 204
kabbalah, 311, 326
Judea-Christian, 203

PLACES OF INTEREST

Chelsea Hotel in New York, 405
Hyde Park, 399
Island Records, 397
National Gallery, 275
Reading Valley Festival, 402
Roebuck, 403
Ronnie Scott's, 397
Stonehenge, 280
the Everyman, 97, 98
The Globe, 143
the Roundhouse, 398
the Ruff Tuff Creampuff Estate Agency, 402
Watkins bookshop, 94
World's End, 401

R

RELIGIONS

Buddhism, 398

REMEDIES

Acetanilidum, 259
Aceticum acidum, 258
Aconitum napellus, 4, 48
Agnus castus, 425
Allium sativa, 259
Amber, 310
Ambra grisea, 66
Amethyst, 304, 310
Anacardium orientale, 66, 240, 258
Anagyris, 259
Apis, 40
Apomorphine, 127
Apple, 325
Aralia racemosa, 258
Argentum nitricum, 4, 66, 258
Arnica, 99, 124, 130, 154, 177, 254, 267, 277, 416, 425, 426
Arsenicum album, 79, 187, 258, 422
Aspidosperma, 259
Aurum metallicum, 68, 69, 333, 442
Ayahuasca, 276
Baryta carbonica, 258
Belladonna, 155, 258, 332, 412
Bellis perennis, 243, 426
Berberis, 44
Berlin Wall, 161, 276
Blatta orientalis, 259
Brassica, 309
Bromium, 259
Bryonia, 261, 336
Butterfly, 432
Cadmium sulphuratum, 42
Calcarea carbonica, 43, 79, 101, 169, 258, 323
Calcarea iodata, 258
Calcarea phosphorica, 44, 258
Calcarea silicata, 258
Cancer, 73
Candida albicans, 244, 245
Cannabis, 40, 41, 52
Carcinosin, 36, 42, 71, 72, 101, 258, 260, 279, 324, 375, 389, 390, 424, 425
Carduus marianus, 128
Cassia sophera, 259
Causticum, 40, 258, 332
Chamomilla, 47, 260
Chelidonium, 266
Chicken, 107
China sulphuricum, 435
Chionanthus virginica, 259

Chocolate, 28, 246, 309
Cocculus indicus, 127, 258
Cortisone, 40, 41, 375
Crataegus oxyacantha, 259
Crotalus cascavella, 28
Crotalus horridus, 134, 403
Cuprum metallicum, 332
Diabetes, 73
Diamond (Adamas), 274, 335
Digitalis, 182
Drosera, 331
Eagle (Haliaeetus leucocephalus), 28, 310
Echinacea, 346
Eel serum (Serum anguillae ichthyotoxinum), 259
Epiphegus, 259
Ergotinum, 259
Eriodictyon, 259
Fat, 76
Ferrum phosphoricum, 259
Fire (Ignis alcoholis), 309
Folliculinum, 216, 323, 348, 349, 425
Fox, 107
Franciscaea uniflora, 258
Gaertner, 101
Genisis, 321
Germanium, 431, 432
Ginseng, 258
Graphites, 258
Haloperidol, 292
Hepar sulphuris calcareum, 242, 244, 258
Hydrastis, 266
Hydrogen, 309
Hyoscyamus, 176, 292
Hypericum, 243
Ignatia amara, 79, 258, 401
Indium metallicum, 259
Iodium, 44, 258
Iris versicolor, 259
Jaborandi, 131
Jade, 431, 436
Jet, 276
Kali arsenicosum, 258
Kali bichromicum, 256, 262
Kali bromatum, 258
Kali carbonicum, 186, 258, 347, 348
Kali iodatum, 258
Kali nitricum, 258
Kali phosphoricum, 65, 258
Kalmia latifolia, 259
Lac defloratum, 259
Lac humanum, 276, 321
Lac leoninum, 432
Lachesis muta, 27, 28, 53, 57, 258

Latrodectus mactans, 325, 326
Lilium tigrinum, 258
Lobelia inflata, 44
Lycopodium, 33, 113, 141, 218, 241, 258, 369, 370
Lycopus virginicus, 259
Magnesia carbonica, 258
Magnesia muriatica, 183, 258
Magnesia phosphorica, 163
Malaria officinalis, 47, 435
Medorrhinum, 71, 401
Melilotus officinalis, 259
Menispernum canadense, 259
Menynanthes trifoliate, 259
Mercury (Mercurius solubilis), 48, 169, 287
Moldavite, 276
Morgan, 65, 101
Myrica cerifera, 266
Natrum carbonicum, 258
Natrum muriaticum, 52, 105, 106, 171, 176, 186, 218, 258, 260, 261, 264, 299, 328, 425, 435, 447
Natrum phosphoricum, 28, 33, 65
Natrum sulphuricum, 130, 171
Nelsons' Travel Combination remedy, 127
Neptunium, 432
Nitricum acidum, 169, 258, 336
Nux vomica, 79, 120, 127, 240, 258, 274, 345, 375
Obsidian, 276
Oleum animale aethereum dippeli, 259
Onosmodium virginianum, 259
Opium, 50, 122, 290, 412
Oxygenium, 422
Ozonum, 432
PC1, 73
Petroleum, 258
Phosphoricum acidum, 258
Phosphorus, 27, 44, 176, 258, 266
Pimpinella saxifraga, 258
Pituitary Gland, 323
Placenta humana, 6
Plastic (Polystyrenum), 432
Platina, 208
Platinum metallicum, 297
Plutonium nitricum, 196
Pothos foetidus, 259
Psorinum, 258
Pulsatilla nigricans, 43, 258, 314
Pyrogenium, 131, 134
Rauwolfia serpentina, 259
Raven (Corvus corax), 432
Rhus toxicodendron, 31, 43, 113, 258, 296
Ricinus communis, 129

RNA remedy, 276
Robinia pseudacacia, 186
Salmon (Onchorynchus tschawytscha), 431
Saponinum, 259
Sapphire, 431
Scarlet Macaw (Ara Macaw), 28
Scorpion (Androctonos amurreuxi hebraeus), 246, 309, 432
Sepia succus, 69, 174, 258, 277
Silica terra, 27, 241, 258
Spartium scoparium, 259
Staphysagria, 42, 125, 127, 172
Stellaria media, 258
Stramonium, 145, 240, 332
Strophanthus hispidus, 259
Sulphur, 36, 37, 55, 56, 58, 65, 101, 169, 196, 258, 265, 291, 344, 347, 348
Swan (Cygnus cygnus), 439
Sycamore seed, 303, 323
Syphilinum, 43, 71, 358
Tabacum, 127
Tamoxifen, 53, 173, 217
Tarentula hispanica, 28
The Crucifixion, 275
The Sphinx, 275
The Temptation, 275
Theridion curassavicum, 127
Thuja occidentalis, 164, 242, 258, 344
Thymus gland, 274
Thyroxine, 53
Triple A, (Ambra grisea, Anacardium orientale, Argentum nitricum, 66
Tuberculinum bovinum, 44, 291, 353, 424
Usnea barbata, 259
Viola, 258
Yucca filamentosa, 259
Zincum, 28, 277
Zincum phosphoricum, 28
Zubeneschamali, 276

S

SCIENCE

biochemist, 380
biochemistry, 365
biochemists, 382, 386
Buckmaster Fuller method, 74
chemist, 380
electron microscope, 241
electron microscopes, 386
materialistic science, 153

physicists, 400
Quantum Physics
   Born-Oppenheimer approximation, 386
   Orbital approximation, 386
   quantum approach, 426
   quantum medicine, 426
   quantum physicists, 386
   quantum physics, 385, 387, 408, 426

Quantum physics, 12
quantum theory, 385, 386
quantum world, 426
subquantum levels, 140
Radiation, 241
   radiation, 442
reductionist Cartesian, 385
science, 311

BIBLIOGRAHY

[1] www.vithoulkas.com/EN/interview_vithoulkas_philosophy.html

[2] Schroyens, Frederik, *Synthesis, Repertorium Homeopathicum Syntheticum*, London Homeopathic Book Publishers, Edition 7.1, 1998

[3] The Homeopathic Symposium www.homeopathicsymposium.com

[4] Hahnemann, Samuel, *Organon of Medicine*, sixth edition translated by William Boericke, Philadelphia 1922, reprinted B Jain, New Delhi, 1997 (referred to throughout the book as the *Organon*)

[5] Close, Stuart, *The Genius of Homoeopathy: Lectures and Essays on Homoeopathic Philosophy*, Boericke and Tafel, Philadelphia 1924, reprinted B Jain, New Delhi, 1996

[6] Brothers Grimm, *Grimm's Fairy Stories*, 1st edition Andrew Dakers, London, 1957, reprinted by Smithmark Publishing, 1988

[7] Mindell, Arnold, *Working With The Dreaming Body,* Independent Publishing Group, 2006

[8] Mindell, Arnold, *Dreaming While Awake: Techniques for 24-Hour Lucid Dreaming*, Hampton Roads Publishing Company Inc, 2000 and 2002

[9] *The Big Issue* www.bigissue.com

[10] Ross, A C Gordon, *Homoeopathy: An Introductory Guide*, Thorsons, Wellingborough, 1976

[11] HPTG - homeopathy training for doctors and veterinary surgeons www.hptg.org

[12] Hawkins, Peter and Shohet, Robin, *Supervision in the Helping Professions*, Open University Press, 2000

[13] Kaplan, Brian, *The Homeopathic Conversation, the Art of Taking the Case*, Natural Medicine Press, London 2001

[14] Murphy, Robin, *A Verbatim Transcription of, The Cancer Tapes* (no publishing details)

[15] Murphy, Robin, *Homeopathic Medical Repertory*, Hahnemann Academy of North America, 2nd edition, Durango Colorado, 1998 - 1st edition was in 1993, 2nd was in 1996

[16] Kent, James, Tyler, *Repertory of the Homoeopathic Materia Medica*, 5th edition Heart and Karl, Chicago 1945, reprinted by Homoeopathic Book Service, Sittingbourne, 1993

[17] Gemmell, David, *Everyday Homoeopathy*, Beaconsfield Publishers, Beaconsfield, 1997

[18] Homeopathic Helpline www.homeopathyhelpline.com

[19] *BNF* (British National Formulary) www.bnf.org/bnf

[20] Maughan, Thomas, *Materia Medica*, (never published)

[21] Ramakrishnan, A U and Coulter, Catherine, *A Homoeopathic Approach to Cancer*, Quality Medical Publishing Inc, St Louis, 2001

[22] Chappell, Peter, *The Second Similimum, A Disease-Specific Complement to Individual Treatment*, Homeolinks, The Netherlands, 2005

[23] Chappell, Peter, *Emotional Healing with Homeopathy, Treating the Effects of Trauma,*

North Atlantic Books, Berkeley, 2003

[24] The work of Bert Hellinger www.hellinger.com

[25] Tapes by George Vithoulkas can be found on www.minimum.com

[26] Tapes by Robin Murphy can be found on www.minimum.com

[27] The word *"Bible"* refers to the canonical collections of sacred writings of Judaism and Christianity (Wikipedia)

[28] Clarke, John Henry, *Dictionary of Practical Materia Medica*, 3 volumes, Homoeopathic Publishing Company, London 1900 and 1925

[29] Bach, Edward and Wheeler, Charles, *Chronic Diseases, A Working Hypothesis*, H K Lewis, London, 1925

[30] Vithoulkas, George, *The Stolen Essences*, privately printed, London, no date, reprinted as *Essence of Materia Medica*, B Jain, New Delhi, 1989

[31] Vithoulkas, George, *The Science of Homeopathy*, Athens Society of Homeopathic Medicine, Athens, 1978, reprinted by B Jain, New Delhi, 1997

[32] *Homoeopathic Links, International Journal for Classical Homeopathy*, Netherlands, 1987 to present

[33] Norland, Misha, *The Nature of Influence*, published in Links, www.homeolinks.nl

[34] Lockie, Dr, Andrew, *The Family Guide to Homoeopathy, The Safe Form of Medicine for the Future*, Hamish Hamilton Ltd, 1989

[35] Castro, Miranda, *The Complete Homeopathy Handbook – A Guide to Everyday Health Care*, Papermac - Pan Macmillan Publishers Limited, London, 1991

[36] Tompkins, Peter and Bird, Christopher, *The Secret Life of Plants – a fascinating account of the physical, emotional and spiritual relations between plants and man*, Perennial, 1989 and then 2002

[37] Vermeulen, Frans, *Prisma, The Arcana of Materia Medica Illuminated, Similars and Parallels between Substance and Remedy*, Emryss Publishers, Haarlem, 2002

[38] Hahnemann, Samuel, *The Organon of Medicine*, 6th edition, translated by Jost Künzli, Alain Naudé and Peter Pendleton, J P Tarcher, Los Angeles, 1982, reprinted by Victor Gollancz, London 1986

[39] Boericke, William and Boericke, Oscar, *Pocket Manual of Homoeopathic Materia Medica and Repertory*, Boericke & Runyon, Philadelphia, 1927 9th edition, reprinted by B Jain, New Delhi, 1996

[40] Hahnemann, Samuel, *The Medicine of Experience,* Berlin, 1805 in *The Lesser Writings of Samuel Hahnemann*, translated by Robert E Dudgeon, W Headland, London, 1851

[41] Demarque, Denis, *L'Homoeopathie Medecine de l'Experience*, Éditions Coquemard, Angouleme, 1968

[42] American Institute of Homeopathy, *American Journal of Homeopathic Medicine* www.homeopathyusa.org/journal

[43] Winston, Julian, *The Faces of Homoeopathy*, Great Auk Publishing, 1999

[44] Treuherz, Francis, *Extreme Homeopathy: Matters of Life and Death, The Homeopath*, 24:1, Society of Homeopaths, Northampton, 2005

45 *Ethics of the Fathers (Pirke Avoth)*, a tractate of the Mishnah, translated from the original Hebrew by Herbert Danby, Oxford University Press, Oxford, 1933

46 *The Homeopath*, the journal of the Society of Homeopaths www.homeopathy-soh.org

47 *Code of Ethics and Practice*, Northampton, the Society of Homeopaths, various dates www.homeopathy-soh.org

48 Homeopathic Education Services in California www.homeopathic.com

49 *Homeopathy* formerly *The British Homeopathic Journal* www.elsevierhealth.com/journals

50 *The Harbinger Magazine*, Henry James Senior, editor, Boston 1845-49

51 Emanuel Swedenborg, *Oeconomia Regnum Animalis*, Stockholm. Published as *The Animal Kingdom*, translated by John James Garth Wilkinson, H Bailliere, London, and Otis Clapp Boston, 1844

52 Schmidt, Pierre, *La Genie Epidemique sa Nature – sa Therapeutique*, privately published, Paris, 1929

53 Peter Richard's work www.biolumanetics.net/tantalus

54 Whitney, Jerome, *Vitalistic Medicine from Ancient Egypt to the 21ˢᵗ Century*, Open Door Books, London, 2000

55 The Journal of the Faculty of Homeopaths www.trusthomeopathy.org

56 Coulter, Harris, *Divided Legacy, four volumes*, Wehawken Press and North Atlantic Books, Washington DC, 1973-1995, Wehauken Press 1973, reprinted North Atlantic Books and Homeopathic Educational Services, 1982

57 Hering, Constantine, *Guiding Symptoms of our Materia Medica,* 10 volumes, Estate of Constantine Hering, Philadelphia, 1890

58 Hughes, Richard, *Cyclopaedia of Drug Pathogenesy*, 5 volumes, E Gould, London 1891

59 *Prometheus*, Journal of the Guild of Homeopaths, 1995-2000

60 Compton Burnett, James, *The Best of Burnett*, edited by H L Chitkara, B Jain, New Delhi, 1992

61 Kent, James Tyler, *Lectures on Homoeopathic Philosophy*, Memorial Edition Ehrhart and Karl, Chicago 1929, reprinted B Jain, New Delhi, 1997

62 *Wizard of Oz*, directed by Victor Fleming, 1939

63 Sankaran, Rajan, *The Sensation of Homoeopathy*, Homoeopathic Medical Publishers, Bombay, 2004

64 Watson, Ian, *A Guide to the Methodologies of Homoeopathy*, Cutting Edge Publications, Cumbria, 1995

65 Roberts, Ernest, *Homoeopathy: Principles and Practice*, Winter Press, London, 2001

66 Tyler, Margaret Lucy, *How Not to Do It*, (Paper read at the International Congress 1911), Unwin, London

67 Bailey, Philip, *Homeopathic Psychology*, Personality Profiles of the Major Constitutional Remedies, North Atlantic Books, Berkeley, 1995

68 Payrhuber, Dietmar, *Dimensions of Homeopathic Medicine*, 1998 (English translation), published in Salzburg, Austria

69 Vithoulkas, George, *Materia Medica Viva*, 10 volumes, Homeopathic Book Publishers, London, and International Academy of Classical Homeopathy, Alonissos, 1992-2007

70 Vithoulkas' *Twelve Levels of Health, please refer to The Science of Homeopathy above*

71 *Dogmatism in Homeopathy, Homeopathic Links*, Volume 15, Number 1, Spring 2002, Page 15-16 www.minimum.com/p7/engine2/address.htm (for backdated copies of journals)

72 Vanden Berghe, Fons, (editor), *The Classical Homeopathic Lectures of Vassilis Ghegas*, 12 volumes, HomeoStudy, Genk Belgium 1987-1999

73 Roberts, Herbert A, *The Rheumatic Remedies and Repertory to the Rheumatic Remedies*, Homoeopathic Publishing Company, London, 1939

74 Arberry, A J, *Mystical Poems of Rumi 2 (The Drunkards)*, the University of Chicago Press, 1991

75 Miles, Martin, *Homoeopathy and Human Evolution*, Winter Press, 1992

76 Hahnemann, Samuel, *The Chronic Diseases, Their Peculiar Nature and Homoeopathic Cure*, 2 volumes, translated by Louis H Tafel, Boericke and Tafel, Philadelphia, 1896, reprinted by B Jain, New Delhi, 1997

77 Hahnemann, Samuel, *Materia Media Pura*, 2 volumes, translated by Robert E Dudgeon, Homoeopathic Publishing Society, Liverpool 1880, reprinted by B Jain, New Delhi, 1997

78 *Kabbalah* literally means 'receiving' in the sense of a 'received tradition' and esoterically interprets the Hebrew Bible and classical Jewish texts and practices (Wikipedia)

79 *The Tanya*, Rabbi Shneur Zalman of Liadi, 1797, revised 1814, published as Lessons in Tanya, translated by Levy Weinberg, edited by Uri Kaploun, Kehot Publication Society, New York, 1998. The *Tanya* deals with Jewish spirituality and psychology, from a Kabbalistic (Jewish mystical) point of view (Wikipedia)

80 Swedenborg, *The Swedenborg Concordance, a Complete Work of Reference to the Theological Writings of Emanuel Swedenborg*, The Swedenborg Society, London, 1976

81 *Health Science Press*, Saffron Walden, Essex

82 Clarke, John Henry, *A Clinical Repertory to the Dictionary of Materia Medica*, Homoeopathic Publishing Company, London 1904

83 *Council of Organisations Registering Homeopaths* www.corh.org.uk/pubs/TheStorySoFar.pdf

84 Farrington, E A, *Comparative Materia Medica*, Hahnemann Publishing House, Philadelphia 1873
and
Farrington, E A, *Clinical Materia Medica*, Hahnemann Publishing House, Philadelphia, 1887, reprinted B Jain, New Delhi, 1995

85 Roberts, H A, *Boenninghausen's Therapeutic Pocket Book*, A B Pub, Calcutta, 1935

86 Creasy, Sheilagh, *The Integrity of Homeopathy*, Peter Irl Publishing, Germany, 2007

87 *Dead Poets Society*, directed by Peter Weir, 1989

88 Kent, James Tyler, *Lectures on Homeopathic Materia Medica*, 4th edition Boericke and Tafel Philadelphia, 1932, reprinted by Homoeopathic Book Service, Sittingbourne, 1989

89 Choudhuri, N M, *A Study on Materia Medica with Repertory*, B Jain, New Delhi, 1983

90 Banerjea, Subrata Kumar, *Miasmatic Prescribing, Its Philosophy, Diagnostic Classification, Clinical Tips, Miasmatic Repertory and Miasmatic Weightage of Medicines,* Allen College of Homoeopathy, Chelmsford, 2002

91 Tyler, Margaret L, *Homeopathic Drug Pictures,* C W Daniel, Saffron Walden, first published in 1942

92 Nash, Eugene Beauharnais *Leaders in Homoeopathic Therapeutics,* Boericke and Tafel Philadelphia 1899

93 Tyler, Margaret L, *Homeopathic Drug Pictures,* C W Daniel, Saffron Walden, first published in 1942

94 Sharma, Yubraj, *Spiritual Bioenergetics of Homoeopathic Materia Medica,* Academy of Light, London, 2004

95 Heindel, Max, *H P Blavatsky and the Secret Doctrine,* reprinted by Kessinger Publishing 2003

96 National Occupational Standard guidelines can be found at http://www.skillsforhealth.org.uk/view_framework.php?id=111

97 *Caduceus* www.caduceus.info

98 *Positive Health* www.positivehealth.com

99 The *I Ching* is the oldest of the Chinese classic texts. A symbol system designed to identify order in what seem like chance events, it describes an ancient system of cosmology and philosophy that is at the heart of Chinese cultural beliefs (Wikipedia)

100 Hurtak, J J, *The Book of Knowledge: The Keys of Enoch,* Academy for Future Science, 1987

101 Julian, O A, *Materia Medica of New Homoeopathic Remedies,* Beaconsfield Publishers Ltd, Beaconsfield, 1997

102 Temple, Jack, *The Healer,* Element Books Limited, Shaftesbury, 1998

103 Roy, Margaret, *Homoeopathic Acute Prescribing, a Text for Practitioners, First Aid and Self Help,* Scottish College of Homoeopathy, Biggar, Scotland, 2005

104 Allen, H C, *Allen's Key Notes and Characteristics of the Materia Medica with Nosodes (Keynotes and Comparisons with Some of the Leading remedies),* B Jain, New Delhi, 1986

105 Scholten, Jan, *Secret Lanthanides, Road to Independence,* Stichting Alonnissos, Utrecht, 2005

106 Sherr, Jeremy, *The Dynamics and Methodology of Homoeopathic Provings,* 2nd edition Dynamis School, Malvern, 1997

107 Bach, Richard, *Bridge Across Forever,* Pan Books, London, 1985

108 Gibson, D M, *First Aid Homoeopathy in Accidents and Ailments,* British Homoeopathic Association, London, 1983

109 *The Lancet,* Volume 366, 27 August 2005 www.thelancet.com

110 *The Lancet,* www.thelancet.com

111 *Killed by Homeopathy? Daily Mail,* Tuesday 6 September 2005 pages 40-41

112 Marais, Eugene, *The Soul of the White Ant,* Human and Rousseau, 2006

[113] Zukav, Gary, *Dancing Wu Li Masters: An Overview of the New Physics*, Rider and Co, 1991, Harper Perennial Modern Classics, 2001

[114] Shakespeare, William, Hamlet Act 1 Scene 3, 1600

[115] *House of Lords Select Committee on Science and Technology, Complementary and alternative medicine: session 1999 - 2000, Sixth Report, Science and Technology Committee Publications* www.parliament.the-stationery-office.co.uk/pa/ld199900/ldselect/ldsctech/123/12301.htm

[116] *The Role of Complementary and Alternative Medicine in the NHS, An Investigation into the Potential Contribution of Mainstream Complementary Therapies to Healthcare in the UK*, led by Christopher Smallwood, 2005, known as the *Smallwood Report* www.freshminds.co.uk

[117] *The Prince's Foundation for Integrated Health Response to the Review of UK Health Research (Cooksey Review)* www.hm-treasury.gov.uk/media/347/C8/cooksey2006_princesfoundationforintegratedhealth.pdf

[118] *First Class Mail*, Intranet communication system for the Society of Homeopaths

[119] *The Talmud* is a record of rabbinic discussions pertaining to Jewish law, ethics, customs and history (Wikipedia)

[120] McTaggart, Lynne, *The Field*, Harper Collins Publishers Limited, 2003

[121] Shakespeare, William, The Tempest Act 4 Secne 1, circa 1610

[122] Lewis, C S, *The Chronicles of Narnia - The Lion, the Witch and the Wardrobe*, Puffin Books, London, 1970

[123] The *Bhagavad Gita* is an ancient Sanskrit text written in a poetic form that is traditionally chanted; hence the title, which translates to 'the Song of the Divine One'. The Bhagavad Gita is revered as sacred by the majority of Hindu traditions and especially so by followers of Krishna. In general speech it is commonly referred to as *The Gita* (Wikipedia)

[124] *Within you without you*, Harrison, George, from the album Sgt Pepper's Lonely Hearts Club Band, Northern Songs Ltd, 1967

[125] *Far from the Madding Crowd*, directed by John Schlesinger, 1967

[126] *Modesty Blaise*, directed by Joseph Losey, 1966

[127] Saunders, Nicholas, *Alternative London*, Saunders, London, 1970

[128] Saunders, Nicholas, *Alternative England and Wales*, Saunders, London, 1975

[129] Heathcote Williams, *Whale Nation*, Jonathan Cape, London, 1988

[130] *The Great Rock 'n Roll Swindle*, directed by Julien Temple, 1981

[131] Clarke, John Henry, *The Prescriber, A Dictionary of the New Therapeutics*, 9th edition, Homoeopathic Publishing Company, London, 1946, reprinted Health Science Press, Saffron Walden, 1983

[132] Lilienthal, Samuel, *Homoeopathic Therapeutics*, 4th edition Boericke and Tafel, Philadelphia 1907, reprinted B Jain, New Delhi, 1998

[133] Tarnas, Richard, *The Passion of the Western Mind - Understanding The Ideas That Have Shaped Our World View*, Ballantine Books, USA, 1991 and 1993, Pimlico, 1996

[134] Swimme, Brian, and Berry, Thomas, *The Universe Story,* Harper Collins, San Francisco, 1994

[135] Goswami, Amit, *The Quantum Doctor: A Physicist's Guide to Health and Healing,* Hampton Roads Publishing Company Incorporated, 2004

[136] Hahnemann, Samuel, *Organon of the Medicinal Art,* 6th edition, edited and annotated by Wenda Brewster O'Reilly, Birdcage Books, Washington, 1996

[137] *What The Bleep Do We Know?* www.thebleep.co.uk

[138] Coelho, Paulo, *The Alchemist,* most recent reprint Harper Collins, 2006

[139] Bohjalian, Chris, *The Law of Similars*, Harmony Books, New York, 1999

[140] Sherr, Jeremy, *Dynamic Materia Medica, Syphilis - A Study of the Syphilitic Miasm through Remedies*, Dynamis Books, Malvern, 2002

[141] Shine, Michelle, *What About Potency?* Food For Thought, London, 2004

NOTES

NOTES